Adult Craniopharyngiomas

Emmanuel Jouanneau • Gérald Raverot
Editors

Adult Craniopharyngiomas

Differences and Lessons
from Paediatrics

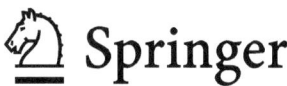 Springer

Editors
Emmanuel Jouanneau
Skull Base and Pituitary Neurosurgical
Department
Hôpital Pierre Wertheimer
"Groupement Hospitalier Est" Hospices
Civils de Lyon
"Claude Bernard" Lyon 1 University
Lyon
France

Gérald Raverot
Endocrinology Department
Reference Center for Rare Pituitary
Diseases HYPO
"Groupement Hospitalier Est" Hospices
Civils de Lyon
"Claude Bernard" Lyon 1 University
Lyon
France

ISBN 978-3-030-41175-6   ISBN 978-3-030-41176-3   (eBook)
https://doi.org/10.1007/978-3-030-41176-3

This Springer imprint is published by the registered company Springer Nature Switzerland AG
The registered company address is: Gewerbestrasse 11, 6330 Cham, Switzerland

Foreword 1

The clinical history of the craniopharyngioma begins with the extraordinary French Neurologist, Joseph Jules Francois Felix Babinski, who, in 1900, described a patient with "dystrophic adiposity and sexual infantilism" who was found to have a cystic lesion in the area of the pituitary. In his 1912 monograph, *The Pituitary Body*, Harvey Williams Cushing described lesions that arose from the embryonic craniopharyngeal duct; however, he had not at this time encountered any of these cysts and tumors surgically. Many different names had been given to the tumors that we currently identify as craniopharyngiomas (a term coined in 1931 by the Philadelphia Neurosurgeon, Charles H. Frazier). In his 1932 monograph on brain tumors treated surgically, Cushing described 92 craniopharyngiomas, recording poor outcomes with regard to morbidity and mortality. In fact, Cushing had called these tumors "the most formidable of intracranial tumors" and also wrote that "Craniopharyngiomas are the most baffling problem which confronts the Neurosurgeon." Today, this remains relatively unchanged!

Although much has been written about the management of childhood craniopharyngiomas, these tumors are also problems in adults, and there are different considerations, nuances, and technical aspects in considering the management of adult craniopharyngiomas, which is the focus of this innovative and extraordinarily helpful volume. In fact, there are some studies that contend that in addition to presentations in childhood, the age-specific incidence of craniopharyngiomas increases as the population ages.

This well-conceived and contemporary book includes contributions from acknowledged experts in neurosurgery, endocrinology, pathology, epidemiology, pediatrics, medicine, neuroradiology, neuro- and radiation-oncology, and genetic and molecular biology. Their varying points of view emphasize the complexity of the subject and its potential and future solutions. They emphasize the necessity of a "Team Approach" and the collaboration of different specialties and scientists in addressing the challenges that this disease presents. Surely, their analysis of the pediatric experience offers us a platform from which to translate the lessons learned to the improvement of managing craniopharyngiomas in the adult population.

In a concise and targeted fashion, this book is the foundation of a pathway to the future and for further success in the management of our patients with this fascinating and multifaceted entity of the craniopharyngioma.

Edward R. Laws
Department of Neurosurgery
Harvard Medical School, Brigham and Women's Hospital
Boston, MA, USA

Foreword 2

The ideal management of craniopharyngiomas is still unresolved and controversially discussed, despite a century of studies and remarkable evolutions of imaging, surgery, and radiation techniques. Harvey Cushing once called them the "most forbidding of the intracranial tumors" for their association with hypothalamic disturbances and for their tendency to recur. Still, to date, there are many obstacles in their management: For individual surgeons, it is difficult to gain experience with these lesions since they are rare disorders, with most of them treated in specialized centers. However, even these centers do not see more than a handful of such patients every year. Some of them report excellent treatment results and a high proportion of surgical resections.

Surgery of craniopharyngiomas is not only a matter of surgical skills and expertise. The threat of hypothalamic injury with its sequelae, such as uncontrollable gain of weight, is a much-feared effect of aggressive removal. Data from nationwide studies reveal that the mortality and morbidity associated with treatment can be worse than the effects that the tumor itself produces. On one side, there has been an enormous evolution in operative procedures: The extended transsphenoidal approach is one of the novel achievements, which allows extracting tumors that are not suitable for transsphenoidal surgery by conventional microscopic techniques a few years ago. The role of transcranial approaches is thus diminished. However, in some instances, the entire battery of craniotomies needed. Several different philosophies of surgeons remain as how to proceed with craniopharyngiomas: Some argued for most radical extraction in each and every patient and dwell on their microsurgical skills. Others advised just to relieve the mass effect by the most minimally invasive procedures available and recommend observation or adjuvant irradiation. Some apply a more differentiated approach in their patients tailored to the individual tumor and the patients' specific situation, respectively, with a variable extent of resection. To date, such an individualized strategy is preferred and referred to as "precision" medicine. It is undoubtedly advantageous, if an individual tumor can be completely extracted without untoward side effects.

On the other side is the threat of treatment-induced hypothalamic damage. The concept of not damaging the hypothalamus with horrible sequelae and major impairment of quality of life is based on the availability of prognostic scales, which provide us with some estimation of the likelihood of hypothalamic damage derived from the imaging patterns of size, composition, and localization of the tumors upon their presentation. There are meanwhile several scales available, deriving from different centers. At least to some degree of probability, we can predict the patients at major risks. After all, we have radiotherapy as yet, and hopefully in the future medical treatments will become available for the different types of craniopharyngiomas. The molecular differential diagnosis between adamantinomatous and papillary craniopharyngioma is to date no more just based on microscopic morphological features but molecular characteristics, such as the wnt-pathway is disrupted or a BRAF V600 mutation can be detected. Consequently, there should be appropriate drugs which interfere with signal disruptions, and in a few case reports the positive effect of appropriate drug administrations has been documented.

The outstanding experience and expertise of specialized pathological, radiological, surgical, medical, and irradiation issues is collected in this volume. The state-of-the-art knowledge is well reflected and may be used for reference purposes. As such, it is the result of a novel approach to cover all aspects of craniopharyngioma in one book. Even to date, we have limited long-term outcome data from the adult patient population. There are obviously major differences in the management of adult and pediatric patients, and essentially this book is dedicated to have these issues addressed.

This book will help in clinical decision making and finding appropriate management for the individual patient as cooperation of specialists from many medical fields, such as pathology, neuroradiology, medicine, pediatrics, neurosurgery, and molecular biology, is beneficial. It clearly reveals the key to proper patient management of this rare type of tumor, which is interdisciplinary cooperation and team-based individualized patient care.

Michael Buchfelder
Department of Neurosurgery
University Hospital Erlangen
Erlangen, Germany

Acknowledgement

M.D.I. has been supported by the Exchange in Endocrinology Expertise (3E) program of the European Union of Medical Specialists (UEMS), Section and Board of Endocrinology.

Contents

Histopathology and Molecular Pathology of Craniopharyngioma in Adults

Alexandre Vasiljevic and Chiara Villa

1.1 Introduction

Craniopharyngioma (CP) is a rare epithelial tumor of the central nervous system affecting 1.7 patients per 1,000,000 person-years [1]. This neoplasm affects the sellar and parasellar region and causes significant morbidities despite having benign histopathological features. This may be explained by its development in close relationship with critical anatomical structures, such as the optic chiasm and hypothalamic–pituitary axis. CP follows a bimodal age distribution with a peak incidence in children aged 0–19 years and adults aged 40–79 years [1]. CP was first recognized as a distinct entity by the Austrian pathologist Jakob Erdheim (1874–1937) who used the term "hypophyseal duct tumor" (*Hypophysenganggeschwülste*) [2]. At that time, Erdheim already identified two main types of CP: adamantinomatous and squamous papillary. He also hypothesized that these tumors originated from ectodermal embryonic remnants of the primitive mouth or *stomodeum*. Indeed during development, the hypophyseal duct connects the stomodeum to an evagination called Rathke's pouch, from which the anterior pituitary lobe is derived.

A. Vasiljevic (✉)
Centre de Pathologie et de Neuropathologie Est, Groupement Hospitalier Est, Hospices Civils de Lyon, Bron, France

Faculté de Médecine Lyon Est, Université Lyon 1, Lyon, France

INSERM U1052, CNRS UMR5286, Cancer Research Centre of Lyon, Lyon, France
e-mail: alexandre.vasiljevic@chu-lyon.fr

C. Villa
Department of Pathological Cytology and Anatomy, Foch Hospital, Suresnes, France

INSERM U1016, CNRS UMR8104, Paris Descartes University, Cochin Institute, Paris, France

Department of Endocrinology, University of Liège, CHU de Liège, Liège, Belgium
e-mail: cm.villa@hopital-foch.org

© Springer Nature Switzerland AG 2020
E. Jouanneau, G. Raverot (eds.), *Adult Craniopharyngiomas*,
https://doi.org/10.1007/978-3-030-41176-3_1

The 2016 World Health Organization (WHO) classification of tumors of the central nervous system distinguishes two types of CP: adamantinomatous craniopharyngioma (ACP) and papillary craniopharyngioma (PCP) [3]. These are two distinct entities that are characterized by distinct epidemiology, morphology, and molecular pathology [4].

1.2   Adamantinomatous Craniopharyngioma

ACP is the most frequently occurring pathological subtype of CP. It predominantly affects children but may also be observed in adults [5]. Macroscopically, ACP shows both solid and cystic components. Cysts are filled with a lipid-rich fluid, often referred to as "motor-oil." White chalky areas, corresponding to calcifications, and brownish areas, corresponding to old hemorrhages, are frequently observed macroscopically. ACPs generally have irregular and infiltrative borders that render safe surgical removal challenging.

1.2.1   Histopathology

1.2.1.1 Histopathological Features
ACPs display a characteristic microscopic appearance that is usually easy to recognize [3, 6–8]. ACPs are composed of complex epithelial nests with solid and cystic areas (Fig. 1.1a). The neoplastic epithelium shows a characteristic organization (Fig. 1.1b). A layer of palisading columnar epithelial cells surrounds the periphery of the epithelial nests (*palisading epithelium*) (Fig. 1.1b, c). This is sometimes described as "picket fence"-like. At low magnification, the cells of this basal layer usually appear more basophilic than the upper layers. A few mitotic figures may be observed here. A low-cellular layer, known as the *stellate reticulum,* lies above the palisading epithelium (Fig. 1.1b, d). This layer is similar to the *stellate reticulum* found in the developing enamel organ. Nodules of "wet keratin" are a pathognomonic feature of ACP. These correspond to aggregates of anuclear squamous "ghost cells" that have lost their nuclear basophilic staining (Fig. 1.1e). Especially at the edge of invasion, the neoplastic epithelium shows round clusters of cells also known as "whorls" or "morules" (Fig. 1.1f). By immunohistochemistry, the nuclear expression of β-catenin is typically observed in these cellular aggregates (see molecular pathology below) (Fig. 1.1f).

1.2.1.2 Regressive Changes and Surrounding Nervous Tissue
ACPs usually undergo extensive regressive changes that may in some cases completely obscure the epithelial component. These changes are frequently found around aggregates of "wet keratin" (Fig. 1.2a). They include calcifications (Fig. 1.2b), macrophagic phagocytosis of cholesterol clefts by multinucleated foreign-body giant cells (Fig. 1.2c, d), necrotic debris, and chronic inflammatory infiltrates. Hemosiderin deposits are common as a result of focal hemorrhages

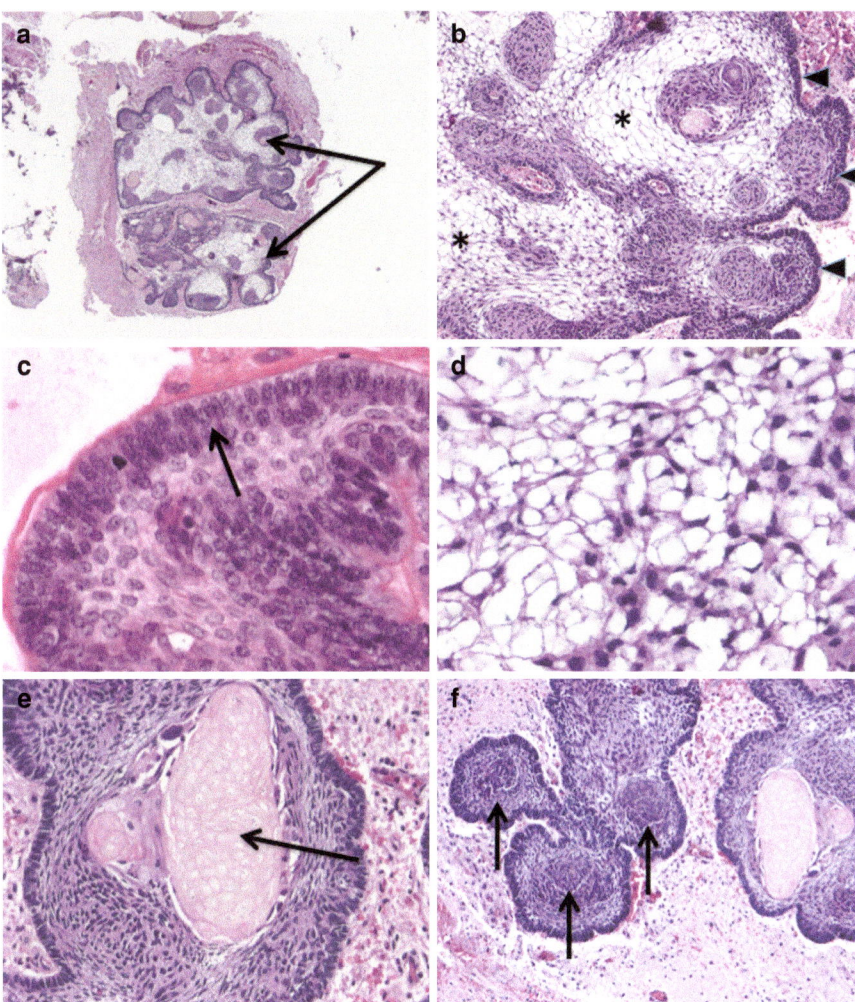

Fig. 1.1 Adamantinomatous craniopharyngioma (ACP): histopathological features (1). (**a**) ACPs are composed of complex epithelial structures with irregular borders (arrows) (hematoxylin, phloxine, saffron (HES) staining; original magnification (OM) ×25). (**b**) ACPs are characterized by an outer layer of palisading columnar cells that are arranged like a "picket fence" (arrowheads). The inner part of the epithelial nest is composed of a loose network of star-shaped cells, the *stellate reticulum* (asterisks) (HPS; OM ×100). (**c**) The palisading layer is composed of basophilic columnar cells (arrow). Mitotic figures may be observed here (HPS; OM ×400). (**d**) The *stellate reticulum* is composed of stellate cells with thin processes in a loose stroma (HPS; OM ×400). (**e**) One typical feature of ACP is "wet keratin" (arrow). It is composed of aggregates of squamous "ghost" cells that have lost their basophilic staining (HPS; OM ×200). (**f**) At the edge of invasion of the nervous tissue, ACPs frequently show round clusters of cells termed "morules" or "whorls" (arrows) (HPS; OM ×100)

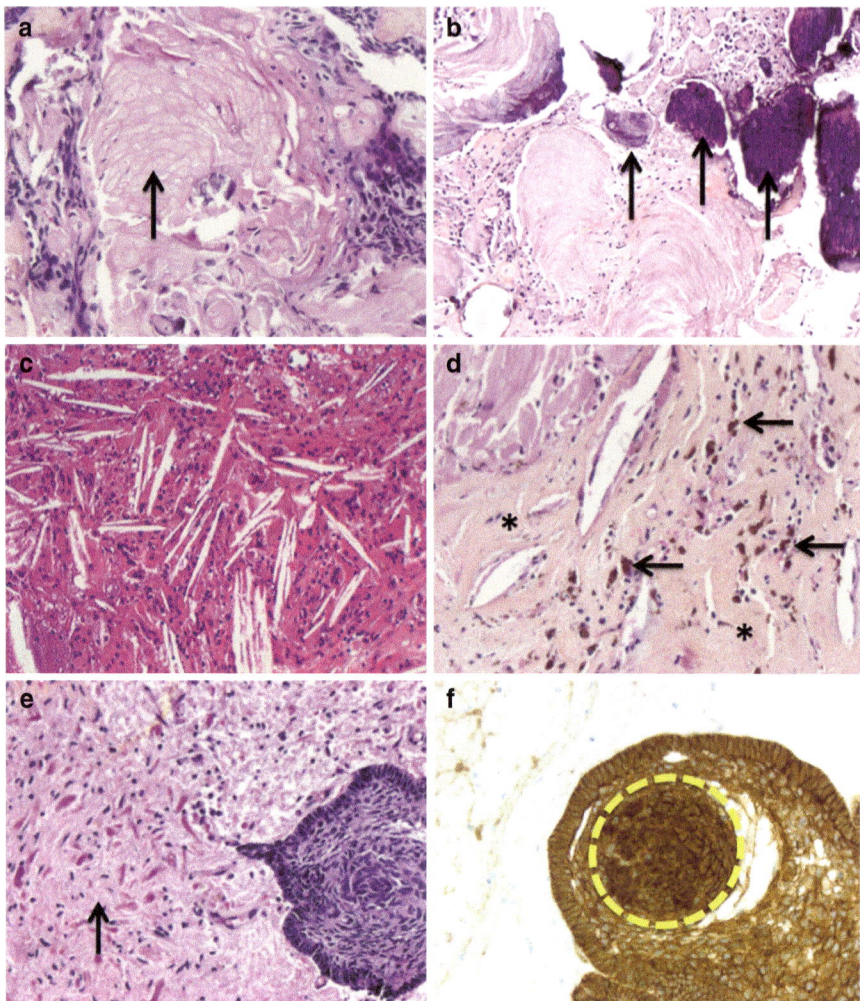

Fig. 1.2 Adamantinomatous craniopharyngioma (ACP): histopathological features (2). (**a**) Aggregates of "wet keratin" are a specific feature of ACP (arrow). These are often surrounded by inflammatory infiltrates composed of macrophages, lymphocytes, and plasma cells (hematoxylin, phloxine, saffron (HPS) staining; original magnification (OM) ×200). (**b**) "Wet keratin" is often associated with calcifications (arrows) (HPS; OM ×100). (**c**) Cholesterol clefts with a foreign-body giant cell reaction are a frequent finding (HPS; OM ×100). (**d**) Other regressive changes include fibrosis (asterisks) and deposits of hemosiderin pigment (arrows) related to chronic hemorrhage (HPS; OM ×200). (**e**) At the interface between ACP and nervous tissue, a florid piloid gliosis is typically found and may be mistaken for pilocytic astrocytoma (arrow) (HPS; OM ×200). (**f**) Nuclear immunoexpression of β-catenin is only seen in discrete clusters of cells that correspond to "morules" or "whorls" (yellow circle) (anti-β-catenin immunohistochemistry; OM ×200)

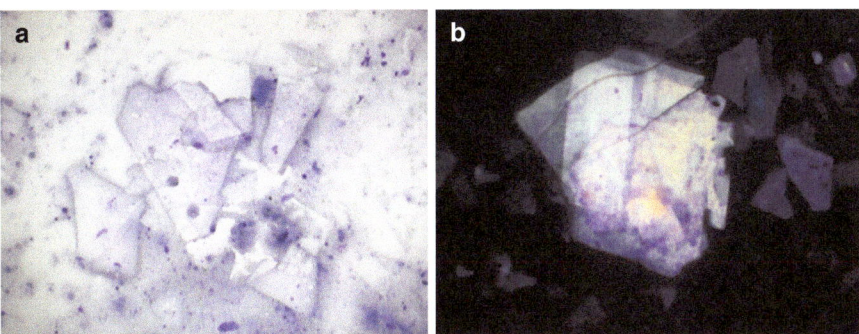

Fig. 1.3 Intraoperative examination of cystic fluid in an adamantinomatous craniopharyngioma. (**a**) The fresh intraoperative observation of the cystic fluid of ACP typically shows rhomboid crystals that correspond to cholesterol crystals (toluidine blue, original magnification (OM) ×400). (**b**) These crystals are birefringent under polarized light (OM ×400)

(Fig. 1.2d). Areas of fibrosis may also be observed (Fig. 1.2d). In ACP, cysts are filled with a cholesterol-rich fluid that has been described macroscopically as appearing like "motor-oil." The intraoperative examination, under polarized light, of cystic fluid from an ACP may reveal birefringent rhomboid crystals that are evocative of the diagnosis (Fig. 1.3a, b).

ACP is often characterized by irregular borders with interdigitations that invade the adjacent nervous tissue [9]. These ill-delineated and infiltrative borders are thought to account for the difficulty in surgical removal of these tumors (Fig. 1.1f). At the interface between the tumor and the nervous tissue, a florid piloid gliosis is typical and may mimic a pilocytic astrocytoma (Fig. 1.2e).

1.2.2   Molecular Pathology

Mutations of the *CTNNB1* gene coding for β-catenin are found in 76.1–100% of ACP cases, highlighting the role of the canonical Wnt/β-catenin pathway in the pathogenesis of this tumor [4, 10–13]. β-catenin is a pivotal element of the Wnt (Wingless integration site) canonical pathway, a tightly regulated signaling cascade which is involved in various cellular processes such as development and homeostasis [14, 15].

Mutations of the β-catenin gene consist mostly of missense mutations and, more rarely, small deletions. They affect exon 3, especially at/or adjacent to serine 33 (codons 32–34), at/or adjacent to serine 37 (codons 36–37), and at threonine 41. These serine/threonine sites mostly represent phosphorylation sites for glycogen synthase 3 (GSK3) [4, 13, 16].

In the absence of Wnt ligands, β-catenin is physiologically phosphorylated by the so-called destruction complex [17]. This is an assembly of multiple proteins that includes Axin, Adenomatous Polyposis Coli (APC), Casein Kinase 1 (CK1), and

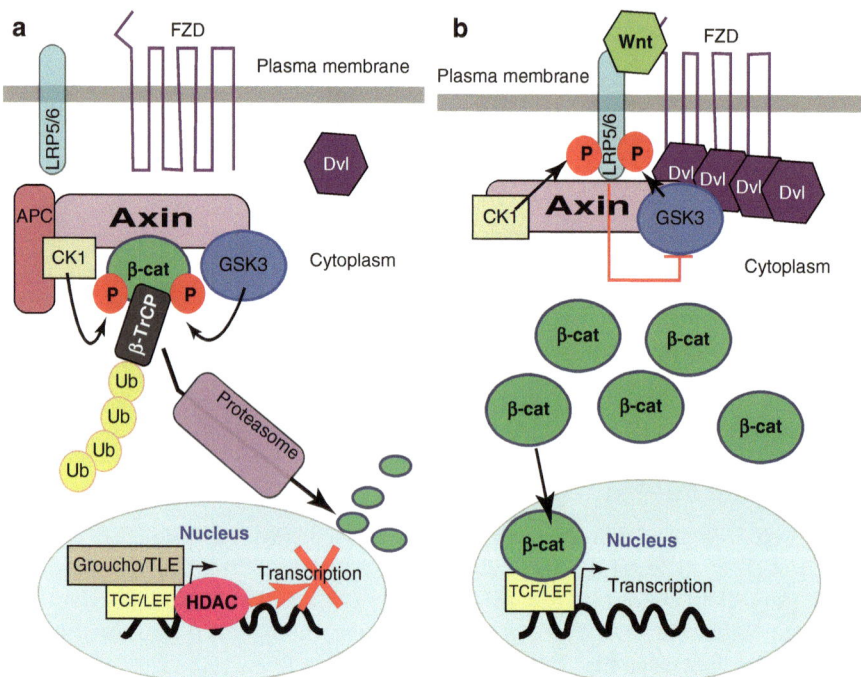

Fig. 1.4 Wnt/β-catenin pathway and adamantinomatous craniopharyngioma: schematic view. (**a**) In the absence of Wnt ligands, β-catenin is phosphorylated by two kinases of the destruction complex, namely GSK3 and CK1. This phosphorylation allows the recognition of β-catenin by β-TrCP which catalyzes its poly-ubiquitination for targeted degradation by the proteasome. In this situation, there is no translocation of β-catenin to the nucleus. TCF/LEF transcription factor and groucho/TLE co-repressor form a repressive complex that recruits histone deacetylases. These enzymes repress the transcription of β-catenin target genes by "closing" the chromatin. (**b**) The binding of Wnt ligands to Frizzled and LRP5/6 leads to the polymerization of Dvl and the recruitment of Axin to the plasma membrane. The phosphorylation of LRP5/6 by GSK3 and CK1 allows the stabilization of β-catenin by various mechanisms, including an inhibition of the catalytic site of GSK3. In this situation, β-catenin accumulates in the cytoplasm, translocates to the nucleus, and binds to TCF/LEF activating the transcription of target genes. In adamantinomatous craniopharyngioma, mutations in the serine/threonine phosphorylation sites for GSK3 prevent the degradation of β-catenin by the proteasome. *APC* Adenomatous Polyposis Coli, *β TrCP* beta transducin repeats-containing protein E3-ubiquitin ligase, *CK1* Casein Kinase 1, *Dvl* dishevelled, *FZD* Frizzled receptor, *Groucho/TLE* groucho/transducin-like enhancer, *GSK3* glycogen synthase kinase 3, *HDAC* histone deacetylase, *LRP5/6* low density lipoprotein receptor-related protein 5/6 (co-receptor), *TCF/LEF* T cell factor/lymphoid enhancer factor, *Wnt* wingless integration site

GSK3 (Fig. 1.4a). The destruction complex first phosphorylates serine 45 via CK1 (α isoform) and then threonine 41 and two serines (Ser33 and Ser37) via the action of GSK3 (β isoform). The phosphorylation of these two serines is required for the proper recognition of β-catenin by the E3-ubiquitin ligase β-TrCP (beta-transducin repeats-containing protein). β-catenin is ubiquitinated by β-TrCP and then targeted to the proteasome where it is degraded. This system prevents any accumulation of free β-catenin in the cytoplasm and nucleus, and thus target genes of β-catenin remain inactive [14].

The binding of Wnt ligands to Frizzled receptor and its coreceptor LRP5/6 (low density lipoprotein receptor-related protein 5/6) leads to the polymerization of Dishevelled (Dvl) and the recruitment of Axin to the plasma membrane (Fig. 1.4b) [18]. Kinases GSK3 and CK1 that are bound to Axin phosphorylate LRP5/6 resulting in the stabilization of β-catenin by the inhibition of its phosphorylation. Multiple mechanisms are involved in the inhibition of β-catenin phosphorylation [18]. GSK3 may be directly inhibited by the phosphorylated motif of LRP5/6. GSK may be sequestered by endocytosis of the Wnt receptor complex into multivesicular bodies thus preventing any interaction with cytosolic β-catenin. The phosphorylation of LRP5/6 also creates a docking site for Axin; this then reinforces the recruitment of Axin to the Wnt-Frizzled-LRP5/6 complex. The end result is the stabilization and accumulation of β-catenin in the cytoplasm and its translocation to the nucleus, where it interacts with TCF/LEF (T cell factor/lymphoid enhancer factor) transcription factors and activates the transcription of various target genes, such as *MYC* and *CCND1* [16].

In ACP, mutations of the phosphorylation sites of β-catenin prevent the degradation of β-catenin and allow its cytosolic accumulation and nuclear translocation. In this situation, the Wnt/β-catenin is activated in the absence of Wnt ligands. By immunohistochemistry, the mutations can be shown to cause nucleocytoplasmic accumulation of β-catenin. This accumulation is not observed in all of the tumoral cells, only in discrete cellular clusters ("whorls") (Fig. 1.2f).

1.2.3   ACP and Odontogenesis

ACPs share histopathologic features with odontogenic tumors, especially calcifying odontogenic cysts [19]. This close morphological similarity highlights the relationship between ACP and tooth development and is in keeping with the embryological origin of this tumor from the primitive mouth. Furthermore, CPs containing fully developed tooth-structures have been reported in rare cases, thus emphasizing the link between ACP and odontogenesis [20].

How Does a Tumor Resembling the Developing Tooth Develop in the Pituitary Region? Erdheim relied on the work of the German Martin Heinrich Rathke (1793–1860) to propose an embryological explanation for this dilemma [2]. Formation of the pituitary gland results from the encounter of two different structures. The neurohypophysis is derived from an evagination of the floor of the diencephalon. The adenohypophysis is derived from Rathke's pouch, an invagination of the roof of the *stomodeum*, located rostrally to the buccopharyngeal membrane. Rathke's pouch is thus an ectodermal structure derived from the primitive mouth [21]. The buccohypophyseal duct is a transient structure that connects Rathke's pouch to the *stomodeum* and closes in the early stages of development [22]. The formation of this canal depends on Sonic Hedgehog signaling. The identification of squamous epithelial nests in the *pars tuberalis* of pituitary specimens at autopsy led Erdheim to connect CP development to pituitary embryology. According to Erdheim, these nests represented remnants of the buccohypophyseal canal and were candidates to be precursors of CP. According to others, these nests result from the squamous metaplasia of adenohypophyseal cells [23]. This hypothesis is notably consistent with the absence of such nests in young patients and their observation in older patients [24]. The development of CPs from metaplastic squamous nests (metaplastic theory) was suggested as an alternative to the development of CPs from remnants of Rathke's pouch (embryonic theory) [5].

There is no definite proof that human ACP derives from remnants of Rathke's pouch. However, some studies using genetically engineered mouse models are consistent with the development of pediatric ACP from undifferentiated precursor cells of Rathke's pouch. These studies also suggest that adult ACP could arise from SOX2-positive stem cells of the adult pituitary gland [25, 26].

ACP development recapitulates odontogenesis (Fig. 1.5). Tooth development results from complex epithelial–mesenchymal interactions [27]. The developing tooth follows highly regulated morphogenetic stages: dental lamina, dental placode,

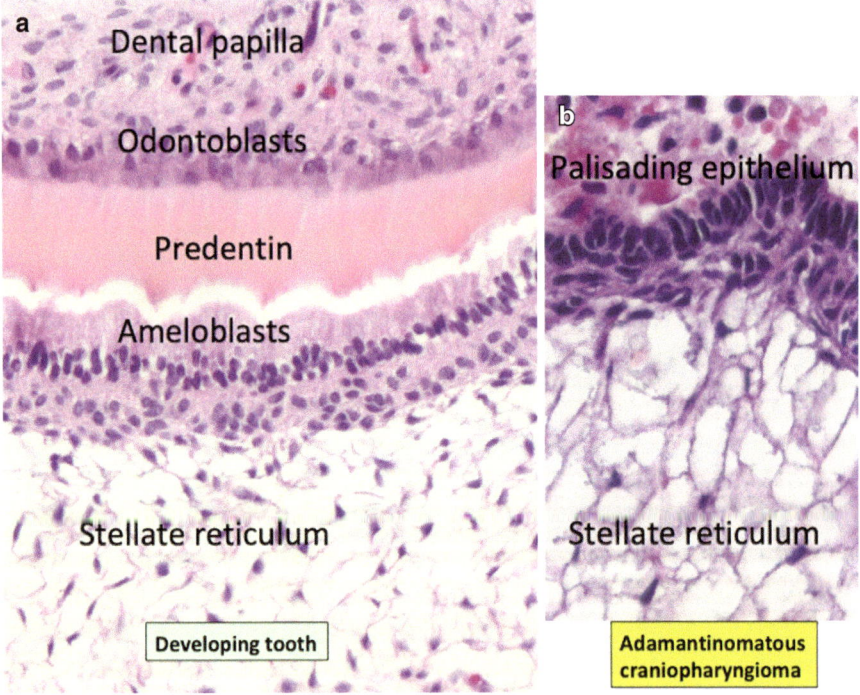

Fig. 1.5 Adamantinomatous craniopharyngioma and odontogenesis. (**a**) At the late cap-stage, the developing dental organ is composed of a layer of odontoblasts covering the dental papilla and secreting predentin, an inner enamel epithelium corresponding to ameloblasts, an outer enamel epithelium, and a *stellate reticulum* located between the two latter layers. (**b**) ACPs histologically resemble the developing enamel organ. The palisaded epithelium is reminiscent of the inner enamel epithelium (ameloblasts) and a typical *stellate reticulum* is found above

bud-stage, cap-stage, and bell-stage. At the cap-stage, the dental organ is composed of various structures, some of which are also found in ACP (Fig. 1.5). The upper part of the dental organ is the enamel organ. It is composed of an inner enamel columnar epithelium and an outer enamel cuboidal epithelium, both delineating the *stellate reticulum* (Fig. 1.5a). The *stellate reticulum* is a network of star-shaped interconnected cells lying in a loose stroma. The condensed ectomesenchyme, located under the enamel organ, is the dental papilla. The inner enamel epithelium corresponds to the ameloblastic layer and overlays the *stratum intermedium.* Odontoblasts differentiate from the cells of the papilla that are adjacent to the inner enamel epithelium. These cells will produce predentin then later dentin, while ameloblasts will synthesize enamel. At the cap-stage, a signaling center termed the enamel knot appears. It is a cluster of cells located in the center of the inner enamel epithelium. These cells produce several molecular signals that promote cellular proliferation and control cuspal patterning and thus the morphogenesis of the tooth crown [27]. The signal molecules secreted by the enamel knot act on epithelial and mesenchymal cells in the vicinity in a paracrine manner.

A transcriptomic study of different cellular compartments in ACP has reinforced the hypothesis of a link between ACP and odontogenesis [28]. This study showed similar molecular signatures of the ACP β-catenin-positive cell clusters and enamel knots of the developing tooth. Similarly, the molecular signature of the palisading epithelium was enriched with genes of the cap-stage enamel epithelium. These findings led the authors to propose a model where the β-catenin-positive "whorls" and the palisading epithelium are the pathological counterparts of the enamel knot and the inner enamel epithelium, respectively (Fig. 1.5b). Similar to the enamel knot in the developing tooth, the β-catenin-positive "whorls" act through complex paracrine signaling on neighboring cells, promoting their proliferation [25].

1.3   Papillary Craniopharyngioma

PCP occurs almost exclusively in adults, with a mean age of 44.7 years [29]. In children, PCPs have been only rarely reported [30]. PCPs are mostly suprasellar and macroscopically, are composed of solid and cystic areas [31]. The cysts contain a viscous yellow fluid [29]. Contrary to ACPs, PCPs are usually well-delineated from the surrounding nervous tissue allowing for easier surgical removal.

1.3.1   Histopathology

At low magnification, the tumor shape appears "cauliflower"-shaped. They show large peripheral protrusions that explain the "papillary" macroscopic appearance (Fig. 1.6a) [3, 7, 8, 29]. These protrusions are composed of fibrovascular cores covered by a well-differentiated non-keratinizing squamous epithelium (Fig. 1.6b). The squamous epithelium does not show a granular layer of cells filled with basophilic keratohyalin granules as is seen in epidermoid or dermoid cysts (Fig. 1.6c).

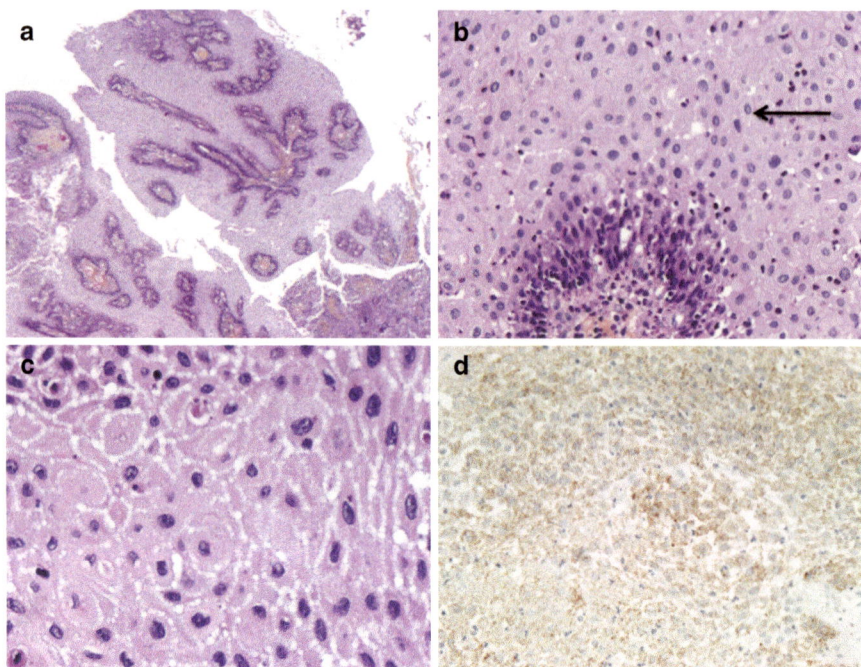

Fig. 1.6 Papillary craniopharyngioma (PCP): histopathological features. Hematoxylin, phloxine, saffron (HES) staining. (**a**) PCP is characterized by an architecture that is grossly papillary (original magnification (OM) ×25). (**b**) The papillae are covered by a bland squamous epithelium (arrow) without a palisading layer or "wet keratin" (OM ×200). (**c**) The squamous neoplastic cells are regular, without any significant atypia. They are connected by junctions (OM ×400). (**d**) Mutated BRAF^{V600E} protein can be detected by immunohistochemistry (anti-BRAF^{V600E} immunohistochemistry, OM ×100)

Neither is the epithelium covered by a layer of "dry keratin" (lamellated anuclear eosinophilic scales). The fibrous stroma of the papillae is usually infiltrated by a small number of chronic inflammatory cells. Stromal hyalinized "whorls" may be found and should not be mistaken for aggregates of "wet" keratin which are seen in ACP [29].

Compared with ACP, there is no palisading epithelium, no "wet keratin," nor *stellate reticulum*. Degenerative changes such as fibrosis, necrosis, calcifications, cholesterol, and hemosiderin deposits are also typically absent.

The mutated BRAF^{V600E} protein may be detected in PCP by immunohistochemistry (Fig. 1.6d; see also molecular pathology below).

1.3.2 Molecular Pathology

The molecular pathology of PCP is characterized by an overactivation of the mitogen-activated protein (MAP) kinase pathway as a result of BRAF V600E mutation. A V600E mutation in the *BRAF* gene is found in 77–100% of PCP cases [4, 12, 13, 32–34]. In normal cells, the binding of growth factors, such as EGF (epidermal growth factor), to receptor tyrosine kinases activates a RAS protein (from RAt Sarcoma) (KRAS, NRAS, and HRAS) by conversion of its inactive guanosine diphosphate (GDP)-bound form into an active guanosine triphosphate (GTP)-bound form [35] (Fig. 1.7a). This conversion is mediated by guanine nucleotide exchange factors such as SOS1 (Son Of Sevenless 1). The activated RAS protein will then initiate the sequential phosphorylation of RAF (rapidly accelerated fibrosarcoma) (ARAF, BRAF, and CRAF), MEK1/2 (MAPKinase-ERK-kinase 1/2), and ERK1/2 (extracellular signal-regulated kinase 1/2) [36]. ERK translocates into the nucleus and phosphorylates various transcription factors, notably resulting in cellular proliferation.

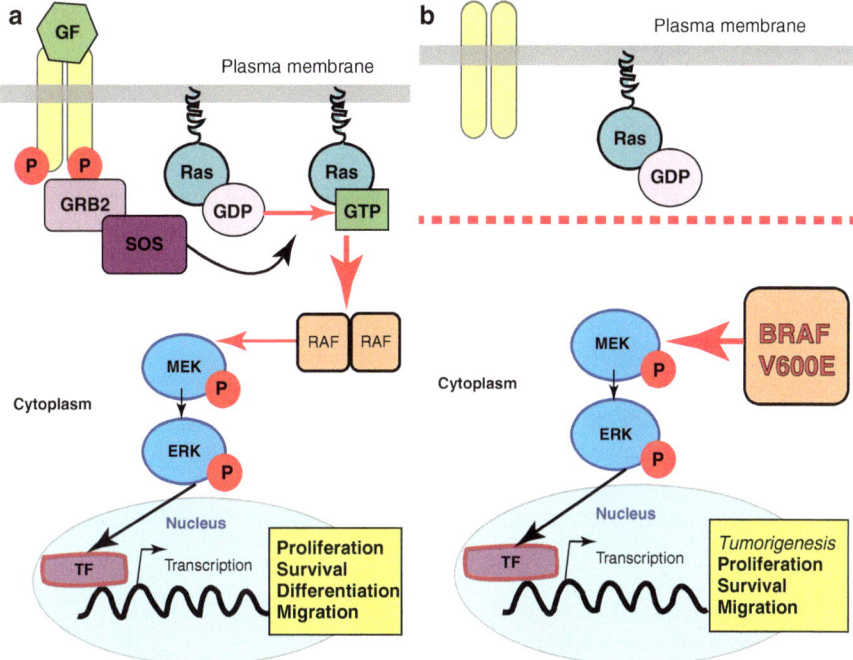

Fig. 1.7 MAPKinase pathway in papillary craniopharyngioma. (**a**) Under physiological conditions, growth factors or mitogens bind to receptor tyrosine kinases, leading to their dimerization and autophosphorylation. This phosphorylation recruits GRB2 and SOS. SOS catalyzes the transformation from an inactive GDP-bound RAS protein to an active GTP-bound RAS protein. RAS then activates the RAF proteins which form dimers. RAF phosphorylates MEK which in turn phosphorylates ERK. ERK is then translocated to the nucleus where it activates the transcription of various genes involved in proliferation. (**b**) In papillary craniopharyngioma, extracellular stimuli are not required to activate the MAPKinase pathway. The BRAF[V600E] protein is constitutively active and phosphorylates MEK, which in turn can activate the downstream signaling cascade. *ERK* extracellular signal-regulated kinase, *GDP* guanosine diphosphate, *GRB2* growth factor receptor bound-protein 2, *GTP* guanosine triphosphate, *MEK* MAPK-ERK-kinase, *RAF* rapidly accelerated fibrosarcoma, *RAS* rat sarcoma, *SOS* Son of Sevenless

The V600E mutation is a class I BRAF mutation resulting in the substitution of a glutamic acid (E) for a valine (V) at position 600. Monomers of BRAF^{V600E} are able to constitutively activate the MAPKinase pathway via the phosphorylation of ERK1/2 (Fig. 1.7b). This activation is independent of RAS signaling [36]. In PCP, the activation of the MAPKinase pathway in SOX2-positive cells of the basal layer may play a role in tumoral growth and impaired differentiation towards pituitary-cell lineages [37].

The presence of BRAF^{V600E} mutated protein can be detected by immunohisto-chemistry using the VE1 antibody [4]. A few case reports show a significant tumoral response of BRAF V600E-mutated PCP under treatment with BRAF inhibitor or a combination of BRAF/MEK inhibitors [38–40].

In order to preoperatively detect BRAF-mutated craniopharyngioma, Fujio and colleagues have suggested three clinical factors that show a high interobserver agreement: age (older than 18 years), absence of calcifications visible on CT scan, and supradiaphragmatic location of the tumor [41].

1.3.3 Origin of PCP

Erdheim suggested that ACP and PCP both developed from squamous nests in the *pars tuberalis,* assuming that they were remnants of the hypophyseal duct (embryonic theory) [2]. In odontogenic tumors, ameloblastomas are characterized by frequent BRAF V600E mutations [19]. This is a feature, in common with PCP, that may favor an embryological view of its development, similar to ACP. However, ameloblastomas and PCP are histologically different. The development of PCP from metaplastic squamous epithelial nests of the *pars tuberalis*, as previously discussed for ACP, is an alternative explanation [5]. A dual model of CP pathogenesis has also been suggested: the embryonic theory for ACP and the metaplastic theory for PCP [5, 8].

Goblet cells and ciliated cells that are reminiscent of Rathke's cleft cyst are occasionally observed in PCP. This finding has raised the question of a link between Rathke's cleft cyst and PCP [42, 43].

1.4 Mixed and Collision Tumors

CPs may rarely be associated with other types of tumors such as gonadotroph adenoma [44], olfactory neuroblastoma [45], or silent pituitary adenoma subtype 3 (now termed plurihormonal Pit1-positive adenoma) [46].

1.5 Malignant Transformation in Craniopharyngiomas

Malignant transformation of CPs is an exceedingly rare event [47–49]. Malignant CPs are usually secondary tumors. They typically develop in patients previously treated by radiation therapy for recurrent ACP. Malignant CPs show histopathological features of squamous carcinoma.

1.6   Differential Diagnosis

1.6.1   ACP and Pilocytic Astrocytoma

ACP, being surrounded by florid piloid gliosis, may be misdiagnosed as a pilocytic astrocytoma when tissue sampling does not include the epithelial component. This may be the case when only a limited biopsy has been performed. In this situation, the comparison with the imaging data is essential. If the tumor is calcified and does not involve the optic nerves, the diagnosis of pilocytic astrocytoma should be carefully considered.

1.6.2   PCP and Rathke's Cleft Cyst with Squamous Metaplasia

A Rathke's cleft cyst may undergo extensive squamous metaplasia and be misdiagnosed as a PCP, especially if remnants of the cyst lining are not found. In this situation, the identification of a BRAF V600E mutation by immunohistochemistry or sequencing is useful to confirm the diagnosis of PCP [50].

1.6.3   ACP and Sellar Xanthogranuloma

Xanthogranuloma (XG) is a clinico-pathological entity described in 1999 by Paulus and colleagues [51]. XGs are characterized by the accumulation of cholesterol clefts surrounded by foreign-body giant cells, infiltrates of lymphocytes, plasma cells, and macrophages, hemosiderin deposits, necrotic debris, and, more rarely, calcifications. They differ from ACPs in several features: the cholesterol granulomatous reaction is more diffuse; in a proportion of cases, a cyst-like squamous or cuboidal epithelium may be observed; they affect young adults with a mean age of 27.4 years; XGs are smaller and show a prominent intrasellar involvement with patients showing severe endocrinological dysfunction. The prognosis in the case of XG is favorable as complete surgical removal is more frequent when compared to ACP. Histologically, XGs do not exhibit palisading epithelium, stellate reticulum, and "wet keratin". The finding of ciliated cells in XG has raised the possibility of a link with Rathke's cleft cyst. Some authors have suggested that XGs mostly correspond to the last stage of chronic inflammation in Rathke's cleft cyst. In these cases, the inflammatory changes are so prominent that the cyst lining is often no longer recognizable [52, 53].

1.6.4   ACP Versus PCP

ACP and PCP are classically seen as distinct entities with non-overlapping histopathological and molecular features. The distinction between ACP and PCP is usually straightforward on histology. However, BRAF V600E mutation can be rarely found in ACP with a *CTNNB1* mutation [32].

1.6.5 Cystic ACP and Rathke's Cleft Cysts

Rathke's cleft cyst may undergo secondary changes, especially in the case of rupture/leakage/hemorrhage. These changes include cholesterol clefts. Differentiation can be based upon nuclear accumulation of β-catenin [54]. However, the nucleocytoplasmic immunopositivity is focal in ACP. The recognition of "wet keratin" in a cystic lesion confirms the diagnosis of ACP and is inconsistent with a Rathke's cleft cyst.

1.7 Conclusion

Histologically, craniopharyngiomas are divided into two distinct pathological subtypes: adamantinomatous craniopharyngioma and papillary craniopharyngioma. These two subtypes differ not only in their histopathological features but also in their molecular pathogenesis. From a molecular point of view, ACP recapitulates tooth development. They are characterized by *CTNNB1* mutations that result in nuclear accumulation of β-catenin in discrete clusters of cells ("whorls" or "morules"). In contrast, PCP is driven by a BRAF V600E mutation that causes activation of the MAPKinase pathway. This molecular abnormality may be targeted by treatment with MAPKinase inhibitors (BRAF inhibitor ± MEK inhibitors).

References

1. Zacharia BE, Bruce SS, Goldstein H, Malone HR, Neugut AI, Bruce JN. Incidence, treatment and survival of patients with craniopharyngioma in the surveillance, epidemiology and end results program. Neuro-Oncology. 2012;14:1070–8.
2. Pascual JM, Rosdolsky M, Prieto R, Straubeta S, Winter E, Ulrich W. Jakob Erdheim (1874-1937): father of hypophyseal-duct tumors (craniopharyngiomas). Virchows Arch. 2015;467:459–69.
3. Bulsei R, Rushing EJ, Giangaspero F, Paulus W, Burger PC, Santagata S. Craniopharyngioma. In: Louis DN, Hiroko O, Wiestler OD, Cavenee WK, editors. WHO classification of tumours of the central nervous system. 4th ed. Lyon: IARC; 2016. p. 324–8.
4. Holsken A, Sill M, Merkle J, Schweizer L, Buchfelder M, Flitsch J, Fahlbusch R, Metzler M, Kool M, Pfister SM, von Deimling A, Capper D, Jones DT, Buslei R. Adamantinomatous and papillary craniopharyngiomas are characterized by distinct epigenomic as well as mutational and transcriptomic profiles. Acta Neuropathol Commun. 2016;4:20.
5. Muller HL. Craniopharyngioma. Handb Clin Neurol. 2014;124:235–53.
6. Szeifert GT, Sipos L, Horvath M, Sarker MH, Major O, Salomvary B, Czirjak S, Balint K, Slowik F, Kolonics L, et al. Pathological characteristics of surgically removed craniopharyngiomas: analysis of 131 cases. Acta Neurochir. 1993;124:139–43.
7. Zada G, Lin N, Ojerholm E, Ramkissoon S, Laws ER. Craniopharyngioma and other cystic epithelial lesions of the sellar region: a review of clinical, imaging, and histopathological relationships. Neurosurg Focus. 2010;28:E4.
8. Larkin SJ, Ansorge O. Pathology and pathogenesis of craniopharyngiomas. Pituitary. 2013;16:9–17.
9. Kawamata T, Kubo O, Hori T. Histological findings at the boundary of craniopharyngiomas. Brain Tumor Pathol. 2005;22:75–8.

10. Sekine S, Shibata T, Kokubu A, Morishita Y, Noguchi M, Nakanishi Y, Sakamoto M, Hirohashi S. Craniopharyngiomas of adamantinomatous type harbor beta-catenin gene mutations. Am J Pathol. 2002;161:1997–2001.

11. Buslei R, Nolde M, Hofmann B, Meissner S, Eyupoglu IY, Siebzehnrubl F, Hahnen E, Kreutzer J, Fahlbusch R. Common mutations of beta-catenin in adamantinomatous cranio-pharyngiomas but not in other tumours originating from the sellar region. Acta Neuropathol. 2005;109:589–97.

12. Brastianos PK, Taylor-Weiner A, Manley PE, Jones RT, Dias-Santagata D, Thorner AR, Lawrence MS, Rodriguez FJ, Bernardo LA, Schubert L, Sunkavalli A, Shillingford N, Calicchio ML, Lidov HG, Taha H, Martinez-Lage M, Santi M, Storm PB, Lee JY, Palmer JN, Adappa ND, Scott RM, Dunn IF, Laws ER Jr, Stewart C, Ligon KL, Hoang MP, Van Hummelen P, Hahn WC, Louis DN, Resnick AC, Kieran MW, Getz G, Santagata S. Exome sequencing identifies BRAF mutations in papillary craniopharyngiomas. Nat Genet. 2014;46:161–5.

13. Goschzik T, Gessi M, Dreschmann V, Gebhardt U, Wang L, Yamaguchi S, Wheeler DA, Lauriola L, Lau CC, Muller HL, Pietsch T. Genomic alterations of adamantinomatous and papillary craniopharyngioma. J Neuropathol Exp Neurol. 2017;76:126–34.

14. Zhan T, Rindtorff N, Boutros M. Wnt signaling in cancer. Oncogene. 2017;36:1461–73.

15. Ghosh N, Hossain U, Mandal A, Sil PC. The Wnt signaling pathway: a potential therapeutic target against cancer. Ann N Y Acad Sci. 2019;1443:54–74.

16. Gao C, Wang Y, Broaddus R, Sun L, Xue F, Zhang W. Exon 3 mutations of CTNNB1 drive tumorigenesis: a review. Oncotarget. 2018;9:5492–508.

17. Stamos JL, Weis WI. The beta-catenin destruction complex. Cold Spring Harb Perspect Biol. 2013;5:a007898.

18. MacDonald BT, He X. Frizzled and LRP5/6 receptors for Wnt/beta-catenin signaling. Cold Spring Harb Perspect Biol. 2012;4:a007880.

19. Gomes CC, de Sousa SF, Gomez RS. Craniopharyngiomas and odontogenic tumors mimic normal odontogenesis and share genetic mutations, histopathologic features, and molecular pathways activation. Oral Surg Oral Med Oral Pathol Oral Radiol. 2019;127:231–6.

20. Muller C, Adroos N, Lockhat Z, Slavik T, Kruger H. Toothy craniopharyngioma: a literature review and case report of craniopharyngioma with extensive odontogenic differentiation and tooth formation. Childs Nerv Syst. 2011;27:323–6.

21. Dubois PM, Elamraoui A. Embryology of the pituitary gland. Trends Endocrinol Metab. 1995;6:1–7.

22. Khonsari RH, Seppala M, Pradel A, Dutel H, Clement G, Lebedev O, Ghafoor S, Rothova M, Tucker A, Maisey JG, Fan CM, Kawasaki M, Ohazama A, Tafforeau P, Franco B, Helms J, Haycraft CJ, David A, Janvier P, Cobourne MT, Sharpe PT. The buccohypophyseal canal is an ancestral vertebrate trait maintained by modulation in sonic hedgehog signaling. BMC Biol. 2013;11:27.

23. Asa SL, Kovacs K, Bilbao JM. The pars tuberalis of the human pituitary. A histologic, immunohistochemical, ultrastructural and immunoelectron microscopic analysis. Virchows Arch A. 1983;399:49–59.

24. Luse SA, Kernohan JW. Squamous-cell nests of the pituitary gland. Cancer. 1955;8:623–8.

25. Martinez-Barbera JP, Andoniadou CL. Paracrine role of stem cells in pituitary tumors: a focus on adamantinomatous craniopharyngioma. Stem Cells. 2016;34:268–76.

26. Apps JR, Martinez-Barbera JP. Genetically engineered mouse models of craniopharyngioma: an opportunity for therapy development and understanding of tumor biology. Brain Pathol. 2017;27:364–9.

27. Som PM, Miletich I. Review of the embryology of the teeth. Neurographics. 2018;8:369–93.

28. Apps JR, Carreno G, Gonzalez-Meljem JM, Haston S, Guiho R, Cooper JE, Manshaei S, Jani N, Holsken A, Pettorini B, Beynon RJ, Simpson DM, Fraser HC, Hong Y, Hallang S, Stone TJ, Virasami A, Donson AM, Jones D, Aquilina K, Spoudeas H, Joshi AR, Grundy R, Storer LCD, Korbonits M, Hilton DA, Tossell K, Thavaraj S, Ungless MA, Gil J, Buslei R, Hankinson T, Hargrave D, Goding C, Andoniadou CL, Brogan P, Jacques TS, Williams HJ, Martinez-Barbera JP. Tumour compartment transcriptomics demonstrates the activation of inflammatory

and odontogenic programmes in human adamantinomatous craniopharyngioma and identifies the MAPK/ERK pathway as a novel therapeutic target. Acta Neuropathol. 2018;135:757–77.

29. Crotty TB, Scheithauer BW, Young WF Jr, Davis DH, Shaw EG, Miller GM, Burger PC. Papillary craniopharyngioma: a clinicopathological study of 48 cases. J Neurosurg. 1995;83:206–14.

30. Borrill R, Cheesman E, Stivaros S, Kamaly-Asl ID, Gnanalingham K, Kilday JP. Papillary craniopharyngioma in a 4-year-old girl with BRAF V600E mutation: a case report and review of the literature. Childs Nerv Syst. 2019;35:169–73.

31. La Corte E, Younus I, Pivari F, Selimi A, Ottenhausen M, Forbes JA, Pisapia DJ, Dobri GA, Anand VK, Schwartz TH. BRAF V600E mutant papillary craniopharyngiomas: a single-institutional case series. Pituitary. 2018;21:571–83.

32. Larkin SJ, Preda V, Karavitaki N, Grossman A, Ansorge O. BRAF V600E mutations are characteristic for papillary craniopharyngioma and may coexist with CTNNB1-mutated adamantinomatous craniopharyngioma. Acta Neuropathol. 2014;127:927–9.

33. Marucci G, de Biase D, Zoli M, Faustini-Fustini M, Bacci A, Pasquini E, Visani M, Mazzatenta D, Frank G, Tallini G. Targeted BRAF and CTNNB1 next-generation sequencing allows proper classification of nonadenomatous lesions of the sellar region in samples with limiting amounts of lesional cells. Pituitary. 2015;18:905–11.

34. Yoshimoto K, Hatae R, Suzuki SO, Hata N, Kuga D, Akagi Y, Amemiya T, Sangatsuda Y, Mukae N, Mizoguchi M, Iwaki T, Iihara K. High-resolution melting and immunohistochemical analysis efficiently detects mutually exclusive genetic alterations of adamantinomatous and papillary craniopharyngiomas. Neuropathology. 2018;38:3–10.

35. Simanshu DK, Nissley DV, McCormick F. RAS proteins and their regulators in human disease. Cell. 2017;170:17–33.

36. Yaeger R, Corcoran RB. Targeting alterations in the RAF-MEK pathway. Cancer Discov. 2019;9:329–41.

37. Haston S, Pozzi S, Carreno G, Manshaei S, Panousopoulos L, Gonzalez-Meljem JM, Apps JR, Virasami A, Thavaraj S, Gutteridge A, Forshew T, Marais R, Brandner S, Jacques TS, Andoniadou CL, Martinez-Barbera JP. MAPK pathway control of stem cell proliferation and differentiation in the embryonic pituitary provides insights into the pathogenesis of papillary craniopharyngioma. Development. 2017;144:2141–52.

38. Aylwin SJ, Bodi I, Beaney R. Pronounced response of papillary craniopharyngioma to treatment with vemurafenib, a BRAF inhibitor. Pituitary. 2016;19:544–6.

39. Brastianos PK, Shankar GM, Gill CM, Taylor-Weiner A, Nayyar N, Panka DJ, Sullivan RJ, Frederick DT, Abedalthagafi M, Jones PS, Dunn IF, Nahed BV, Romero JM, Louis DN, Getz G, Cahill DP, Santagata S, Curry WT Jr, Barker FG. Dramatic response of BRAF V600E mutant papillary craniopharyngioma to targeted therapy. J Natl Cancer Inst. 2016;108:djv310.

40. Rostami E, Witt Nystrom P, Libard S, Wikstrom J, Casar-Borota O, Gudjonsson O. Recurrent papillary craniopharyngioma with BRAFV600E mutation treated with neoadjuvant-targeted therapy. Acta Neurochir. 2017;159:2217–21.

41. Fujio S, Juratli TA, Arita K, Hirano H, Nagano Y, Takajo T, Yoshimoto K, Bihun IV, Kaplan AB, Nayyar N, Fink AL, Bertalan MS, Tummala SS, Curry WT Jr, Jones PS, Martinez-Lage M, Cahill DP, Barker FG, Brastianos PK. A clinical rule for preoperative prediction of BRAF mutation status in craniopharyngiomas. Neurosurgery. 2018;85(2):204–10.

42. Okada T, Fujitsu K, Miyahara K, Ichikawa T, Takemoto Y, Niino H, Yagishita S, Shiina T. Ciliated craniopharyngioma--case report and pathological study. Acta Neurochir. 2010;152:303–6.

43. Schlaffer SM, Buchfelder M, Stoehr R, Buslei R, Holsken A. Rathke's cleft cyst as origin of a pediatric papillary craniopharyngioma. Front Genet. 2018;9:49.

44. Karavitaki N, Scheithauer BW, Watt J, Ansorge O, Moschopoulos M, Llaguno AV, Wass JA. Collision lesions of the sella: co-existence of craniopharyngioma with gonadotroph adenoma and of Rathke's cleft cyst with corticotroph adenoma. Pituitary. 2008;11:317–23.

45. Chang KC, Jin YT, Chen RM, Su LJ. Mixed olfactory neuroblastoma and craniopharyngioma: an unusual pathological finding. Histopathology. 1997;30:378–82.

46. Moshkin O, Scheithauer BW, Syro LV, Velasquez A, Horvath E, Kovacs K. Collision tumors of the sella: craniopharyngioma and silent pituitary adenoma subtype 3: case report. Endocr Pathol. 2009;20:50–5.
47. Kristopaitis T, Thomas C, Petruzzelli GJ, Lee JM. Malignant craniopharyngioma. Arch Pathol Lab Med. 2000;124:1356–60.
48. Ishida M, Hotta M, Tsukamura A, Taga T, Kato H, Ohta S, Takeuchi Y, Nakasu S, Okabe H. Malignant transformation in craniopharyngioma after radiation therapy: a case report and review of the literature. Clin Neuropathol. 2010;29:2–8.
49. Nomura S, Aihara Y, Amano K, Eguchi S, Chiba K, Komori T, Kawamata T. A rare case of malignant craniopharyngioma reactive to adjunctive stereotactic radiotherapy and chemotherapy: case report and literature review. World Neurosurg. 2018;117:332–8.
50. Schweizer L, Capper D, Holsken A, Fahlbusch R, Flitsch J, Buchfelder M, Herold-Mende C, von Deimling A, Buslei R. BRAF V600E analysis for the differentiation of papillary craniopharyngiomas and Rathke's cleft cysts. Neuropathol Appl Neurobiol. 2015;41:733–42.
51. Paulus W, Honegger J, Keyvani K, Fahlbusch R. Xanthogranuloma of the sellar region: a clinicopathological entity different from adamantinomatous craniopharyngioma. Acta Neuropathol. 1999;97:377–82.
52. Kleinschmidt-DeMasters BK, Lillehei KO, Hankinson TC. Review of xanthomatous lesions of the sella. Brain Pathol. 2017;27:377–95.
53. Fujio S, Takajo T, Kinoshita Y, Hanaya R, Arimura H, Sugata J, Sugata S, Bohara M, Hiraki T, Yoshimoto K, Arita K. Sellar xanthogranuloma: a quest based on nine cases assessed with anterior pituitary provocation test. World Neurosurg. 2019;130:e150–9.
54. Hofmann BM, Kreutzer J, Saeger W, Buchfelder M, Blumcke I, Fahlbusch R, Buslei R. Nuclear beta-catenin accumulation as reliable marker for the differentiation between cystic craniopharyngiomas and rathke cleft cysts: a clinico-pathologic approach. Am J Surg Pathol. 2006;30:1595–603.

John R. Apps and Juan Pedro Martinez-Barbera

2.1 Genetically Engineered Mouse Models (GEMMS) of Craniopharyngioma

2.1.1 Adamantinomatous Craniopharyngioma

Adamantinomatous craniopharyngiomas (ACPs) harbour activating point mutations in exon three of the *CTNNB1* gene, leading to a failure of ubiquitin mediated destruction of the protein β-catenin, and as a consequence the over-activation of the Wnt pathway [1–4] (Fig. 2.1). Despite the presence of the mutation throughout the epithelial tumour, activation of the pathway, as evidenced by nuclear β-catenin immunostaining (Fig. 2.2) and the expression of downstream targets such *Lef1* and *Axin2*, are limited to a small proportion of cells, either single cells or often correlating with epithelial whorls and known as clusters [5, 6].

Genetically engineered mouse models have been generated by expressing a functionally equivalent form of mutant β-catenin to that found in human ACP leading to the activation of the Wnt pathway [7]. Cre recombinase-mediated excision of exon 3 of *CTNNB1* results in the deletion of the degradation domain of β-catenin without affecting its transcriptional activating properties. In other words, this mutant β-catenin protein can act as a transcriptional activator and promote the expression of

J. R. Apps
Cancer Research UK Clinical Trials Unit (CRCTU), Institute of Cancer and Genomic Sciences, University of Birmingham, Birmingham, UK

Developmental Biology and Cancer, Birth Defects Research Centre, UCL Great Ormond Street Institute of Child Health, University College London, London, UK
e-mail: j.apps@ucl.ac.uk

J. P. Martinez-Barbera (✉)
Developmental Biology and Cancer, Birth Defects Research Centre, UCL Great Ormond Street Institute of Child Health, University College London, London, UK
e-mail: j.martinez-barbera@ucl.ac.uk

© Springer Nature Switzerland AG 2020
E. Jouanneau, G. Raverot (eds.), *Adult Craniopharyngiomas*,
https://doi.org/10.1007/978-3-030-41176-3_2

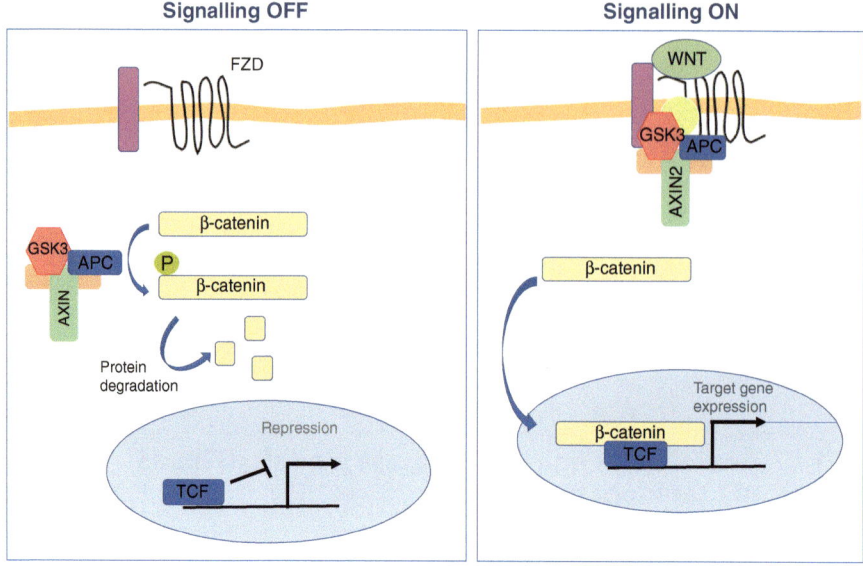

Fig. 2.1 Schematic representation of the WNT/β-catenin pathway. In the absence of WNT ligands, β-catenin is targeted for proteosomal destruction through phosphorylation of amino acids encoded in exon 3 by the Axin/GSK3β/APC destruction complex. Upon ligand binding, the destruction complex is sequestered to the cell membrane, facilitating translocation of β-catenin to the nucleus and activation of transcription. Mutation of the phosphorylation domain renders β-catenin resistant to degradation, resulting in increased half-life of the mutant protein and over-activation of the WNT pathway

Fig. 2.2 Histomorphological features of mouse and human ACP. (**a**) Haematoxylin and eosin staining of mouse and human tumours showing the presence of microcystic changes (stellate reticulum; arrows) and whorl-like nodular structures (cell clusters; arrowheads). (**b**) Immuno-histochemistry with a specific anti-β-catenin antibody showing the presence of cell clusters with nucleocytoplasmic accumulation of β-catenin (arrows). Reproduced with permission from [6]

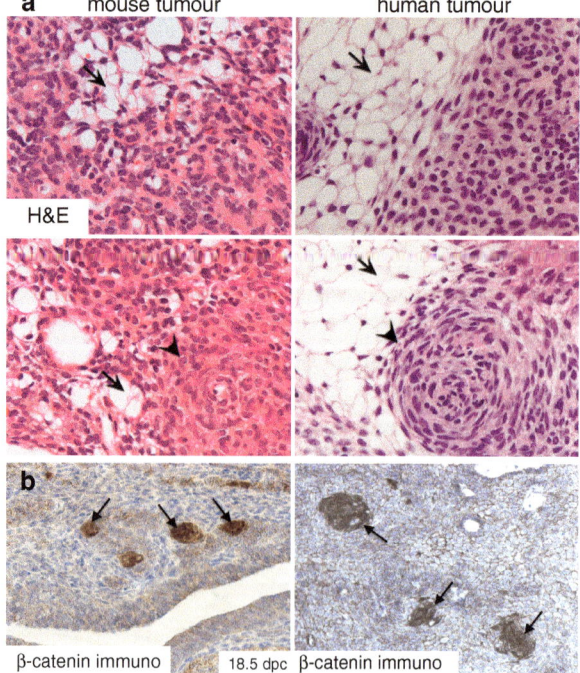

target genes but its degradation is impaired. We will refer to this form of mouse β-catenin as well as the human β-catenin expressed in human tumours as oncogenic β-catenin. Using specific Cre recombinase-expressing mouse lines, two main models of ACP have been developed: the embryonic and the inducible models [6, 8]. Like in human ACP, the presence of cell clusters that accumulate nucleocytoplasmic β-catenin has been demonstrated within the developing tumours in both mouse models (Fig. 2.2b).

2.1.2 Embryonic Model of Human ACP

In the embryonic model (*Hesx1*[Cre/+]; *Ctnnb1*[lox(ex3)/+]), oncogenic β-catenin is activated using Cre recombinase expressed from the *Hesx1* gene promoter. *Hesx1* is a developmental gene that is expressed in the embryonic precursors of the anterior pituitary, which form Rathke's pouch [9]. Lineage tracing has demonstrated that these precursors give rise to all of the hormone-producing cells in the adult pituitary gland [6, 10, 11]. These mice develop enlarged dysfunctional pituitaries during embryonic development, characterised by enlargement and a particular deficit of some cell types (e.g. growth hormone-producing cells, i.e. somatotrophs). A high proportion of the mice die at birth, due to upper airway obstruction, but those that survive are smaller (growth hormone deficient) and go on to develop cystic-solid tumours, resulting in death at around 6 months of age [6, 12].

As in human tumours, despite the presence of the mutation in all cells, the developing pituitaries of these mice are characterised by isolated clusters showing nucleocytoplasmic β-catenin accumulation. These clusters express markers of WNT pathway activation, e.g. *Lef1*, *Axin2*, but lack markers of hormone-producing cell differentiation and a proportion express the pituitary stem cell marker SOX2 [13, 14]. Highlighting a need for the tumour-initiating mutation to occur in an undifferentiated cell type, activation of the WNT pathway in more committed precursors or differentiated hormone-producing cells does not lead to the formation of clusters and is non-tumourigenic [6].

Andoniadou et al. used a mouse line reporting WNT pathway activation to isolate these cluster cells by flow-activated cell sorting and perform expression analysis comparing cluster versus non-cluster pituitary tissue [15]. This identified the high expression of many secreted factors by the cluster cells, including sonic hedgehog (SHH) and members of the fibroblast growth factor (FGF), transforming growth factor β (TGFβ) and bone morphogenic protein (BMP) families of growth factors, as well as many inflammatory mediators such as cytokines and chemokines. These findings were confirmed by in situ hybridisation in human tumours and comparison with RNA sequencing of human clusters, collected by laser capture microdissection. This confirmed shared gene signatures between murine and human clusters [16]. Moreover, many of the genes/pathways that were identified as dysregulated in the murine model have been later confirmed to be expressed in human ACP [17–21]. This suggests a strong homology both histologically and molecularly between mice and human clusters.

Late-stage tumours also have some similarities with human ACP. They are frequently cystic, often haemorrhagic and have areas of microcystic change, similar to the stellate reticulum seen in human ACP [6, 12]. Imaging of the mouse models has also identified similar features on multi-parametric MRI to human ACP, most notably an absence of reduction in signal intensity of cystic fluid on FLAIR imaging, suggestive of similarities between the cysts contents in mouse and human ACP [12].

Serial MRI of the embryonic model has characterised a non-linear growth pattern, with tumour and cyst expansion after a long period of relative quiescence [12]. In contrast to human ACP, murine ACPs have not been observed to calcify, and the degenerative changes of ghost cells/wet keratin have not been observed, nor the finger-like protrusions seen in a proportion of ACP [22]. The reasons of these differences are not understood, but may reflect species-specific differences.

2.1.3 Inducible Model of Human ACP

It is now established that SOX2+ve cells in the adult pituitary represent a stem cell population showing both self-renewal properties and capacity to differentiate into all lineages of the anterior pituitary [8, 23]. In the inducible model of ACP ($Sox2^{creERT2+/-}$; $Ctnnb1^{lox(exon3)/+}$), oncogenic β-catenin was specifically expressed in the SOX2+ve cell population using a tamoxifen inducible Cre recombinase (*CreERT2*). Similar to the embryonic model, activation of the WNT pathway in these SOX2 positive cells from 6 weeks of age led to the development of nucleocytoplasmic-accumulating β-catenin cell clusters and subsequent development of undifferentiated tumours (synaptophysin and hormone negative) [8]. As with the embryonic model, these clusters have also been shown to produce a range of soluble factors (e.g. inflammatory mediators and other growth factors) [24, 25]. Gene expression analyses of purified cluster cells from both mouse models and human tumours have revealed that clusters are molecularly similar [25]. These experiments support further the validity of the mouse models and raise important questions about the function of these secreted factors or the nature of the cluster cells.

2.2 Stem Cell Paracrine Tumourigenesis: A Novel Mechanism of Somatic Stem Cells Contribution to Tumour Formation

The detailed analyses performed in the mouse models have revealed a surprising mechanism underlying tumour formation. Lineage tracing of the SOX2+ve cells upon expressing oncogenic β-catenin, using yellow fluorescent protein (YFP), revealed that the tumours of the inducible model were not derived from the SOX2+ve cells and did not carry the activating β-catenin mutation [8]. The cell clusters were

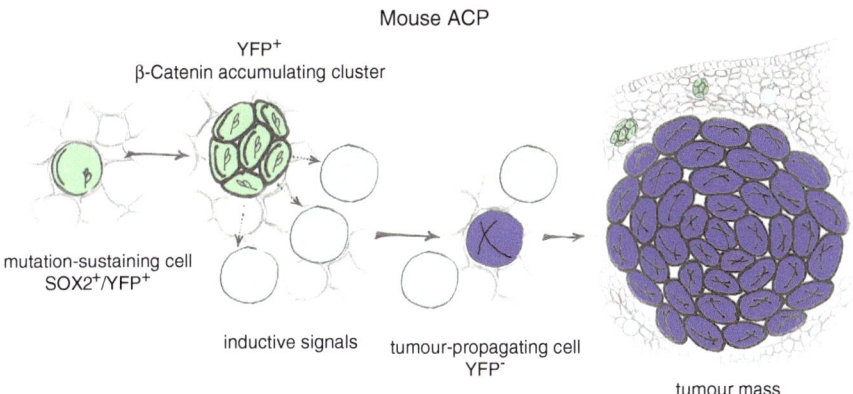

Fig. 2.3 Paracrine model of involvement of pituitary stem cells in tumourigenesis. When targeted to express oncogenic β-catenin, SOX2+ cells (green) accumulate nucleocytoplasmic β-catenin, proliferate transiently, stop dividing and form clusters. Clusters secrete signals to the surrounding cells to induce cell transformation and tumour growth from a cell that is not derived from the targeted SOX2+ stem cell. Reproduced with permission from [8]

derived from the targeted cells, therefore demonstrating that the origin of the clusters is a SOX2+ve stem cell. However, the tumours were derived from a different cell lineage. This was surprising because in other organs, somatic stem cells have been shown to be the cancer-initiating cells when targeted with oncogenic insults [26–28] (Fig. 2.3)

Subsequent lineage tracing of the embryonic model using both YFP and TdTomato, under the Rosa26 locus, has also confirmed that $Hesx1^{Cre/+}$; $Ctnnb1^{lox(ex3)/+}$ tumours are not derived from the $Hesx1$-expressing cell lineage and that tumour cells are non-recombined and do not contain the mutated $CTNNB1$ gene [24]. Further investigation has shown that the cellular microenvironment is modified by the presence of the clusters with infiltration and expansion of cell not normally detected in the pituitary gland and drastic alteration in components of the extracellular matrix (ECM) [24]. Because these microenvironment changes take place weeks before the appearance of the tumour mass or the detection of tumour cells with high-proliferative index, it is likely that they play an instructive role in tumour initiation. Exome sequencing of late-stage tumours in the embryonic model has also confirmed the acquisition of somatically acquired mutations, therefore demonstrating that the cell masses in the mouse models are tumours. Specifically, we identified 272 mutations in 15 murine tumours (average 18.13 mutations per tumour) [24].

Therefore, the tumours form in a paracrine manner in both mouse models, whereby the cells (e.g. SOX2+ve) targeted with the oncogenic insult (e.g. β-catenin) are bestowed with tumour-inducing potential. We have proposed the concept of paracrine tumourigenesis based on these observations [8], an idea that has been observed in mouse models of other tumour/cancers such as liver, skin, brain and leukaemia

[28–33]. This concept challenges a more traditional understanding of cancer as a cell autonomous process and suggests that paracrine signalling may be critical in cell transformation and tumour initiation [28, 34]. The initiation of tumours/cancer requires not only the genetic heterogeneity in the control of gene expression, either at the level of DNA mutations or epigenetics, but importantly a pro-tumourigenic microenvironment that promotes and fuels the expansion of the tumour-initiating cells. The mouse models of ACP are helping understand better the pathogenesis of craniopharyngioma and in addition, are ideal tools to unravel the mechanisms involved in paracrine tumourigenesis in cancer initiation.

2.3   Childhood-Onset Craniopharyngioma is a Developmental Disorder

These mouse models have demonstrated that ACPs develop from *CTNNB1* mutations in either embryonic or adult stem cells. Such mutations result in the formation of cluster of stem cells which create a pro-tumourigenic cellular microenvironment leading to tumour development several weeks later. We have estimated that there is a latency period of around 18 weeks after birth before murine tumours are detectable by MRI [12], suggesting that children fated to develop craniopharyngioma may be born harbouring cell clusters in the pituitary without a proper tumour mass. The observation by Professor Hermann Muller's group that childhood patients with craniopharyngioma have a reduced height standard deviation score (SDS) score at one year of age gives support to this idea that childhood-onset craniopharyngioma is a developmental disorder [35]. In fact, somatotrophs are the most affected cell type in the embryonic model [6]. Moreover, rare cases of congenital craniopharyngioma tumours have been described [36]. This evidence suggests that *CTNNB1* mutation may occur in pituitary progenitors during development or early life. In contrast, it is plausible to speculate that adult-onset craniopharyngioma may result from mutation in SOX2+ve adult pituitary stem cells, as shown in the inducible ACP murine model. Consistent with exome sequencing approaches in human ACP, which have failed to identify additional recurrent mutations to *CTNNB1*, the research from the mouse models suggests that *CTNNB1* mutations alone are sufficient to induce ACP tumourigenesis when targeting the correct cells.

Recent expression profiling of human ACP samples has begun to decipher the histologically observed relationship between ACP pathogenesis and the developing tooth and tooth tumours such as calcifying odontogenic cysts. Analyses of gene expression profiles and specific markers such as the ectodysplasin receptor (EDAR) suggest that ACP clusters are molecularly similar to the enamel knot, a critical signalling structure whose paracrine activities are required for normal tooth development [16]. This is consistent with the idea that clusters are signalling hubs influencing tumour growth and invasive behaviour [37, 38]. The histological similarities between ACP tumourigenesis and tooth development have been known for over 100 years [39]; however, these recent gene expression data provide a molecular paradigm to understand those similarities. We have proposed that similar to the paracrine role of the enamel knot during tooth development, i.e. instructing a complex signalling crosstalk with surrounding enamel epithelia and dental mesenchyme, the ACP cell clusters' activities may also control tumour cell behaviour and proliferation [16]. Moreover, mouse models of normal tooth development and disease models may inform about pathways that could be tumourigenic in ACP. For example, patients with Costello syndrome carry mutations in *HRAS* resulting in the over-activation of the MAPK/ERK pathway and show abnormal tooth formation due to increased proliferation and irregular orientation of tooth epithelial cells [40]. Of note, inhibition of the MAPK/ERK pathway (Fig. 2.4) using specific drugs rescues this phenotype by reducing proliferation and improving epithelial cell dynamics. Likewise, the inhibition of the MAPK/ERK pathway has recently been shown to reduce proliferation and induce apoptosis in mouse and human ACP in vitro [16].

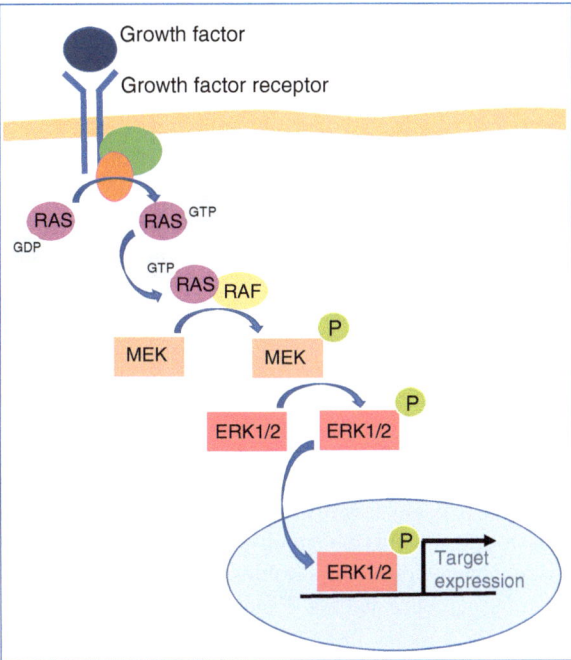

Fig. 2.4 Schematic representation of the MAPK pathway. Growth factor binding to tyrosine kinase receptor complexes results in exchange of GDP for GTP on RAS proteins and subsequent interaction with RAF. Activated RAF triggers a cascade of phosphorylation leading to phosphorylation of MEK, which subsequently phosphorylates ERK. Activated ERK translocates to the nucleus to activate the transcription of target genes involved in multiple processes including cell proliferation and survival. In cancer, the pathway can be activated by increased ligand expression, mutation or amplification of growth factor receptors or activating mutations in RAS or RAF

2.4   Cluster Cells Are Molecularly Similar and Share a Signature of Cellular Senescence

An important question derived from the research in mouse models is what are the cluster cells and what are the underpinnings on the tumour-inducing potential? Comprehensive molecular and immunohistochemical profiling of clusters in both human and murine cluster cells have shown clusters to exhibit all the markers of senescence, specifically: markers of (1) cell cycle arrest (Ki67 and phospho-histone 3 negative); (2) DNA damage and activation of a DDR (p21, p16, p53, yH2AX, pDNA-PKcs, PARP1, pATM); (3) increased lysosomal content (GLB1, LAMP1, LAMP2, lysozyme C) and activation of the NF-kB pathway (pIKB, RELA/p65, NEMO) and (4) the gene expression profile of oncogene induced senescence by using gene-set enrichment analysis (GSEA) [24].

While senescence has traditionally been considered an anti-cancer mechanism, a pro-tumourigenic aspect is also increasingly appreciated [34]. These result from the paracrine activities of the senescence associated secretory phenotype (SASP), a loosely defined range of secretory signals, including pro-inflammatory cytokines, growth factors and ECM modifiers that can be pro-tumourigenic. Specifically, senescent cells have been shown to be capable of driving (1) growth and proliferation of tumour cells; (2) tumour angiogenesis, invasion and metastasis; (3) cellular reprogramming and emergence of tumour-initiating cells and (4) local immuno-suppressive microenvironments. Therefore, it is plausible to hypothesise that the activities of the senescent cluster cells may drive tumour initiation and growth of ACP in both mouse and human models.

To assess functionally this hypothesis, we have genetically modified the SASP in the embryonic and inducible models and assessed the effects in tumour development (Fig. 2.5). In a set of experiments, we have shown that while generation of senescent clusters in young mice is always tumourigenic, this is not the case when clusters are formed in aged mice. Specifically, activation of oncogenic β-catenin in 1-month-old mice led to the formation of 48 tumours in all mice used ($n = 15$), but only to 5 tumours in 6–9-month-old mice ($n = 17$; only 3 mice affected) [24]. Analysis of the SASP activities of the clusters revealed a lower expression of SASP factors in older relative to younger mice. In a second set of experiments, we generated a new mouse model where the WNT pathway is activated by deleting the *Apc* gene encoding adenomatous polyposis coli, leading to the stabilisation of wild-type β-catenin rather than the expression of oncogenic β-catenin. Stabilisation of wild-type β-catenin results in weaker induction of senescence and SASP and failure to develop tumours [24]. These experiments support the concept that senescence and SASP are instrumental in the non-cell autonomous tumourigenesis observed in the mouse models of ACP.

2.5   Papillary Craniopharyngioma and Adamantinomatous Craniopharyngioma are Distinct Tumour Entities

Papillary craniopharyngiomas (PCPs) are mostly tumours of the adults [41]. As in ACPs, PCPs do not show any sign of endocrine differentiation, i.e. lack of expression of hormones or cell-lineage markers and are negative for neuroendocrine

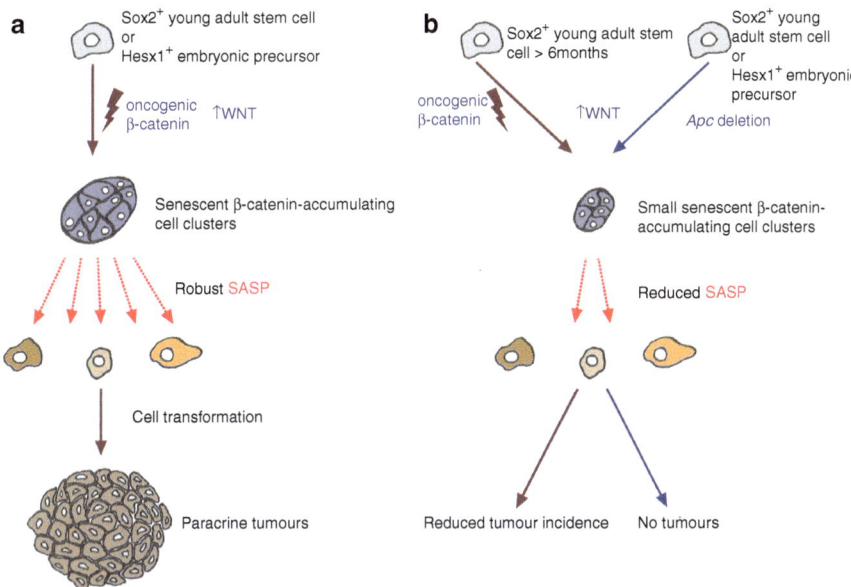

Fig. 2.5 Senescent cells through the SASP can induce tumour formation. (**a**) Targeting Sox2+ stem cells from young adults, or Hesx1+ embryonic precursors to express oncogenic β-catenin, results in the formation of senescent cell clusters and a robust SASP. This leads to cell transformation and generation of the cell of origin of the paracrine tumours; thus, the tumours are not derived from the mutation-sustaining cells. (**b**) In contrast, the expression of oncogenic β-catenin in Sox2+ stem cells of older mice leads to a reduced tumour incidence or the failure to produce tumours. In addition, upregulation of the WNT pathway through the deletion of Apc in young adult stem cells or embryonic precursors also fails to induce tumours. In all cases described in B, there is attenuated senescence and SASP activation. Reproduced with permission from [24]. This article is licensed under a Creative Commons Attribution 4.0 International License

markers (e.g. synaptophysin). Molecularly, PCPs are associated with activating *BRAF-V600E* mutation rather than *CTNNB1* mutations [42]. Contrary to ACP, where the effect of the *CTNNB1* mutations is the accumulation of nucleocytoplasmic β-catenin in specific cells (clusters and dispersed single cells), the expression of oncogenic *BRAF-V600E* is observed broadly throughout the PCP tumours [42, 43]. The consequence of BRAF-V600E expression is the over-activation of the MAPK/ERK pathway (Fig. 2.4). However, unexpectedly, despite the broad expression of BRAF V600E protein, only a small population of epithelial tumour cells activate the MAPK/ERK pathway as assessed by expression of phospho-ERK1/2, a read out of activated pathway [43]. These cells express SOX2 but not any pituitary differentiation marker. Moreover, the vast majority of Ki-67+ cycling cells are contained within the SOX2+ve cell compartment suggesting that activated MAPK/ERK bestows proliferative capacity upon a small subpopulation of SOX2+ve cells while impairing their differentiation. Supporting these data, murine studies have shown that the activation of the MAPK/ERK pathway by the expression of *Braf-V600E* in SOX2 embryonic progenitors results in a drastic increase in the proliferation potential of these cells, elevated clonogenic potential and failure to differentiate into hormone-producing cells [43]. In these mouse models, markers of senescence have not been observed (unpublished data), suggesting a more cell-autonomous role in these tumours of the oncogenic driver (i.e. BRAF-V600E). Unfortunately, these mice die perinatally, which precludes the assessment of tumour formation. Together, these murine experiments suggest that SOX2 stem cells play a critical role in the pathogenesis of both ACPs and PCPs, although by different molecular mechanisms.

2.6   Patient-Derived Xenografts (PDXs) Models of Human Craniopharyngioma

The first xenograft model was described in 1979, with surgical biopsies injected subcutaneously into nude mice and tumours engrafted in most of the mice, even after a second pass of the transplanted tumours. These tumours retained the typical ACP architecture [44]. Further attempts at xenografting were not published until 2006 when Xu et al. injected suspensions of ACP and PCP tumour cells subcutaneously in nude mice with engraftment success rate of 28% for ACP and 18% for PCP. Microvascular development and proliferation were observed [45].

More recently, orthotopic intracranial injections of ACP-dissociated tumours have been developed by Stache et al. [46]. In this model, pieces of tumour are directly injected using a stereotactic frame into the cerebral cortex of immunodeficient mice and with careful selection of three cases up to 100% engraftment success has been reported [46]. These patient-derived xenografts maintain their tissue architecture and histological serial analysis has shown the presence of cell clusters at the leading edge of tumour invasion, as observed histologically and by micro-CT analysis in human ACP [37]. Further analysis of these xenograft models by MRI has revealed that xenografts recapitulate radiographic features, including calcification, of their original tumours as well as evolution of histological features over time. MRI assessment has revealed increased tumour volumes of the engrafted tumour over time, suggesting slow growth of these tumours [12, 47]. Together with the GEMMS, PDXs are helpful models to perform preclinical studies to assess treatment response to novel therapeutic strategies (Table 2.1).

2.7   Therapeutic Lessons from Mouse Models

The availability of these models has enabled the in vivo and *ex vivo* testing of novel therapeutic agents against ACP. A therapeutic trial in the embryonic GEMM ACP model has recently been published testing the efficacy of inhibiting the sonic hedgehog (SHH) pathway [48]. This pathway has been suggested as a potential target by several groups based on its activation in the tumour cells and the expression of SHH ligand in the cell clusters, in keeping with their function as signalling hubs [15, 18, 20, 21]. Pharmacokinetic and pharmacodynamics experiments have confirmed that the small molecular smoothened inhibitor vismodegib could effectively inhibit the

Table 2.1 Summary of preclinical murine models of human adamantinomatous craniopharyngioma

	GEMMs	PDXs
Tumour origin	Mouse	Human
Availability	Easy	Difficult
Tumour location	Orthotopic (sellar)	Orthotopic (cerebral hemispheres) or heterotopic
Growth	Fast (weeks) Cystic and solid	Slow (months) Solid only
Preserved cellular architecture	Partial	Identical
BBB penetrance problems	No/unlikely	Yes (if transplanted in brain)
Tumour–immune cells interactions	Yes	No (immunocompromised host)
Therapeutic endpoints for testing novel agents	Survival, MRI response, histological Tissues can also be tested *ex vivo*	MRI response, histological Survival curves not defined

BBB Blood–brain barrier, *GEMMs* genetically engineered mouse models, *NA* not applicable, *PDXs* patient-derived xenografts

pathway in murine ACP by inhibiting the function of the protein smoothened (SMO) [49]. Such inhibition has been shown to delay tumourigenesis in some cancer models [50, 51]. Surprisingly at first, inhibition of the pathway results in an increased mortality among treated mice [48]. Review of MRI shows an acceleration of tumour growth and histologically treated mice tumours exhibit higher proliferation rates as assessed by elevated Ki-67 expression. Further studies have confirmed a similar effect in human ACP tissue, both in a xenograft model and in tissue explants, where treatment with vismodegib results in increased tumour proliferation. Analysis of the embryonic model subsequently highlighted that vismodegib-mediated SHH pathway inhibition leads to a significant increase in numbers of clonogenic tumour cells, i.e. cells capable of expansion in vitro. Interestingly, pro-tumourigenic actions of SHH pathway inhibition have been observed in other tumour types, e.g. pancreatic and colorectal cancer [52–55]. The common feature between these cancers and ACP is that the activation of the SHH pathway is achieved in a ligand-dependent manner, i.e. by the secretion of an excess of hedgehog ligands, rather than by mutations in the SHH receptor or transducer proteins such as PTCH1 or SMO [48]. These adverse results of SHH pathway inhibition highlight the need for preclinical testing of novel therapies prior to testing in patients, and suggest that SHH pathway inhibition should be avoided in ACP patients.

A recently identified targetable pathway in both ACP and PCP is the MAPK/ERK pathway [16, 42]. In PCPs, the use of MAPK/ERK inhibitors has shown promising results and instigated clinical trials [56–59]. In PCP, the activation of the pathway is caused by mutations in BRAF-V600E, a component of the signalling cascade. In human ACP, the MAPK/ERK pathway is not activated directly due to any oncogenic mutation in the pathway components, but rather it is the result of the expression of several ligands, such as FGFs, epidermal growth factor (EGF) and platelet-derived growth factor (PDGF) in the cell clusters [15, 16]. To test the efficacy of inhibition of this pathway, *ex vivo* cultures of murine pituitaries have been grown with and without the presence of the MEK inhibitor trametinib. These experiments have shown a significant reduction in proliferation and a drastic increase in apoptosis in a dose-dependent manner, a finding further validated and confirmed in *ex vivo* cultures of human ACP [16]. The *ex vivo* culture ACP tumour samples provides a faster and easily reproducible method to screen therapeutic agents provide a basis on which to further evaluate the efficacy of MAPK pathway inhibition in ACP in preclinical trials.

In addition to purely treating with single targeted agents, therapeutic testing of murine models can also combine with other treatment modalities. For instance, radiotherapy is an effective treatment against craniopharyngioma, which could be combined with other chemical therapies such as MAPK/ERK inhibition (apps) or inflammatory modulators (e.g. blocking interleukin 1 (IL1) or IL6 signalling) [16, 17]. Moreover, new emerging senolytic therapies may be relevant to treat human ACP tumours, which contain senescent cluster cells, and the mouse models are ideal tools to test these [24, 60].

2.8   Conclusion

In the last decade, the combination of molecular studies and development of murine modes has led to a significant leap in our understanding of the pathogenesis of craniopharyngioma. Discoveries in the murine models are challenging and advancing our understanding of the developmental and cellular processes underlying tumourigenesis, not only in craniopharyngioma, but also more widely in other tumour types. For the first time, targeted therapies are being evaluated across a range of models, providing hope for the successful use of such agents to treat patients with craniopharyngioma. We anticipate that some of these novel treatments will be proven to reduce tumour burden and made available to patients through clinical trials in the next 5 years.

Acknowledgement JPMB is a Great Ormond Street Hospital Children's Charity Principal Investigator. JRA is funded by a Cancer Research UK Clinical Trials Fellowship.

References

1. Buslei R, et al. Common mutations of beta-catenin in adamantinomatous craniopharyngiomas but not in other tumours originating from the sellar region. Acta Neuropathol. 2005;109:589–97. https://doi.org/10.1007/s00401-005-1004-x.
2. Kato K, et al. Possible linkage between specific histological structures and aberrant reactivation of the Wnt pathway in adamantinomatous craniopharyngioma. J Pathol. 2004;203:814–21. https://doi.org/10.1002/path.1562.
3. Sekine S, et al. Craniopharyngiomas of adamantinomatous type harbor beta-catenin gene mutations. Am J Pathol. 2002;161:1997–2001.

4. Oikonomou E, et al. Beta-catenin mutations in craniopharyngiomas and pituitary adenomas. J Neuro-Oncol. 2005;73:205–9. https://doi.org/10.1007/s11060-004-5232-z.
5. Buslei R, et al. Nuclear beta-catenin accumulation associates with epithelial morphogenesis in craniopharyngiomas. Acta Neuropathol. 2007;113:585–90. https://doi.org/10.1007/s00401-006-0184-3.
6. Gaston-Massuet C, et al. Increased Wingless (Wnt) signaling in pituitary progenitor/stem cells gives rise to pituitary tumors in mice and humans. Proc Natl Acad Sci U S A. 2011;108:11482–7. https://doi.org/10.1073/pnas.1101553108.
7. Apps JR, Martinez-Barbera JP. Genetically engineered mouse models of craniopharyngioma: an opportunity for therapy development and understanding of tumor biology. Brain Pathol. 2017;27:364–9. https://doi.org/10.1111/bpa.12501.
8. Andoniadou CL, et al. Sox2(+) stem/progenitor cells in the adult mouse pituitary support organ homeostasis and have tumor-inducing potential. Cell Stem Cell. 2013;13:433–45. https://doi.org/10.1016/j.stem.2013.07.004.
9. Hermesz E, Mackem S, Mahon KA. Rpx: a novel anterior-restricted homeobox gene progressively activated in the prechordal plate, anterior neural plate and Rathke's pouch of the mouse embryo. Development. 1996;122:41–52.
10. Andoniadou CL, et al. Lack of the murine homeobox gene Hesx1 leads to a posterior transformation of the anterior forebrain. Development. 2007;134:1499–508. https://doi.org/10.1242/dev.02829.
11. Jayakody SA, et al. SOX2 regulates the hypothalamic-pituitary axis at multiple levels. J Clin Invest. 2012;122:3635–46. https://doi.org/10.1172/jci64311.
12. Boult JKR, et al. Preclinical transgenic and patient-derived xenograft models recapitulate the radiological features of human adamantinomatous craniopharyngioma. Brain Pathol. 2017;28(4):475–83. https://doi.org/10.1111/bpa.12525.
13. Martinez-Barbera JP. Molecular and cellular pathogenesis of adamantinomatous craniopharyngioma. Neuropathol Appl Neurobiol. 2015;41(6):721–32. https://doi.org/10.1111/nan.12226.
14. Martinez-Barbera JP. 60 years of neuroendocrinology: biology of human craniopharyngioma: lessons from mouse models. J Endocrinol. 2015;226:T161–72. https://doi.org/10.1530/joe-15-0145.
15. Andoniadou CL, et al. Identification of novel pathways involved in the pathogenesis of human adamantinomatous craniopharyngioma. Acta Neuropathol. 2012;124:259–71. https://doi.org/10.1007/s00401-012-0957-9.
16. Apps JR, et al. Tumour compartment transcriptomics demonstrate the activation of inflammatory and odontogenic programmes in human adamantinomatous craniopharyngioma and identify novel therapeutic targets. Acta Neuropathol. 2018;135:755–77.
17. Donson AM, et al. Molecular analyses reveal inflammatory mediators in the solid component and cyst fluid of human adamantinomatous craniopharyngioma. J Neuropathol Exp Neurol. 2017;76:779–88. https://doi.org/10.1093/jnen/nlx061.
18. Gump JM, et al. Identification of targets for rational pharmacological therapy in childhood craniopharyngioma. Acta Neuropathol Commun. 2015;3:30. https://doi.org/10.1186/s40478-015-0211-5.
19. Gong J, et al. High expression levels of CXCL12 and CXCR4 predict recurrence of adamantinomatous craniopharyngiomas in children. Cancer Biomark. 2014;14:241–51. https://doi.org/10.3233/cbm-140397.
20. Gomes DC, et al. Sonic Hedgehog pathway is upregulated in adamantinomatous craniopharyngiomas. Eur J Endocrinol. 2015;172:603–8. https://doi.org/10.1530/eje-14-0934.
21. Holsken A, et al. Adamantinomatous and papillary craniopharyngiomas are characterized by distinct epigenomic as well as mutational and transcriptomic profiles. Acta Neuropathol Commun. 2016;4:20. https://doi.org/10.1186/s40478-016-0287-6.
22. Martinez-Barbera JP, Buslei R. Adamantinomatous craniopharyngioma: pathology, molecular genetics and mouse models. J Pediatr Endocrinol Metab. 2015;28:7–17. https://doi.org/10.1515/jpem-2014-0442.

23. Rizzoti K, Akiyama H, Lovell-Badge R. Mobilized adult pituitary stem cells contribute to endocrine regeneration in response to physiological demand. Cell Stem Cell. 2013;13:419–32. https://doi.org/10.1016/j.stem.2013.07.006.
24. Gonzalez-Meljem JM, et al. Stem cell senescence drives age-attenuated induction of pituitary tumours in mouse models of paediatric craniopharyngioma. Nat Commun. 2017;8:1819. https://doi.org/10.1038/s41467-017-01992-5.
25. Gonzalez-Meljem JM, Martinez-Barbera JP. Senescence drives non-cell autonomous tumorigenesis in the pituitary gland. Mol Cell Oncol. 2018;5:e1435180. https://doi.org/10.1080/237 23556.2018.1435180.
26. Clevers H. The cancer stem cell: premises, promises and challenges. Nat Med. 2011;17:313–9. https://doi.org/10.1038/nm.2304.
27. He XC, et al. PTEN-deficient intestinal stem cells initiate intestinal polyposis. Nat Genet. 2007;39:189–98.
28. Martinez-Barbera JP, Andoniadou CL. Concise review: Paracrine role of stem cells in pituitary tumors: a focus on adamantinomatous craniopharyngioma. Stem Cells. 2016;34(2):268–76. https://doi.org/10.1002/stem.2267.
29. Lujambio A, et al. Non-cell-autonomous tumor suppression by p53. Cell. 2013;153:449–60. https://doi.org/10.1016/j.cell.2013.03.020.
30. Kode A, et al. Leukaemogenesis induced by an activating beta-catenin mutation in osteoblasts. Nature. 2014;506:240–4. https://doi.org/10.1038/nature12883.
31. Nicholes K, et al. A mouse model of hepatocellular carcinoma: ectopic expression of fibroblast growth factor 19 in skeletal muscle of transgenic mice. Am J Pathol. 2002;160:2295–307. https://doi.org/10.1016/s0002-9440(10)61177-7.
32. Demehri S, Turkoz A, Kopan R. Epidermal notch1 loss promotes skin tumorigenesis by impacting the stromal microenvironment. Cancer Cell. 2009;16:55–66. https://doi.org/10.1016/j.ccr.2009.05.016.
33. Nicolas M, et al. Notch1 functions as a tumor suppressor in mouse skin. Nat Genet. 2003;33:416–21. https://doi.org/10.1038/ng1099.
34. Gonzalez-Meljem JM, Apps JR, Fraser HC, Martinez-Barbera JP. Paracrine roles of cellular senescence in promoting tumourigenesis. Br J Cancer. 2018;118:1283–8. https://doi.org/10.1038/s41416-018-0066-1.
35. Muller HL, Merchant TE, Puget S, Martinez-Barbera JP. New outlook on the diagnosis, treatment and follow-up of childhood-onset craniopharyngioma. Nat Rev Endocrinol. 2017;13:299–312. https://doi.org/10.1038/nrendo.2016.217.
36. Kostadinov S, Hanley CL, Lertsburapa T, O'Brien B, He M. Fetal craniopharyngioma: management, postmortem diagnosis and literature review of an intracranial tumor detected in utero. Pediatr Dev Pathol. 2014;17(5):409–12. https://doi.org/10.2350/14-06-1506-cr.1.
37. Apps JR, et al. Imaging invasion: micro-CT imaging of adamantinomatous craniopharyngioma highlights cell type specific spatial relationships of tissue invasion. Acta Neuropathol Commun. 2016;4:57. https://doi.org/10.1186/s40478-016-0321-8.
38. Apps JR, Martinez-Barbera JP. Molecular pathology of adamantinomatous craniopharyngioma: review and opportunities for practice. Neurosurg Focus. 2016;41:E4. https://doi.org/10.3 171/2016.8.focus16307.
39. Bernstein ML, Buchino JJ. The histologic similarity between craniopharyngioma and odontogenic lesions: a reappraisal. Oral Surg Oral Med Oral Pathol. 1983;56:502–11.
40. Goodwin AF, et al. Abnormal Ras signaling in Costello syndrome (CS) negatively regulates enamel formation. Hum Mol Genet. 2014;23:682–92. https://doi.org/10.1093/hmg/ddt455.
41. Louis DN, Ohgaki H, Wiestler OD, Cavenee WK. World Health Organisation histological classification of tumours of the central nervous system. Lyon: International Agency for Research on Cancer; 2016.
42. Brastianos PK, et al. Exome sequencing identifies BRAF mutations in papillary craniopharyngiomas. Nat Genet. 2014;46:161–5. https://doi.org/10.1038/ng.2868.
43. Haston S, et al. MAPK pathway control of stem cell proliferation and differentiation in the embryonic pituitary provides insights into the pathogenesis of papillary craniopharyngioma. Development. 2017;144:2141–52. https://doi.org/10.1242/dev.150490.

44. Bullard DE, Bigner DD. Heterotransplantation of human craniopharyngiomas in athymic "nude" mice. Neurosurgery. 1979;4:308–14. https://doi.org/10.1227/00006123-197904000-00006.
45. Xu J, et al. Angiogenesis and cell proliferation in human craniopharyngioma xenografts in nude mice. J Neurosurg. 2006;105:306–10. https://doi.org/10.3171/ped.2006.105.4.306.
46. Stache C, et al. Insights into the infiltrative behavior of adamantinomatous craniopharyngioma in a new xenotransplant mouse model. Brain Pathol. 2015;25:1–10. https://doi.org/10.1111/bpa.12148.
47. Holsken A, et al. Characterization of the murine orthotopic adamantinomatous craniopharyngioma PDX model by MRI in correlation with histology. PLoS One. 2018;13:e0197895. https://doi.org/10.1371/journal.pone.0197895.
48. Carreno G, et al. SHH pathway inhibition is protumourigenic in adamantinomatous craniopharyngioma. Endocr Relat Cancer. 2019. https://doi.org/10.1530/erc-18-0538.
49. Wong H, et al. Pharmacokinetic-pharmacodynamic analysis of vismodegib in preclinical models of mutational and ligand-dependent Hedgehog pathway activation. Clin Cancer Res. 2011;17:4682–92. https://doi.org/10.1158/1078-0432.Ccr-11-0975.
50. Sekulic A, et al. Long-term safety and efficacy of vismodegib in patients with advanced basal cell carcinoma: final update of the pivotal ERIVANCE BCC study. BMC Cancer. 2017;17:332. https://doi.org/10.1186/s12885-017-3286-5.
51. Sekulic A, et al. Efficacy and safety of vismodegib in advanced basal-cell carcinoma. N Engl J Med. 2012;366:2171–9. https://doi.org/10.1056/NEJMoa1113713.
52. Lee JJ, et al. Stromal response to Hedgehog signaling restrains pancreatic cancer progression. Proc Natl Acad Sci U S A. 2014;111:E3091–100. https://doi.org/10.1073/pnas.1411679111.
53. Rhim AD, et al. Stromal elements act to restrain, rather than support, pancreatic ductal adenocarcinoma. Cancer Cell. 2014;25:735–47. https://doi.org/10.1016/j.ccr.2014.04.021.
54. Gerling M, et al. Stromal Hedgehog signalling is downregulated in colon cancer and its restoration restrains tumour growth. Nat Commun. 2016;7:12321. https://doi.org/10.1038/ncomms12321.
55. Madison BB, et al. Epithelial hedgehog signals pattern the intestinal crypt-villus axis. Development. 2005;132:279–89. https://doi.org/10.1242/dev.01576.
56. Himes BT, et al. Recurrent papillary craniopharyngioma with BRAF V600E mutation treated with dabrafenib: case report. J Neurosurg. 2018;1:1–5. https://doi.org/10.3171/2017.11.Jns172373.
57. Rostami E, et al. Recurrent papillary craniopharyngioma with BRAFV600E mutation treated with neoadjuvant-targeted therapy. Acta Neurochir. 2017;159:2217–21. https://doi.org/10.1007/s00701-017-3311-0.
58. Brastianos PK, et al. Dramatic response of BRAF V600E mutant papillary craniopharyngioma to targeted therapy. J Natl Cancer Inst. 2016;108:djv310. https://doi.org/10.1093/jnci/djv310.
59. Roque A, Odia Y. BRAF-V600E mutant papillary craniopharyngioma dramatically responds to combination BRAF and MEK inhibitors. CNS Oncol. 2017;6:95–9. https://doi.org/10.2217/cns-2016-0034.
60. Kirkland JL, Tchkonia T, Zhu Y, Niedernhofer LJ, Robbins PD. The clinical potential of senolytic drugs. J Am Geriatr Soc. 2017;65(10):2297–301. https://doi.org/10.1111/jgs.14969.

Epidemiology, Clinical Presentation, and Prognosis of Adult-Onset Craniopharyngioma

3

Romain Manet, Caroline Apra, and Emmanuel Jouanneau

Abbreviations

AO   Adult onset
CO   Childhood onset
CP   Craniopharyngioma
DI   Diabetes insipidus

3.1   History

"Erdheim Tumor, Hypophyseal Epidermoid Tumor, Rathke's pouch tumor, Rathke cleft cyst or tumor, epithelioma, adamantinoma, ameloblastoma, craniopharyngeal pouch tumors—All craniopharyngiomas": *a long journey…*

The first autopsy description comes from a German pathologist, Friedrich Albert Von Zenker (1825–1898), in 1857 [1]. The autopsy revealed a tumor described as a suprasellar tumor containing cholesterol and a squamous epithelial wall.

R. Manet · C. Apra
Pituitary and Skull Base Neurosurgical Department, Neurological Hospital, Hospices Civils de Lyon, Lyon, France
e-mail: omain.manet@neurochirurgie.fr

E. Jouanneau (✉)
Pituitary and Skull Base Neurosurgical Department, Neurological Hospital, Hospices Civils de Lyon, Lyon, France

Claude Bernard University Lyon 1, Lyon, France
e-mail: emmanuel.jouanneau@chu-lyon.fr

© Springer Nature Switzerland AG 2020
E. Jouanneau, G. Raverot (eds.), *Adult Craniopharyngiomas*,
https://doi.org/10.1007/978-3-030-41176-3_3

However, to perfectly understand the origin of the tumor, five decades were required. This elucidation of the tumor consisted of several steps: first, with the discovery of squamous cells in the infundibulum of the pituitary gland by Hubert Von Luschka (1820–1875), that mimic the features of the epithelium of the oral cavity; second, with Martin Rathke (1793–1860), a German anatomist, understanding the role of the evagination of the oral epithelium in the development of the anterior pituitary; thirdly, with Mott and Barret in 1899 followed by J. Erdheim (1874–1937) in 1904, who perfectly described the pathogenesis of craniopharyngiomas (CP).

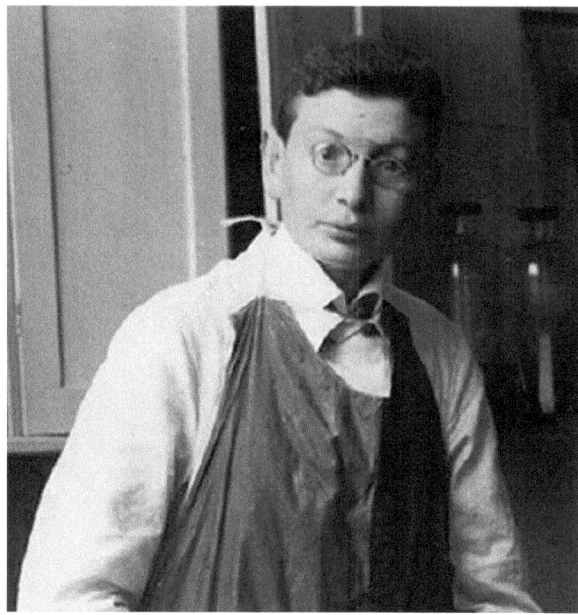

Photograph of Jacob Erdheim, the first to describe the histopathology of craniopharyngiomas

The publication was so impressive that, for decades after, many authors dubbed CP "Erdheim tumors," until CH Frazier, a US surgeon (1870–1936), coined the term CP in 1931, a name that was popularized afterward by H. Cushing, in 1932, in his publication describing more than 2000 cerebral tumors [1].

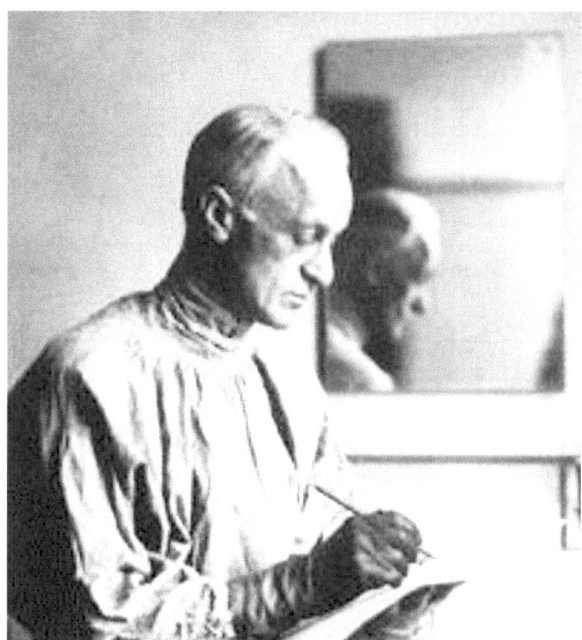

Photograph of Harvey Cushing, the father of modern Neurosurgery, Peter Bent Brigham Hospital, Boston, USA

At the same time, the correlation between the tumor and its clinical presentation was progressively understood. Rupert Boyce and Cecil Beadles in 1893 linked the death of a 35-year-old patient with large suprasellar partially calcified tumors. Mott and Barret in 1893, J. Babinski (1857–1932) and A. Fröhlich (1871–1953), French and Austrian neurologists, respectively, in 1900 and 1901, described the adiposo-genital syndrome termed the Babinski-Fröhlich syndrome. At this point, it was not completely understood which organ was responsible for the symptoms: the pituitary or the hypothalamus. This was the subject of a famous argument between two co-workers: H. Cushing (Neurosurgeon, 1869–1939) and P. Bailey (Neuropathologist and Neurosurgeon, 1892–1973), the latter being opposed to the pituitary being responsible, believing in the role of the hypothalamus. N. Dott (an Irish Neurosurgeon, 1897–1973), and a pupil of H. Cushing, disagreed with his mentor and showed, by his work, the fundamental role of the hypothalamus in controlling, memory, cognition, temperature, feeding behavior as well as endocrine functions.

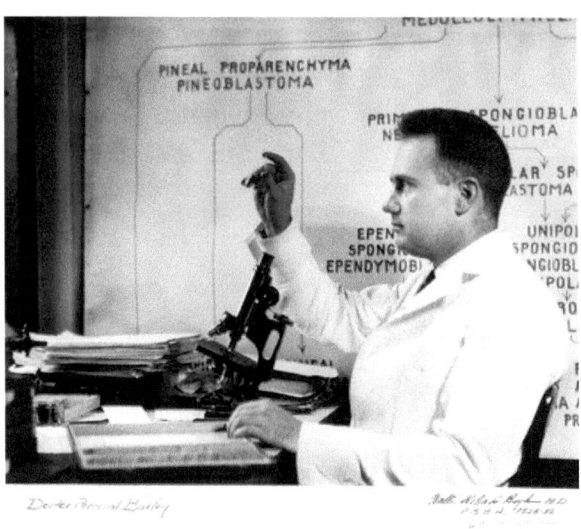

Photograph of Percival Bailey, neuroanatomist, neurologist, neuropathologist, neurosurgeon, co-worker of H. Cushing for the first human brain tumor classification

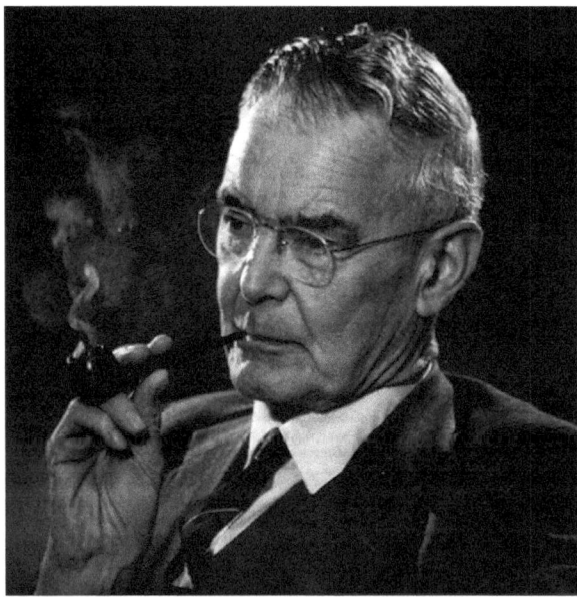

Photograph of Norman Dott, Pupil of H. Cushing, Scottish neurosurgeon in Edinburgh

In terms of surgery, the first attempt at removal of a CP (cystic lesion with visual impairment and DI) is attributed to E. Halstead in Chicago, who took a sublabial nasal approach in 1909. For CP, H. Cushing in his own series of 92 CP patients used the nasal route in some, but preferred a sub-frontal approach for a better visualization of the optic structures in most cases. With his skill, the mortality dropped to

15%. His reports mentioned the poor retrochiasmatic exposition and a splitting technique of the optic chiasm to improve tumor exposure. N. Dott contributed to popularization of a two-step technique with firstly a sub-frontal approach and then a secondary transfrontal transventricular approach to reach the ventricular part of the tumor. His surgical description relates in detail how to improve the control of the retrochiasmatic part, sacrificing the blind optic nerve [2]. Using the transventricular route, he therefore perfectly understood the impact that a sharp dissection of the attached tumor may have on the hypothalamus and already advocated for a partial resection. However, surgical results remained poor until the development of antibiotics (Penicillin in 1944) and corticosteroid use (during the 1950s).

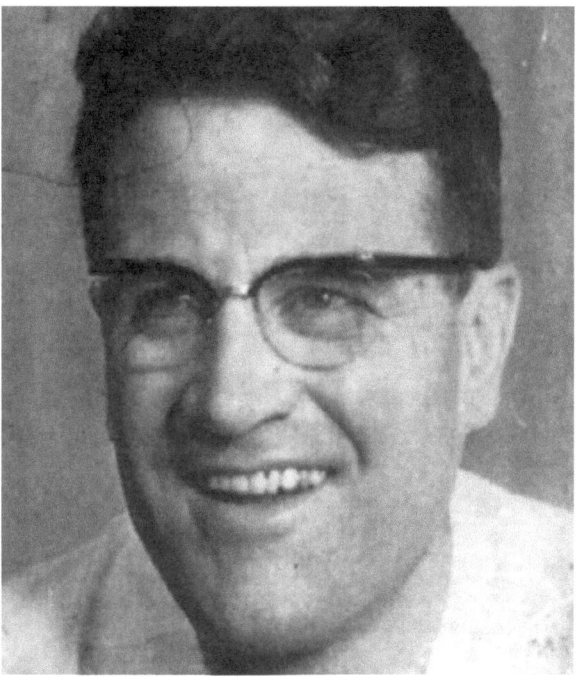

Photograph of Gerard Guiot, Pupil of Norman Dott, French neurosurgeon in Paris (Foch Suresnes Hospital) who re-introduced the transsphenoidal route for pituitary tumors

The following decade produced technical refinements with the introduction of the surgical microscope at the end of the 1950s and modern imaging (the CT scan in 1974 and MRI at the beginning of the 1990s). With G. Guiot (1912–1998 [3]), a French neurosurgeon (a pupil of N. Dott) and J. Hardy (1932– [3]), a Canadian Neurosurgeon, a pupil of G. Guiot, the sublabial route was again used for pituitary diseases including CP. In the three last decades, a new surgical tool, the endoscope which allows extended endonasal approaches, has emerged improving the exposure of the tumor especially for the ventricle and retrochiasmatic parts [4, 5]. Italian and US groups, headed by P. Cappabianca and A. Kassam, respectively, greatly contributed to this surgical advance. Nonetheless, regardless of the efforts made during surgery, microscopic tumor removal remains difficult and recurrences frequent.

We are now entering into the promising era of molecular therapy, and thus expect improvements in the management of CP since the results of surgery and radiotherapy approaches have remained sometimes disappointing to date.

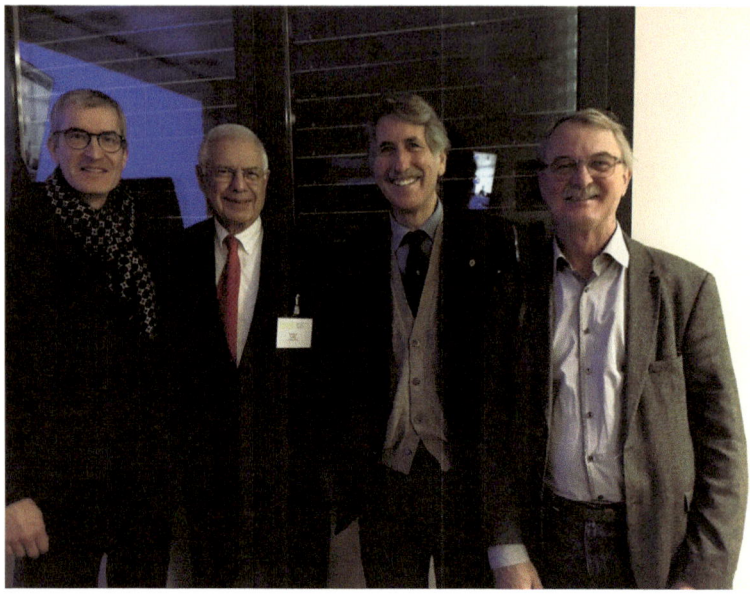

Paolo CAPPABIANCA, one of the Pioneers of Endoscopic Endonasal surgery for Pituitary Tumors, Naples, Italy (from left to right; Emmanuel JOUANNEAU, Edward LAWS, Paolo CAPPABIANCA, Engelbert KNOSP)

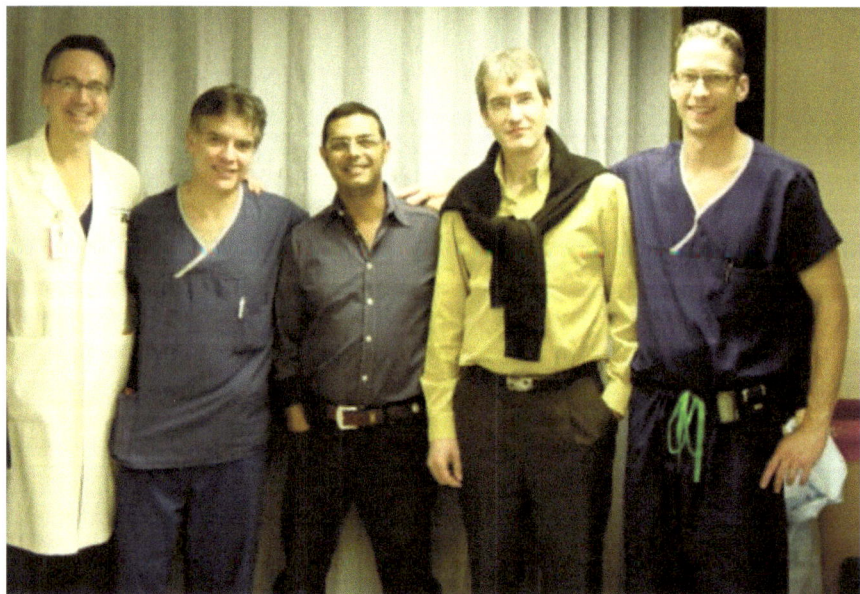

Amin KASSAM, one of the Pioneers of Endoscopic Endonasal surgery for Pituitary Tumors, starting in the same period as the Naples team, Pittsburgh, Pensylvanny, USA (from left to right: Carl SNYDERMAN, Riccardo CARRAU, Amin KASSAM, Emmanuel JOUANNEAU, Paul GARDNER)

After more than a century of worldwide contributions to treatment, the quote from H. Cushing that "CP are the most formidable of intracranial tumors" still remains perfectly true and CPs continue to challenge neurosurgeons.

3.2   Epidemiology of Adult-Onset CP

Because of the rarity of these tumors, their descriptive epidemiology has been established on scarce studies and remains likely incomplete. Only one publication has analyzed cancer registries including adult patients, collecting exhaustive data in a defined area [6]. In this publication, Bunin and colleagues analyzed data from three US registries : (1) the Central Brain Tumor Registry of the United States (CBTRUS) collected data on CP for the years 1990–1993 from ten state cancer registries representing a total catchment area of 26.8 million US citizens; (2) the Greater Delaware Valley Pediatric Tumor Registry (GDVPTR), a population-based registry of pediatric cancer that covers a region in the eastern USA representing approximately 1.8 million <15 year old children, covering a 30-year period (1970–1989); (3) the University of Southern California/Los Angeles County Cancer Surveillance Program (CSP) has collected data on all new intracranial neoplasms diagnosed in California since 1972, which represents a population of almost 10 million people. Overall, the incidence was 0.5–2.0 cases/million/year. The authors reported no gender or racial difference between Caucasians and African Americans. They noted a bimodal age distribution, classically found in the literature, with the maximum incidence rates in children aged 5–14 years and adults in the sixth decade, giving a calculated incidence of 0.2/100,000/year. In adult-onset craniopharyngioma (AO-CP), the peak incidence was found at 65–74 years in CBTRUS and 50–74 years in Los Angeles county data. The lowest incidence occurred among those aged 15–34 years. In our meta-analysis of the literature regarding AO-CP (see below), we found an average age of 43 years (Table 3.2).

The other published epidemiological study, based on registry data, included only pediatric patients [7].

No environmental risk factor for the development of CP has thus far been identified. However, some studies have shown geographical variations in the incidence of these tumors, suggesting possible involvement of environmental factors [8].

Similarly, no genetic predisposing factor has been identified. Only two reports of siblings with craniopharyngiomas have been published [9, 10].

CP refers to a rare embryonic malformation, probably arising from residual Rathke's pouch cells, developing in the sellar and parasellar region. The adamantinomatous type is the most frequent histological diagnosis, even in AO-CP. Squamous papillary tumors are more commonly found in AO-CP than in childhood-onset craniopharyngioma (CO-CP) [11, 12], and represent 25.9% of the AO-CP cases (Table 3.2). Malignant transformation (MT) remains extremely rare, with a recent review finding only 23 reported cases [13]. Squamous cell carcinoma represented the most frequent type (80.96%). The authors reported a median time from initial benign diagnosis to MT was 8.5 years (range, 3–55 years). The median overall survival after MT was 6 months (range, 2 weeks to 5 years).

3.3 Clinical Presentation of Adult-Onset Craniopharyngioma

Morbidity associated with CP is related to tumoral development along the hypothalamo-hypophyseal tract and its proximity to important anatomical features, in particular the opto-chiasmatic and hypothalamic structures.

3.3.1 Our series (Table 3.1)

We recently reviewed the last pure adult-onset CP cases that were newly diagnosed in the department and operated on using an endonasal approach during the last 6 years. To give a clear picture of the initial clinical presentation, we have excluded patients here that were referred or followed-up patients that had been previously treated.

The population is composed of 22 patients (from 51 AO-CP patients in all treated during the same period) with a majority of females (sex ratio F/M = 2.14). The mean age was 58 years (range 18–79) (see Table 3.1).

3.3.1.1 Ophthalmology
Visual impairment was the main complaint in 65% of the population (association of visual acuity and visual field impairment in almost all cases) and only 30% of patients had a normal visual examination.

3.3.1.2 Endocrine Symptoms
Fifty five percent of patients had normal endocrine status, whereas 27% had panhypopituitarism, 18.2% isolated hypogonadism, and 13.6% had diabetes insipidus (DI).

3.3.1.3 Non-specific Symptoms
Surprisingly, headaches were reported by only 9% of our patients in this series. An obstructive hydrocephalus occurred in 9% of patients, requiring immediate CSF shunt.

3.3.1.4 Hypothalamic and Limbic Symptoms
Weight issues were classified as follows: normal when BMI was between 18.5 and 24.9, overweight between 25 and 29.9, obese when greater than 30 (class I: 30–34.9; class II: 35–39.9, and class III: morbid obesity over 40) (World Health Classification).

Interestingly, unexplained weight issues occurring recently prior to diagnosis were frequently reported in our population. At diagnosis, 73% of the patients were overweight with obesity seen in 37% (class I: 23%; class II: 14%). Only 27% were

Table 3.1 Pre-operative

Parameter		Our series ($n = 22$)	
Population		n	%
Sex	Male	7	30
	Female	15	70
Age (years), median		58 (18–79)	
Pre-operative characteristics			
Visual status ($n = 20$)	Normal	6	30
	Visual field abnormalities	11	55
	Unilateral decreased visual acuity	7	35
	Bilateral decreased visual acuity	5	23
	Visual impairment as main complaint	13	65
Endocrine status	Normal	12	55
	Panhypopituitarism	6	27
	Isolated hypogonadism	2	9
	Isolated hyperprolactinemy	2	9
	Diabetes insipidus	4	18
Neurological status	Vertigo	1	5
	Signs of elevated intracranial pressure	2	9
	Headaches	2	9
Cognitive status	Cognitive impairment	5	23
	Slow-down or signs of depression	4	18
Social status	Working	11	50
	Retired	8	36
	Work stoppage	3	14
Weight	BMI <25	6	27
	BMI [25; 30]	8	36
	BMI [30; 35]	5	23
	BMI >35	3	14
Height	Female	161 ± 3	
	Male	176 ± 5	
MRI grading	Grade 0	1	4
	Grade 1	7	32
	Grade 2	14	64

normal weight. The recent occurrence of overweight before diagnosis represented strong evidence of disease-related symptoms. Not surprisingly, statistics was difficult on such a small cohort, with grade 2 of the Puget MRI classification (tumor involving the third ventricle floor) being correlated with overweight except in the case of two grade two patients with normal body weight.

In our retrospective review, pre-operative neuropsychological tests were not performed but clear cognitive dysfunction or depression was noted in, respectively, 23 and 18% of patients without any cause, except in one case who had a prior history of depression. Among the 14 active patients, 3 had stopped work because of a cognitive impact. Once again, these symptoms were related to hypothalamic involvement.

3.3.1.5 Radiology and Histology

In terms of tumor types, using the PUGET classification [14], we found 1 grade 0, 7 grade 1, and 14 grade 2 tumors. Most of the adult tumors were suprasellar-secondary intraventricular and infundibulotuberal tumors and were rarely purely intraventricular or sellar type. We found more adamantinomatous (75%) than papillary tumors (25%).

3.3.2 Literature

A recent meta-analysis of AO-CP management has been published [15]. However, this publication included only a few series with mixed populations of AO-CP and CO-CP patients in which individual data on AO-CP could not be extracted, as well as papers that were quite old.

To avoid these biases, we proceeded to perform a similar literature review using Medline and Embase databases, to analyze epidemiology and clinical presentation of AO-CP, including recent series reporting individual data on AO-CP patients, published in the last 20 years, and excluding all articles with undifferentiated mixed populations of CO-CP and AO-CP or populations of CO-CP. We aggregated the results of our series of 22 patients with data from 15 AO-CP studies, representing a total of 709 patients, comprised of 56.1% of males, with a mean age of 42.7 years. Details of this analysis are shown in Table 3.2.

3.3.2.1 Ophthalmology

As is the case in CO-CP, visual disorders represent the most common findings in AO-CP. Visual field impairment is found in 60–85% and visual acuity impairment in 40–74% [30, 31]. In our meta-analysis, we found an overall rate of 68.9% of visual defects (Table 3.2). Some authors reported higher percentages of visual impairment in AO-CP than CO-CP (85% vs 59%) [31] while others did not [30, 32]. Blindness remains rare (3% of AO-CP), whereas optic atrophy affects 15% of patients [30].

3.3.2.2 Endocrine

At clinical presentation of AO-CP, symptoms of pituitary failure are frequent: half of the patients have at least one endocrine manifestation [32]. Most of the time, patients present partial deficiencies (73%); galactorrhea was found in 8% of patients at the time of diagnosis of AO-CP, impaired sexual function in 28%, and menstrual disorders in 57% of female patients [30]. Complete anterior panhypopituitarism at diagnosis has been reported in only 12% of AO-CP, complete panhypopituitarism was found in only 3%, and ADH deficiency in 6% of AO-CP [31]. In our meta-analysis, we found an overall rate of 29.9% of anterior pituitary failure (partial or complete) and 17.9% of diabetes insipidus (Table 3.2). Endocrine dysfunction appears to be more frequent in children [29].

3.3.2.3 Hypothalamic and Limbic Symptoms

In addition to the resulting pituitary dysregulation, hypothalamic impairment can lead to dysfunction of feeding and drinking, arousal (wakefulness and attention),

3 Epidemiology, Clinical Presentation, and Prognosis of Adult-Onset…   45

Table 3.2 Epidemiology and clinical presentation in series including individual data on patients with AO-CP

Series	N	Average age	Male sex%	Histo: papillary%	Visual impairment	Anterior pituitary impairement	DI	Hypothalamic impairment	Headache	Hydro
Balde et al. [16]	35	44.7	75	NA	37.1	37.1	5.7	5.7	31.4	NA
Bosnjak et al. [17]	8	63	50	NA	87.5	12.5	0	NA	NA	12.5
Dandurand et al. [15]	22	46.7	55	45.4	95.6	22.7[a]	NA	4.5	36.4[b]	NA
Eldevik et al. [18]	24	38.5	41.7	33.3	NA	NA	NA	NA	NA	NA
Frank et al. [19]	9	44.9	44.4	NA	77.8	88.9	0	NA	NA	NA
Gardner et al. [20]	16	54.9	62.5	NA	87.5	37.5	12.5	NA	NA	NA
Jung et al. [21]	41	45.8	57.8	26.8	63.8	26	10.9	NA	24.4	0
Kim et al. [22]	16	40	75	NA	100	100	56.3	NA	NA	NA
Kim et al. [23]	146	41.4	59.6	34.9	66.4	51.4[a]	NA	NA	52	19.2
Lee et al. [24]	90	43.3	55.5	NA	66.7	5.5	26.7	NA	50	NA
Lee et al. [25]	82	42	64.3	23.5	78.1	11	12.2	19.5	40.2	NA
Leng et al. [26]	21	48.3	38	17.6	81	66.7	23.8	NA	14.3	4.2
Lopez-Serna [27]	153	32.4	51.6	16.3	66.7	70.5[a]	NA	NA	11.7[c]	NA
Norris et al. [28]	8	29	62.5	NA	50	87.5	25	NA	50	12.5
Wang et al. [29]	16	32.2	43.8	18.2	NA	75	18.8	NA	50	NA
Our series	22	58	31.8	23.8	70	45.2	18	73	9	9
Overall	709	42.7	56.1	25.9	68.9	29.9	17.9	21.7	42.3	13.4

[a]Unspecified endocrinopathies (mixed anterior and posterior pituitary failure)
[b]Headache + hydrocephalus
[c]Headache + intracranial hypertension syndrome

energy balance, memory, circadian rhythm, panting, sweating, and autonomic nervous system regulation (blood pressure, heart rate, and gastro-intestinal tract stimulation).

Our own series provides evidence of frequent hypothalamic signs (weight issues in 73% and cognitive impairment in 41%). In our meta-analysis, the percentages are clearly lower, with an overall rate of 21.7% with hypothalamic dysfunction (Table 3.2).

Overweight and obesity represent the more common findings in hypothalamic damage. Disruption of responses to leptin and insulin within the hypothalamic arcuate nucleus (located in the median eminence), responsible for controlling satiety, hunger, and regulating energy balance, results in hyperphagia, autonomic imbalance, reduction of energy expenditure, and hyperinsulinemia [33]. In these patients, obesity may also be influenced by behavioral disorders, mood alterations, and increased anxiety-related personality traits [34]. The weight gain is generally refractory to usual dietary or lifestyle interventions and to pharmacotherapy. Bariatric surgery has been proposed as a treatment alternative but its effectiveness remains uncertain [35]. Prevalence of obesity in AO-CP is unequivocal. In a large series that differentiated CO-CP ($n = 112$) and AO-CP ($n = 112$) [31], authors found significantly less obesity in AO-CP than in CO-CP. Only 16% were obese at diagnosis (Class I obesity ($30 < BMI < 35$): 10%; Class II obesity ($35 < BMI < 40$): 4%; Class III obesity ($BMI \geq 40.0$): 2%), 39% were overweight but not obese, and 41% had normal weight. In contrast, in another large series, overweight and obesity were more prevalent in AO-CP (52%) compared with CO-CP patients (40%)[36]. In our series, we also found significantly more overweight and obese patients. Compulsive behavior seemed, however, to be less frequent. Thus, AO-CP series are probably not large enough to draw definitive conclusions.

The opposite situation, of anorexia/weight loss, is rarely seen affecting only 2–8% of AO-CP patients [30, 31].

Surprisingly, hypothalamic data on AO-CP are scarce in the literature, especially regarding cognitive functions.

3.3.2.4 Other Symptoms

Headache is a common symptom at diagnosis of CP, reported in up to 36–63% of adult-onset CP patients [30–32]. These are most of the time non-specific; intracranial hypertension has been described in only 15% of AO-CP [32]. Only one study found significantly less headaches in adult-onset CP than in childhood onset CP (56 vs 78%) [30]. In our meta-analysis, we found an overall rate of 42.3% with headache at presentation (Table 3.2), while in our series, the frequency of headaches is low and related to hydrocephalus.

Hydrocephalus is significantly less common in patients with AO-CP than CO-CP (18% vs 40%) [31]. Tumoral resection can be sufficient to restore functional CSF flow; however, CSF shunting is often necessary. In our meta-analysis, we found an overall rate of hydrocephalus at diagnosis of 13.4% (Table 3.2).

Other findings such as neurological deficits or an altered level of consciousness remain very unusual at clinical presentation but are probably underestimated because of a small cohort in which that aspect was not really addressed.

3.4   Long-Term Morbidity and Mortality in Treated Adult-Onset CP

The long-term morbidity and mortality in CP is dependent on intrinsic factors (related to the tumor characteristics) and extrinsic factors (related to treatment modalities). Morbidity includes hypopituitarism, hypothalamic impairment, visual, neurological, and cognitive deficits, as well as increased cardiovascular risk and reduced bone health, resulting in a significant reduction in quality of life (QoL) [37].

3.4.1   Morbidity

Management of CP must be directed by therapeutic outcomes rather than surgical parameters. *Optimal surgical management of AO-CP remains controversial.* In particular, it is still unclear if GTR is better than STR associated with radiotherapy. In their meta-analysis, Dandurand et al. found a recurrence rate that was slightly lower in gross total resection (GTR) than in subtotal resection (STR) completed by radiotherapy (RXT), though this did not reach significance (OR: 0.63, 95% CI: 0.33–1.24, $p = 0.18$) [9]. Thus, the aggressiveness of surgical resection should be adapted from case to case, taking into account the balance between risk of recurrence and risk of post-operative sequelae. The impact of the surgical route (endonasal or cranial approach) on long-term prognosis has never been precisely reported although some authors [38] have shown better results with the ventral approach than with the cranial route. There should be, therefore, no dogma in the field and the choice should aim for the shortest direct route and adequate exposure of the tumor interface and critical structures [39]. Lastly, surgery for recurrence is associated with higher morbidity and mortality [9].

3.4.1.1 Endocrine Morbidity
The surgical management of the pituitary stalk that influences endocrine outcome remains uncertain. Post-operative hypopituitarism is consistent and complete when the stalk is resected during surgery. Some authors suggest that in about 50% of cases, the stalk is not invaded by the tumor and thus recommend its anatomical preservation: in a retrospective study of 122 surgical cases (mixture of children and adult patients), Van Effenterre et al. reported a surgically preserved stalk in 54 patients using a cranial microscopic approach; at 1 year follow-up, 30% of them had a panhypopituitarism, 33% had a partial deficiency, and 37% had intact pituitary function (30% had total tumor removal

and 7% had partial tumor removal) [40]. However, other authors have suggested that preserving the pituitary stalk does not guarantee intact endocrinological functions post-operatively, and the surgical strategy should focus on the quality of the resection (GTR) in order to avoid a tumor remnant [41]. Thus in another study, stalk preservation was achieved in 24 patients out of 39 (61.5%); post-operatively 14 (58.3%) had a persistent complete pituitary insufficiency, 2 (8.3%) had incomplete pituitary insufficiency, and 8 (33.3%) had preserved pituitary function [13]. In this series, the rate of recurrence was similar in patients who had stalk preservation (25%) and in patients who underwent stalk section (26.7%). Finally, the possibility of preserving the pituitary is related to the origin of the tumor (sellar, suprasellar secondary intraventricular, intraventricular tumors where preservation can be tried, and infundibulotuberal tumors where is no possibility of preservation) and to the experience of the surgeon as well. In a more simple way, preserving the stalk does not override tumor treatment, even if we know the endocrine outcome is likely worse.

Long-term endocrine morbidity remains definitely high. In recent publications, the prevalence of complete anterior pituitary insufficiency was reported to be as high as 89 % [10], with specific TSH, GH, ACTH, gonadotropin insufficiencies, and DI in 86%, 91%, 92% 93.5%, and 81% of cases, respectively [42]. Hypopituitarism, by itself, has been reported to impact QoL [43] and is associated with an overall excess mortality, with a standardized mortality ratio (SMR) of 1.55 [44]. This excess mortality particularly affects women and young patients.

3.4.1.2 Ophthalmologic Morbidity

Visual impairment in AO-CP was reported to be as high as 40–47% at 10 years follow-up [30, 45], and visual field impairment up to 63% [46]. However, endonasal surgery may have a better visual outcome than cranial surgery and, in our own experience, the visual results were good in more than 90% of patients, who were able to resume normal activities.

3.4.1.3 Hypothalamic Morbidity

Overall, the high morbidity and poor prognosis associated with CP significantly reduce the quality of life (QoL) of patients. As previously mentioned, the primary sequelae affecting patients' QoL are visual impairment and endocrine deficits but hypothalamic lesions also caused overweight issues, neuropsychological deficits, and emotional instability [37]. Quite surprisingly, few data have been reported showing hypothalamic outcomes in AO-CP to date. This reduction in QoL has been found to be more pronounced in AO-CP than in CO-CP, with no gender difference [36]. In the AO-CP group, authors reported a strong correlation between BMI and QoL reduction. Our own data has shown, however, that almost all patients, with the exception of 2, resumed normal daily activities or work at the same level despite overweight issues after surgery. Cognitive functions have been significantly improved as well. This highlights that further studies are warranted for AO-CP in large prospective series.

Post-operative hypothalamic morbidity is also correlated with the severity of adhesions which can be evaluated pre-operatively on MRI [47]. Readers should refer to the specific chapter in this book by Prieto et al. Adamantinomatous subtypes would be more infiltrative, limiting the possibility of achieving GTR, whereas papillary subtypes may have a better outcome and fewer cases of recurrence [48].

3.4.2 Mortality

Craniopharyngioma accounts for the highest mortality of all tumors arising from the sellar region, with women more affected than men [49, 50]. The standardized morbidity ratio (SMR) was reported to be as high as 19.4 [50].

The overall survival rates in recent publications are reported as between 89 and 94% at 5 years, 85 and 90% at 10 years, and 62 and 76% at 20 years [30, 40, 42, 51].

Female sex, hydrocephalus, hypothalamic damage, incomplete tumor resection, tumor recurrence, repeated surgery, radiotherapy, panhypopituitarism, and obesity were found to be risk factors for excess mortality [30, 31, 42, 45, 49].

This mortality is highly dependent on the age at diagnosis: survival being better among children than AO-CP patients. In the US national cancer database analysis, 5-year survival rates were reported to be 99%, 80%, and 38% when diagnosis was made in patients who were aged <20 years, 20–64 years, and >65, respectively [6]. In a large national population-based study [52] the reported 5-, 10-, and 15-year survival rates were lower for AO-CP (86%, 82%, and 64%, respectively) in comparison to CO-CP (100%, 96%, and 89%). In this study, authors found an average of 9.6 years of life lost in patients with AO-CP.

Endocrine impairments have a negative impact on mortality: patients without hormonal deficiency have only 2.3 years of life lost compared with patients with hypopituitarism and/or DI who lost 18.5 years of life [52].

Several studies showed higher mortality for women compared to men [30, 31, 42, 45, 49], possibly resulting from the fact that women with hypopituitarism not only have unsubstituted hypogonadism but may also have an unfortunate exposure to the combinations of estrogens and progestogens.

Long-term overall vascular morbidity has been found to be significantly higher in CP patients in comparison with the general population (22% vs 4.8–8%), with 16% incidence of cerebrovascular accidents and 6% of myocardial infarctions, compared with 1–3.2% and 3.8–4.8%, respectively, in the general population [45]. Patients with CP have a 3–19-fold higher cardiovascular mortality in comparison to the general population [45, 49, 50]. Female gender, in particular premenopausal estrogen-deficient patients, appears to be significantly more affected than men by cardiovascular morbidity and mortality (SMR is twofold higher in females) [45, 49].

The literature does not provide robust data to determine the potential contribution of tumor size, tumor site, or surgical approach on mortality in patients with CP [53].

Post-operative mortality ranges from 0 to 16.9% [40] in cases of primary surgery and up to 10.5–40.6% in procedures on recurrent tumors [54, 55]. Our own experience demonstrated that in older patients with severe pre-operative morbidity factors (mainly cardiovascular morbidity associated with severe obesity), the rate of mortality is very high bringing into question a palliative approach rather than a curative one.

3.5   Modern Management of CP Improves Prognosis?

The introduction of MRI in the 1990s has undoubtedly transformed the management of CP. Precise evaluation of tumor size, location, and extent allows for a good evaluation of the expected difficulties and probability of successful radical surgical excision. In particular, MRI evaluation of the potential tumoral adhesions (in particular, invasion of the hypothalamus and anatomical situation of the optic chiasm) could help to confirm the most feasible surgical route and anticipate the individual surgical risks [47].

Progress in diagnosis and management of CP has resulted in a significant improvement of prognosis. In a population-based study (period 1951–1982, Finland), the analysis of 5-year survival rate after diagnosis for patients diagnosed in the 1970s, 1980s, and 1990s was reported as 73%, 91%, and 98%, respectively [56]. However, interpretation of these findings must be nuanced. For example, in a comparison of patients treated before or after 1987 for CP, Olsson et al. found no difference in prevalence of myocardial or cerebral infarctions among CP patients.

3.6   Conclusion

In summary, AO-CP are rare sellar/suprasellar tumors (accounting for 4% of our adult pituitary cases per year). Their management and prognosis slightly differ from CO-CP with more sellar-suprasellar tumors, accessible by endonasal extended transtubercular approaches. At the time of diagnosis, endocrine, visual, and/or cognitive morbidity is present in more than two thirds of cases. The literature provides only poor data on hypothalamic dysfunction and alteration of quality of life in AO-CP patients, pre- and post-operatively, and further studies are therefore warranted. The long-term morbidity remains high, depending on the tumor characteristics and treatment modalities. However, our own data seems to indicate that despite hypothalamic issues, social integration of patients may be better than that of children. The mortality related to AO-CP is higher than in CO-CP, in particular in young patients and women, and remains a concern for surgery in obese patients with negative prognostic factors and repeat surgery.

References

1. Barkhoudarian G, Laws ER. Craniopharyngioma: history. Pituitary. 2013;16(1):1–8.
2. Prieto R, Pascual JM. Norman M. Dott, master of hypothalamic craniopharyngioma surgery: the decisive mentoring of Harvey Cushing and Percival Bailey at Peter Bent Brigham Hospital. J Neurosurg. 2017;127(4):927–40.
3. Patel SK, Husain Q, Eloy JA, Couldwell WT, Liu JK. Norman Dott, Gerard Guiot, and Jules Hardy: key players in the resurrection and preservation of transsphenoidal surgery. Neurosurg Focus. 2012;33(2):E6.
4. Cappabianca P, Alfieri A, de Divitiis E. Endoscopic endonasal transsphenoidal approach to the sella: towards functional endoscopic pituitary surgery (FEPS). Minim Invasive Neurosurg. 1998;41(2):66–73.

5. Kassam AB, Gardner PA, Snyderman CH, Carrau RL, Mintz AH, Prevedello DM. Expanded endonasal approach, a fully endoscopic transnasal approach for the resection of midline suprasellar craniopharyngiomas: a new classification based on the infundibulum. J Neurosurg. 2008;108(4):715–28.
6. Bunin GR, Surawicz TS, Witman PA, Preston-Martin S, Davis F, Bruner JM. The descriptive epidemiology of craniopharyngioma. J Neurosurg. 1998;89(4):547–51.
7. Haupt R, Magnani C, Pavanello M, Caruso S, Dama E, Garrè ML. Epidemiological aspects of craniopharyngioma. J Pediatr Endocrinol Metab. 2006;19(Suppl 1):289–93.
8. Stiller CA, Nectoux J. International incidence of childhood brain and spinal tumours. Int J Epidemiol. 1994;23(3):458–64.
9. Boch AL, van Effenterre R, Kujas M. Craniopharyngiomas in two consanguineous siblings: case report. Neurosurgery. 1997;41(5):1185–7.
10. Green AL, Yeh JS, Dias PS. Craniopharyngioma in a mother and daughter. Acta Neurochir. 2002;144(4):403–4.
11. Burger Burger PC, Scheithauer BW, Vogel FS. Surgical pathology of the nervous system and its coverings. 3rd ed. New York: Churchill Livingstone; 1991.
12. Samii M, Tatagiba M. Craniopharyngioma. In: Kaye AH, Laws Jr ER, editors. Brain tumors: an encyclopedic approach. New York: Churchill Livingstone; 1995. p. 873–94.
13. Sofela AA, Hettige S, Curran O, Bassi S. Malignant transformation in craniopharyngiomas. Neurosurgery. 2014;75(3):306–14.
14. Puget S, Garnett M, Wray A, et al. Pediatric craniopharyngiomas: classification and treatment according to the degree of hypothalamic involvement. J Neurosurg. 2007;106(1 Suppl): 3–12.
15. Dandurand C, Sepehry AA, Asadi Lari MH, Akagami R, Gooderham P. Adult craniopharyngioma: case series, systematic review, and meta-analysis. Neurosurgery. 2018;83(4): 631–41.
16. Baldé NM, Diallo MM, Poirier J-Y, Sow MS, Brassier G, Lorcy Y. Long-term outcome of the adult onset craniopharyngiomas. Ann Endocrinol. 2007;68(2–3):186–90.
17. Bosnjak R, Benedicic M, Vittori A. Early outcome in endoscopic extended endonasal approach for removal of supradiaphragmatic craniopharyngiomas: a case series and a comprehensive review. Radiol Oncol. 2013;47(3):266–79.
18. Eldevik OP, Blaivas M, Gabrielsen TO, Hald JK, Chandler WF. Craniopharyngioma: radiologic and histologic findings and recurrence. AJNR Am J Neuroradiol. 1996;17(8):1427–39.
19. Frank G, Pasquini E, Doglietto F, Mazzatenta D, Sciarretta V, Farneti G, Calbucci F. The endoscopic extended transsphenoidal approach for craniopharyngiomas. Neurosurgery. 2006;59(1 Suppl 1):75–83.
20. Gardner PA, Kassam AB, Snyderman CH, Carrau RL, Mintz AH, Grahovac S, Stefko S. Outcomes following endoscopic, expanded endonasal resection of suprasellar craniopharyngiomas: a case series. J Neurosurg. 2008;109(1):6–16.
21. Jung T-Y, Jung S, Choi J-E, Moon K-S, Kim I-Y, Kang S-S. Adult craniopharyngiomas: surgical results with a special focus on endocrinological outcomes and recurrence according to pituitary stalk preservation. J Neurosurg. 2009;111(3):572–7.
22. Kim EH, Ahn JY, Kim SH. Technique and outcome of endoscopy-assisted microscopic extended transsphenoidal surgery for suprasellar craniopharyngiomas. J Neurosurg. 2011;114(5):1338–49.
23. Kim Y-H, Kim C-Y, Kim JW, Kim YH, Han JH, Park C-K, Paek SH, Oh CW, Kim DG, Jung H-W. Longitudinal analysis of visual outcomes after surgical treatment of adult craniopharyngiomas. Neurosurgery. 2012;71(3):715–21.
24. Lee MH, Kim S-H, Seoul HJ, Nam D-H, Lee J-I, Park K, Kim J-H, Kong D-S. Impact of maximal safe resection on the clinical outcome of adults with craniopharyngiomas. J Clin Neurosci. 2012;19(7):1005–8.
25. Lee EJ, Cho YH, Hong SH, Kim JH, Kim CJ. Is the complete resection of craniopharyngiomas in adults feasible considering both the oncologic and functional outcomes? J Korean Neurosurg Soc. 2015;58(5):432–41.

26. Leng LZ, Greenfield JP, Souweidane MM, Anand VK, Schwartz TH. Endoscopic, endonasal resection of craniopharyngiomas: analysis of outcome including extent of resection, cerebrospinal fluid leak, return to preoperative productivity, and body mass index. Neurosurgery. 2012;70(1):110–23.
27. Lopez-Serna R, Gómez-Amador JL, Barges-Coll J, Nathal-Vera E, Revuelta-Gutiérrez R, Alonso-Vanegas M, Ramos-Peek M, Portocarrero-Ortiz L. Treatment of craniopharyngioma in adults: systematic analysis of a 25-year experience. Arch Med Res. 2012;43(5):347–55.
28. Norris JS, Pavaresh M, Afshar F. Primary transsphenoidal microsurgery in the treatment of craniopharyngiomas. Br J Neurosurg. 1998;12(4):305–12.
29. Wang L, Ni M, Jia W, Jia G, Du J, Li G, Zhang J, Wang Z. Primary adult infradiaphragmatic craniopharyngiomas: clinical features, management, and outcomes in one Chinese institution. World Neurosurg. 2014;81(5–6):773–82.
30. Karavitaki N, Brufani C, Warner JT, Adams CBT, Richards P, Ansorge O, Shine B, Turner HE, Wass JAH. Craniopharyngiomas in children and adults: systematic analysis of 121 cases with long-term follow-up. Clin Endocrinol. 2005;62(4):397–409.
31. Wijnen M, van den Heuvel-Eibrink MM, Janssen JAMJL, et al. Very long-term sequelae of craniopharyngioma. Eur J Endocrinol. 2017;176(6):755–67.
32. Gautier A, Godbout A, Grosheny C, et al. Markers of recurrence and long-term morbidity in craniopharyngioma: a systematic analysis of 171 patients. J Clin Endocrinol Metab. 2012;97(4):1258–67.
33. Lee M, Korner J. Review of physiology, clinical manifestations, and management of hypothalamic obesity in humans. Pituitary. 2009;12(2):87–95.
34. Roemmler-Zehrer J, Geigenberger V, Störmann S, Ising M, Pfister H, Sievers C, Stalla GK, Schopohl J. Specific behaviour, mood and personality traits may contribute to obesity in patients with craniopharyngioma. Clin Endocrinol. 2015;82(1):106–14.
35. Bingham NC, Rose SR, Inge TH. Bariatric surgery in hypothalamic obesity. Front Endocrinol. 2012;3:23.
36. Kendall-Taylor P, Jönsson PJ, Abs R, Erfurth EM, Koltowska-Häggström M, Price DA, Verhelst J. The clinical, metabolic and endocrine features and the quality of life in adults with childhood-onset craniopharyngioma compared with adult-onset craniopharyngioma. Eur J Endocrinol. 2005;152(4):557–67.
37. Müller HL. Diagnostics, treatment, and follow-up in craniopharyngioma. Front Endocrinol. 2011;2:70.
38. Komotar RJ, Starke RM, Raper DMS, Anand VK, Schwartz TH. Endoscopic endonasal compared with microscopic transsphenoidal and open transcranial resection of craniopharyngiomas. World Neurosurg. 2012;77(2):329–41.
39. Liu JK, Sevak IA, Carmel PW, Eloy JA. Microscopic versus endoscopic approaches for craniopharyngiomas: choosing the optimal surgical corridor for maximizing extent of resection and complication avoidance using a personalized, tailored approach. Neurosurg Focus. 2016;41(6):E5.
40. van Effenterre R, Boch A-L. Craniopharyngioma in adults and children: a study of 122 surgical cases. J Neurosurg. 2002;97(1):3–11.
41. Ordóñez-Rubiano EG, Forbes JA, Morgenstern PF, et al. Preserve or sacrifice the stalk? Endocrinological outcomes, extent of resection, and recurrence rates following endoscopic endonasal resection of craniopharyngiomas. J Neurosurg. 2018;1:1–9.
42. Crowley RK, Hamnvik OP, O'Sullivan EP, Behan LA, Smith D, Agha A, Thompson CJ. Morbidity and mortality in patients with craniopharyngioma after surgery. Clin Endocrinol. 2010;73(4):516–21.
43. Ishii H, Shimatsu A, Okimura Y, et al. Development and validation of a new questionnaire assessing quality of life in adults with hypopituitarism: adult hypopituitarism questionnaire (AHQ). PLoS ONE. 2012;7(9):e44304.
44. Jasim S, Alahdab F, Ahmed AT, Tamhane S, Prokop LJ, Nippoldt TB, Murad MH. Mortality in adults with hypopituitarism: a systematic review and meta-analysis. Endocrine. 2017;56(1):33–42.

45. Pereira AM, Schmid EM, Schutte PJ, Voormolen JHC, Biermasz NR, van Thiel SW, Corssmit EPM, Smit JWA, Roelfsema F, Romijn JA. High prevalence of long-term cardiovascular, neurological and psychosocial morbidity after treatment for craniopharyngioma. Clin Endocrinol. 2005;62(2):197–204.
46. Duff J, Meyer FB, Ilstrup DM, Laws ER, Schleck CD, Scheithauer BW. Long-term outcomes for surgically resected craniopharyngiomas. Neurosurgery. 2000;46(2):291–302.
47. Prieto R, Pascual JM, Rosdolsky M, Barrios L. Preoperative assessment of craniopharyngioma adherence: magnetic resonance imaging findings correlated with the severity of tumor attachment to the hypothalamus. World Neurosurg. 2018;110:e404–26.
48. Adamson TE, Wiestler OD, Kleihues P, Yaşargil MG. Correlation of clinical and pathological features in surgically treated craniopharyngiomas. J Neurosurg. 1990;73(1):12–7.
49. Bülow B, Attewell R, Hagmar L, Malmström P, Nordström CH, Erfurth EM. Postoperative prognosis in craniopharyngioma with respect to cardiovascular mortality, survival, and tumor recurrence. J Clin Endocrinol Metab. 1998;83(11):3897–904.
50. Tomlinson JW, Holden N, Hills RK, Wheatley K, Clayton RN, Bates AS, Sheppard MC, Stewart PM. Association between premature mortality and hypopituitarism. West Midlands Prospective Hypopituitary Study Group. Lancet. 2001;357(9254):425–31.
51. Visser J, Hukin J, Sargent M, Steinbok P, Goddard K, Fryer C. Late mortality in pediatric patients with craniopharyngioma. J Neuro-Oncol. 2010;100(1):105–11.
52. Olsson DS, Andersson E, Bryngelsson I-L, Nilsson AG, Johannsson G. Excess mortality and morbidity in patients with craniopharyngioma, especially in patients with childhood onset: a population-based study in Sweden. J Clin Endocrinol Metab. 2015;100(2):467–74.
53. Erfurth EM, Holmer H, Fjalldal SB. Mortality and morbidity in adult craniopharyngioma. Pituitary. 2013;16(1):46–55.
54. Fahlbusch R, Honegger J, Paulus W, Huk W, Buchfelder M. Surgical treatment of craniopharyngiomas: experience with 168 patients. J Neurosurg. 1999;90(2):237–50.
55. Yaşargil MG, Curcic M, Kis M, Siegenthaler G, Teddy PJ, Roth P. Total removal of craniopharyngiomas. Approaches and long-term results in 144 patients. J Neurosurg. 1990;73(1):3–11.
56. Sorva R, Heiskanen O. Craniopharyngioma in Finland. A study of 123 cases. Acta Neurochir. 1986;81(3–4):85–9.

Craniopharyngioma Diagnosis: A Rationale for Accurate MRI Assessment of Tumor Topography and Adhesion to the Hypothalamus

4

Ruth Prieto and José M. Pascual

Abbreviations

3V   Third ventricle
CP   Craniopharyngioma
MBA   Mammillary body angle
MRI   Magnetic resonance imaging
PG   Pituitary gland
PS   Pituitary stalk
TVF   Third ventricle floor

> Gentlemen, I have a confession to make. Half of what we have taught you is in error, and furthermore we cannot tell you which half is it.
> William Osler (1849–1919)

4.1 Introduction. MRI Assessment of Craniopharyngiomas: What Essential Information Should a Neurosurgeon Obtain from It?

The considerable morphological heterogeneity of craniopharyngiomas (CPs) led Harvey Cushing to consider them as the most baffling problem in neurosurgery [1]. Almost a century later, and despite the great progress in neuroradiological techniques in the last few decades, CP treatment remains a challenge even for the most experienced and skilled neurosurgeons [2–5]. A major source of difficulty lies in the exceedingly variable topography and adhesion patterns to the hypothalamus

R. Prieto (✉)
Department of Neurosurgery, Puerta de Hierro University Hospital, Madrid, Spain

J. M. Pascual
Department of Neurosurgery, La Princesa University Hospital, Madrid, Spain

© Springer Nature Switzerland AG 2020
E. Jouanneau, G. Raverot (eds.), *Adult Craniopharyngiomas*,
https://doi.org/10.1007/978-3-030-41176-3_4

55

observed among these lesions. Hypothalamic dysfunction is the major cause of death and serious morbidity associated with CP surgery, including long-term neuro-psychological deficits which severely impair patients' quality of life. Accordingly, a correct preoperative definition of the CP location and the CP-hypothalamus relationships is essential for choosing the most appropriate surgical strategy in each case, one capable of minimizing the risks of hypothalamic injury.

CPs are still considered the model of a "pituitary or suprasellar" lesion in many neurosurgical and neuroradiological texts, even in those published in the MRI era [6, 7]. The widespread and unfortunate use of the term "suprasellar" for CPs dates back to the early twentieth century when the identification of suprasellar shadows represented the fundamental sign for a correct preoperative diagnosis [1, 8]. This imprecise term points to the suprasellar cistern as the anatomical compartment where CPs develop as a general rule. The main concern for neurosurgeons is, however, the hypothalamic deformation caused by the tumor, and even more importantly, the extension and degree of the CP attachment to the hypothalamus. Consequently, the term "suprasellar" should be abandoned and replaced by an accurate definition of CP topography, based on the anatomical position of the hypothalamus relative to the tumor and the morphological/functional status of this vital structure [9, 10]. In this chapter we will discuss the rationale for an accurate preoperative definition of CP topography and the type of CP-hypothalamus adhesion, based on several fundamental radiological signs that can be easily assessed on conventional preoperative MRI studies. This rationale has proven useful to predict the risks of hypothalamic injury associated with the surgical procedure and can help neurosurgeons to anticipate the difficulties that will be encountered during the procedure, facilitating accordingly the proper surgical strategy to be employed in each patient.

4.2   Radiological Diagnosis of Craniopharyngiomas: Historical Development

CPs were identified as a new tumor entity by the Viennese pathologist Jakob Erdheim (1874–1937) in 1904 [11, 12]. These epithelial lesions were found to develop at any point along the hypothalamus–pituitary axis, from the pituitary gland up to the third ventricle (3V). From the outset of CP surgery, a correct preoperative diagnosis of these heterogeneous tumors has been a challenge and the evolution of surgical strategies has been intimately linked to the progressive refinement of neuroradiological methods. The first significant milestone in CP diagnosis was reached in 1905 with the introduction of X-rays in clinical practice by the leading figure of American neurosurgery, Harvey Cushing (1869–1939) [13, 14]. The observation of hyperdense "shadows" above the sella turcica on skull radiographs, a very specific sign of CPs related to the presence of calcifications within the tumor, significantly improved the accuracy of preoperative diagnosis for these tumors [15, 16]. As a result, the number of failed exploratory craniotomies, a relatively common event at the early stage of CP surgery, markedly decreased afterwards [17, 18].

Nevertheless, X-rays did not enable CP diagnosis in all cases, as intracranial calcifications could only be detected in about two-thirds of the patients [15]. In addition, a major limitation of cranial radiographs was the fact that they did not provide precise information about the extension and anatomical relationships of the tumor, data of paramount importance for proper surgical planning [16, 17]. In 1918, the neurosurgeon Walter Dandy (1886–1946) developed at Johns Hopkins the technique of air-ventriculography, a revolutionary diagnostic tool which allowed the clear picture of the cerebral ventricles and their anatomical deformations caused by intracranial lesions [19]. Preoperative definition of the 3V occupation by the tumor decisively influenced the choice of surgical approach to attempt CP removal. Thanks to this technique, Walter Dandy and Harvey Cushing pioneered the use of frontal transventricular and/or transcallosal surgical routes for the excision of CPs developed at or extending into the 3V [8, 18, 20]. Air-ventriculography, however, also had significant limitations, primarily the impossibility of defining the tumors' relative position in relation to the third ventricle floor (TVF) and walls, the neural structures including the hypothalamic nuclei. A 3V filling defect could be either due to CPs pushing the TVF upwards or to lesions that truly occupy the 3V cavity [21–23].

In the early 1960s, the French neurosurgeon Bernard Pertuiset (1920–2000) discussed the impossibility of achieving a reliable preoperative definition of CP topography with the existing neuroradiological methods (angiography and air-ventriculography) and introduced the important topographical concept of a pseudointraventricular location for CPs [21]. This topography corresponded to those tumors apparently growing within the 3V but which in fact originated beneath the ventricle, from suprasellar structures, and caused an upward displacement and progressive inward folding of the TVF during the tumors' growth [21, 24]. The presence of an intact TVF capping the tumor dome would suppose a high risk of hypothalamic injury in cases where a trans-ventricular approach was attempted through this delicate and vital neural structure. These tumors mimicking the occupation of the 3V should be differentiated from those CPs which had invaded the 3V, after breaking through the TVF, as well as from true intraventricular tumors [22]. The introduction of computed tomography (CT) in the late 1970s markedly improved the diagnostic accuracy of CPs and their differentiation from other pituitary and parapituitary lesions, especially due to its high sensitivity to detect minute calcifications [25]. Unfortunately, CT scans did not provide an accurate depiction of the anatomical CP-brain relationships, as this diagnostic tool usually only obtained images through axial sections of the cranium. A clear definition of the position and anatomical disruption of the thin neural layer that forms the 3V boundaries was not possible with CT for most CP cases encroaching upon the 3V at the time of diagnosis [22]. CP topographical classifications based on the relative position of the lesion regarding the optic chiasm, the neural structure of reference in transcranial approaches, persisted in the CT era, with the differentiation of three major categories: prechiasmatic, subchiasmatic, and retrochiasmatic lesions [26–28]. The anatomical position and distortion of the hypothalamus and 3V regarding the tumor was not ascertained preoperatively with CT. This shortcoming commonly led to erroneous topographical diagnosis and inappropriate surgical approaches to CPs in the decades prior to the MRI era.

Since the introduction of MRI in the late 1980s, this diagnostic technique has represented the gold standard for the diagnosis of CPs, particularly because the anatomical relationships of the mass could be observed in the three spatial dimensions [6, 29, 30]. CP classifications employing as fundamental criterium the extension of the mass through the vertical axis and the degree of invasion into the 3V rapidly replaced the prior schemes focused on the chiasm-tumor position [31, 32]. The first topographical CP classification system based on preoperative MRI studies was designed by the French neuroradiologist Charles Raybaud, from The Timone University Hospital in Marseille, who differentiated four basic anatomic regions that could be occupied by the tumor: sellar, suprasellar, infundibulo-tuberal, and 3V [29]. His MRI-based scheme was the first to highlight, as had been previously demonstrated in the seminal necropsy study by Juraj Steno, that a majority of CPs primarily develop and occupy the infundibulo-tuberal region of the TVF [23, 29, 33].

4.3   Origin of Craniopharyngiomas: The Major Determinant of CP-3V Relationships

For a proper MRI assessment of CPs, it is necessary to have a clear knowledge about the precise origin of these lesions because it will determine the specific tumor-3V relationships in each case. The embryogenetic theory proposed originally by Jakob Erdheim at the beginning of twentieth century considered that CPs originated from epithelial remnants of either the Rathke's pouch (the embryonic primordium of the pituitary gland) or an incompletely involuted craniopharyngeal duct (Rathke's pouch's path of migration during the embryo's development) [11, 12]. Recent anatomical and molecular evidence has provided substantial support for this theory [34, 35]. Therefore, CPs may develop at any point along the vertical pituitary–hypothalamic axis, showing a wide range of locations from the sella to the 3V, each with a different CP-hypothalamus relationship [24, 36]. The predominant accumulation of Rathke's pouch remnants at the upper and lower areas of the pars tuberalis, a tongue of adenohypophysial tissue enveloping the pituitary stalk (PS) and infundibulum, supports that the frequency of the different possible tumor locations varies [37]. CPs most commonly originate either at the junction between the pituitary gland (PG) and the PS or at the upper edge of the PS, in close contact with the infundibulum. The midline origin of CPs along the pituitary–hypothalamic axis makes the midsagittal and coronal MR images through the infundibular region the two basic sections to accurately elucidate CP topography [38].

Less than 20% of CPs show minimal or absent adhesions to the hypothalamus, these cases originating either at the dorsal surface of the PG, within the sella turcica, or exclusively within the 3V, from the ependymal layer lining of the 3V cavity [39]. In the former group, the TVF (and the hypothalamic nuclei included within it) is situated above the tumor and separated from its dome by the leptomeningeal layers (arachnoid and pia mater), a fact that noticeably reduces the surgical risk of hypothalamic injury [39]. Conversely, in the subgroup of strictly 3V CPs, the TVF is situated below the tumor and separated from it by the ependymal layer of the

3V. This unusual topography is characterized by a small, patch-like or pedicle-like attachment to the inner surface of the TVF or 3V walls that can be straightforwardly dissected with a relatively low risk of hypothalamic injury [39].

The remaining CP topographies, which represent about 80% of cases overall, have a more intimate relation with the hypothalamus. Half of them corresponds to CPs originated at the infundibulum itself, or within the neural layer of the adjacent region of the tuber cinereum, the two structures that form the TVF [40]. This subgroup of infundibulo-tuberal CPs usually has a subpial development, a fact that eventually triggers a strong reactive gliosis in the nervous tissue around the tumor. This reaction is responsible for the extensive and strong adhesion between the TVF remnants (and hypothalamus) and the tumor. In the other cases (approximately 30%), a tumor originated from the PG or the PS, within the suprasellar cistern, may either displace the TVF upwards, mimicking an intraventricular position, or break through the TVF and invade the 3V. This latter subgroup grossly encroaches upon the hypothalamus, causing the most severe damage to this vital region [41]. The highest risk of hypothalamic injury will therefore occur when the tumor is either originated within the TVF itself or has secondarily invaded the 3V. In both cases, the hypothalamic nuclei are situated around the bulk of the tumor, and there is no intervening meningeal layer that can be used as a safe dissection plane [39].

4.4 Craniopharyngioma Topography: Usefulness of Current Classification Schemes

Numerous classification schemes for CP topography have been proposed since the definition of this pathological entity [42]. Only a few of them provide valuable information regarding the accurate anatomical relationships between the tumor and the hypothalamus. The first topographical scheme based on anatomopathological CP features was presented by Juraj Steno in 1985 after the thorough study of 30 brain specimens of non-operated CPs from the Burdenko Institute, in Moscow [33]. He noticed that a majority of CPs grew in both the suprasellar cistern and the 3V cavity (extraventricular–intraventricular CPs, 46%). Contrary to the purely extraventricular or purely intraventricular CPs, these extra-intraventricular lesions were found to associate the highest surgical risk due to their strong attachments to the surrounding TVF remnants, usually located around the mid-third or central portion of the tumor [23, 33]. More recently, in 2008, Amin K. Kassam presented a topographical scheme based on the relative position of the tumor regarding the PS-infundibulum complex, the anatomical structures of reference initially found when using the transsphenoidal approach [43]. Four major groups were considered: (1) preinfundibular CPs; (2) transinfundibular CPs or tumors extending into the PS; (3) retroinfundibular CPs; and (4) intraventricular CPs which were situated above an intact PS.

Only a few years ago, the neurosurgical team headed by Songtao Qi at the Nanfang Hospital (Guangzhou, China) presented a topographical scheme based on a thorough analysis of the relationships between the tumor capsule and the meningeal layers of the pituitary–hypothalamic axis, in a series of 195 surgically treated CPs [10]. Four major topographical patterns were identified: (1) infra-diaphragmatic, characterized by the presence of the diaphragma sellae between the tumor and the brain undersurface; (2) extra-arachnoidal, originated in the suprasellar cistern above the diaphragma sellae and separated from the TVF by an arachnoidal layer; (3) intra-arachnoidal; and (4) subarachnoidal-subpial, originated within the nervous tissue of the TVF itself. The subarachnoidal-subpial group was found by the authors to represent as much as 30% of cases in children and 50% in adults, and it was characterized by the lack of any membranous layers between the tumor and the pituitary–hypothalamic axis [5, 10].

The most widely used MRI-based topographic classification for CPs is the one proposed by Christian Sainte-Rose and Stephanie Puget at the Hôpital Necker Enfants Malades in Paris [44, 45]. This scheme is based on the degree of hypothalamic distortion caused by the tumor, as observed with conventional MRI. Three major types of hypothalamic involvement by the tumor were considered: (1) grade 0, in which the hypothalamus had a normal appearance on preoperative MRI scans; (2) grade 1 for cases with a recognizable but displaced hypothalamus; and (3) grade 2, encompassing all tumors which were encroaching upon the region of the hypothalamus, whose anatomical boundaries were not identifiable. Saint-Rose and Puget's scheme assumes that the 3V involvement depends on the progressive expansion of a tumor theoretically originated at the suprasellar region, without taking into consideration that CPs may originate at any point along the pituitary–hypothalamic axis. In fact, the appearance of the TVF on preoperative MRIs is misleading to reliably ascertain the anatomical integrity of this structure. An unidentifiable TVF does not necessarily mean it has been breached or invaded by the tumor. For example, in a series of 17 intraventricular CPs operated on by Songtao Qi et al. at Nanfang hospital, the authors found that 15% of cases in which the TVF was not identified on preoperative MRIs corresponded to purely intraventricular CPs presenting a small pedicle attachment to the intact TVF that allowed a safe and straightforward total removal. On the contrary, a quarter of cases with an identifiable TVF had an undissectible, wide, and dense type of CP adhesion [10].

1.5   CP Topography: A Comprehensive Scheme for Accurate MRI Assessment of Tumor-3V Relationships

In 2004, our group presented a CP topography classification based on the true anatomical relationships between the tumor and the 3V after analyzing a cohort of lesions originally described as "intraventricular" [22]. For this purpose, we correlated the anatomical relationships observed in whole CP specimens from non-operated patients with the pre- and postoperative MRI of operated lesions as well as with the intraoperative findings observed in 105 cases involving the 3V. We were able to identify four major CP topographies depending on the specific type of CP-3V relationship (Fig. 4.1): (1) *suprasellar-pseudointraventricular CPs* (Fig. 4.1B), a category of lesions originated at the pars tuberalis that envelops the PS; these lesions

| Sellar-Suprasellar | S-SS-Pseudo 3V | S-SS-Secondary 3V | Not-Strictly 3V (Infundibulo-Tuberal) | Strictly 3V |

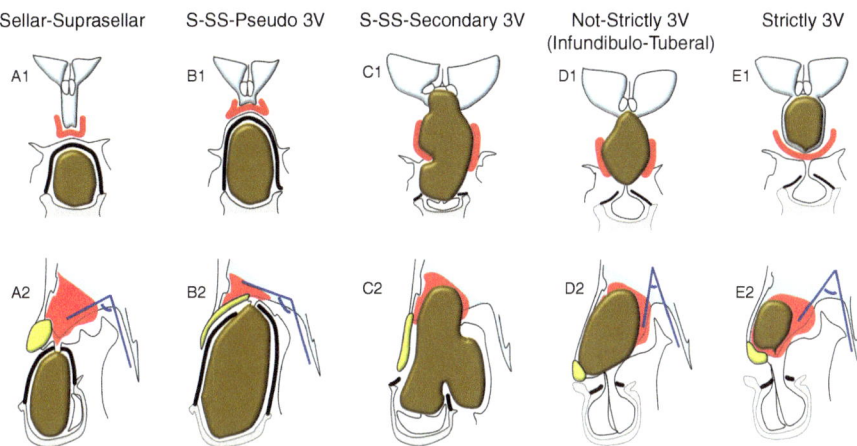

Fig. 4.1 Craniopharyngioma topographical classification based on the tumor origin along the hypophyseal–hypothalamic axis and the tumor-third ventricle relationships [22, 24]. Coronal transinfundibular (upper panel) and midsagittal (lower panel) drawings are shown for the five major categories considered. (**A1–A2**) Sellar-suprasellar category, formed by tumors developed below an intact third ventricle floor. Note that the optic chiasm (yellow) and the mammillary body angle (MBA, blue angle) have a normal appearance and value, respectively. The hypothalamus (in red) is situated above the lesion. (**B1–B2**) Sellar-suprasellar-pseudointraventricular type, which mimics an intraventricular position. Note that the optic chiasm is stretched upward and the MBA has an obtuse value (>90°). The hypothalamus is above the upper pole of the tumor. (**C1–C2**) Sellar-suprasellar-secondary intraventricular category. It includes the CPs which invade the cavity of the third ventricle after breaking through the third ventricle floor. Note that the optic chiasm is stretched forward in front of the tumor and the hypothalamus is positioned around the mid-third or central portion of the lesion. (**D1–D2**) Not-strictly intraventricular or infundibulo-tuberal type, formed by lesions originated within the TVF (infundibulum-tuber cinereum) which predominantly expand into the 3V. Note that the optic chiasm is compressed forward against the tuberculum sellae, the hypothalamus is around the mid-third portion of the tumor and the MBA is hyperacute (<30°). (**E1–E2**) Strictly intraventricular category, which includes the CPs wholly developed within the 3V, above an anatomically intact TVF. Note that the optic chiasm is slightly compressed downward and the hypothalamus is situated below the lower pole of the tumor

grow in the suprasellar cistern and cause an upward displacement of the TVF, mimicking an intraventricular position; (2) *sellar/suprasellar-secondary intraventricular CPs* (Fig. 4.1C), lesions usually originated at the junction between the PG and the PS that initially develop under the 3V but eventually invade the 3V cavity after breaking through the TVF; (3) *infundibulo-tuberal or not-strictly intraventricular CPs* (Fig. 4.1D), tumors developed within the neural layer of the infundibulum/ tuber cinereum, in close contact with the hypothalamic nuclei, which predominantly expand within the 3V at later stages; and (4) *strictly intraventricular CPs* (Fig. 4.1E), tumors primarily developed within the 3V, above an intact TVF. An additional topographical category of CPs without involvement of the 3V must be considered, *the sellar-suprasellar group* (Fig. 4.1A), which includes those tumors originated at the dorsal surface of the PG that exclusively occupy the sellar and/or suprasellar compartments beneath an intact TVF [38].

In contrast to other topographical classifications, ours scheme takes into consideration the type of hypothalamic-CP relationship, which is the critical factor to predict the feasibility of a safe radical removal. Besides being a relatively simple scheme, the importance of this classification lies in the fact that it has proven useful to predict the position and anatomic status of the hypothalamus, as well as the type of tumor adhesion to it.

4.6   The Mammillary Body Angle: A Useful MRI Sign to Ascertain CP Topography

Identification of the TVF can hardly be achieved preoperatively on conventional MRI sequences (T1- and T2-weighted MRI) at the time of diagnosis, because the infundibulum and the tuber cinereum are very thin structures that are usually severely distorted by the tumor once it reaches a size larger than 2–3 cm in diameter. In contrast, the solid consistency of the mammillary bodies makes possible the recognition of these structures on midsagittal MRI scans despite their usually gross displacement and deformation caused by the tumor. Based on this concept, our group defined the mammillary body angle (MBA) as a simple, useful radiological tool to predict the CP topography and the type of 3V distortion caused by the tumor [46]. The MBA is defined as the angle formed by the intersection of a plane tangential to the base of one of the mammillary bodies with the plane tangential to the fourth ventricle floor. This angle can easily be measured on midsagittal MRI scans (Fig. 4.2). In healthy humans without intracranial pathology, the normal MBA value ranges between 50° and 70°. CP growth usually leads to substantial modifications in the MBA, whose specific changes depend on the original site of tumor development. Sellar/suprasellar CPs originated below the TVF cause an upward displacement of the mammillary bodies, shifting the MBA towards an obtuse value (>90°). An obtuse MBA is a strong predictor of the pseudointraventricular CP topography, which mimics an intraventricular position. In contrast, a downward displacement of the mammillary bodies and thus an MBA change towards an acute angle (<90°) is usually observed among CPs with a primarily intraventricular growth. The MBA value becomes even more reduced or hyperacute (<30°) in the case of CPs originated within the TVF itself (infundibulo-tuberal CPs) [46].

4.7   CP Adherence to the Hypothalamus: A Stratification Model to Predict Surgical Risk

Patient outcome following CP removal is related, above all, to the extension and strength of tumor adhesion to the hypothalamus [47]. Preoperative distinction between CPs that can be radically removed from those whose removal would inevitably lead to irreversible hypothalamic injury is one of the most critical aspects of CP surgery. The methodical examination of 500 CPs, including brain autopsy specimens and surgically treated cases, has allowed our group to define the first

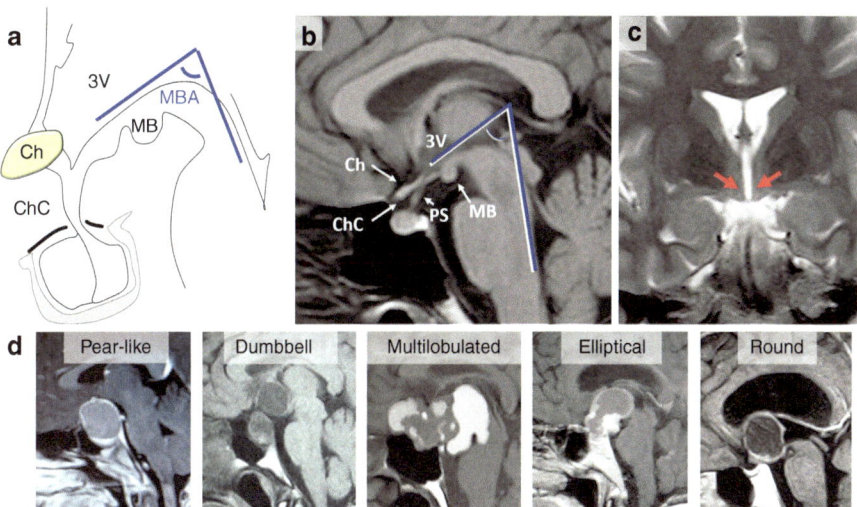

Fig. 4.2 Preoperative assessment of MRI signs which help to define the CP topography according to the CP-3V anatomical relationship. Midsagittal (**a**) scheme, (**b**) T1 weighted MRI scan and coronal-transinfundibular (**c**) MRI scans corresponding to a healthy adult. The seven fundamental radiological variables to define CP topography are: (1) Occupation of the chiasmatic cistern (ChC) by the tumor; (2) Occupation of the third ventricle (3V) by the tumor; (3) Anatomical distortion of the pituitary stalk (PS); (4) Mammillary body angle (MBA) which is the angle formed by the intersection of a plane tangential to the base of the mammillary bodies (MB) with the plane tangential to the fourth ventricle floor; (5) Anatomical distortion of the optic chiasm (Ch); (6) Relative position of the hypothalamus (red arrows) regarding the tumor, better assessed on coronal-transinfundibular MRI sections; (7) Tumor shape (**d**) the five major morphologies displayed by the tumor are shown

comprehensive model to categorize CP adherence [39]. Furthermore, this model can be assessed with conventional MRI studies. The pattern of CP adhesion is determined for each case by three components of the attachment: (1) the anatomical structures attached to the tumor; (2) the morphologic pattern or extent of the attachment; and (3) the adhesion strength. Taking into consideration these three components, CP adhesion can be classified into five increasing levels of severity—mild, moderate, serious, severe, and critical—each obviously associating a higher risk of hypothalamic injury, postoperative morbidity and mortality (Fig. 4.3).

The least severe type of adhesion (level I or mild adhesion) is observed for wholly intrasellar or sellar-suprasellar CPs which are separated from the TVF by a meningeal layer, either the dura mater of the diaphragma sellae or the arachnoid membranes of the chiasm cistern [39]. A slightly higher risk (level II) occurs for strictly intraventricular CPs showing a pedicle (fibrovascular stem) or a sessile (rectangular patch of tumor capsule) attachment to the ependymal lining of the 3V. These small attachments can usually be released. The next level of adherence severity (level III) is found in suprasellar CPs tightly adhered or fused to the pial surface of the infundibulum and/or tuber cinereum, without any intervening arachnoid layer. Attempts to release the tumor from the median eminence/basal

I - Mild   II - Moderate   III - Serious   IV - Severe   V - Critical

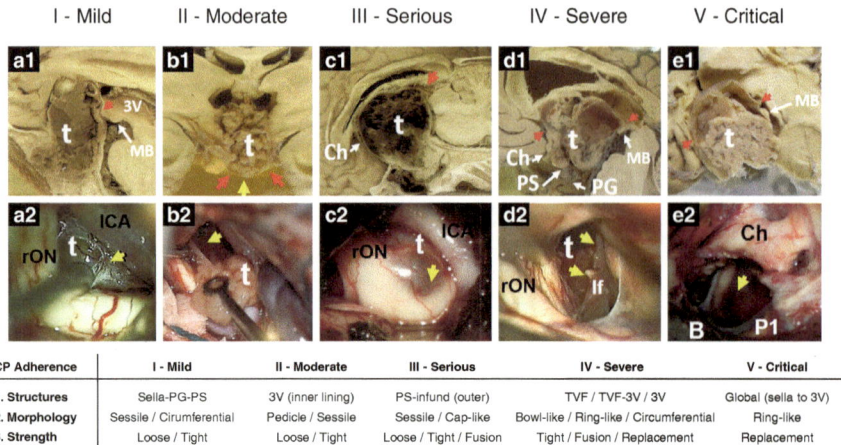

CP Adherence	I - Mild	II - Moderate	III - Serious	IV - Severe	V - Critical
1. Structures	Sella-PG-PS	3V (inner lining)	PS-infund (outer)	TVF / TVF-3V / 3V	Global (sella to 3V)
2. Morphology	Sessile / Cirumferential	Pedicle / Sessile	Sessile / Cap-like	Bowl-like / Ring-like / Circumferential	Ring-like
3. Strength	Loose / Tight	Loose / Tight	Loose / Tight / Fusion	Tight / Fusion / Replacement	Replacement

Fig. 4.3 Craniopharyngioma (CP) adherence severity levels. Upper row shows autopsy specimens of CPs (t) and lower row presents surgical images of the corresponding levels of CP adherence severity as observed in the surgical procedure of cases with the same topography. *Mild CP
adherence (Severity Level I)*: (**a1**) Midsagittal brain section showing the gross specimen of a sellar-
suprasellar CP (t). Red arrow points the upwardly displaced hypothalamus, over the upper pole of
the tumor. MB: mammillary body; 3V: third ventricle. (**a2**) Right pterional view showing the
arachnoid layer (yellow arrow) between the tumor capsule (t) and the right optic nerve (rON). ICA:
internal carotid artery. Moderate CP adherence (Severity level II): (**b1**) Coronal section from an
autopsy brain specimen showing a strictly intraventricular papillary CP (t) with a small basal
attachment (yellow arrow) to the ependymal layer of the intact third ventricle floor (red arrows).
(**b2**) Surgical view of a strictly intraventricular CP (t) through a right pterional approach showing
the pedicle attachment (arrow) to the TVF. Serious CP adherence (Severity level III): (**c1**)
Midsagittal section of a brain specimen showing a suprasellar-pseudointraventricular CP (t) whose
upper pole has displaced the third ventricle floor upward (red arrow). The optic chiasm is stretched
upward over the tumor. (**c2**) Right pterional view showing the tight attachment (arrow) between the
tumor and the upwardly displaced chiasm and third ventricle floor. *Severe CP adherence (Severity
level IV)*: (**d1**) Not-strictly intraventricular or infundibulo-tuberal CP (t). Notice how the MB is the
only visible structure of the third ventricle floor, the chiasm (Ch) is compressed forward in front of
the tumor, the pituitary stalk (PS) is amputated, and the pituitary gland (PG) is intact below the
tumor. Red arrows point to the hypothalamus, fused around the central, mid-portion of the tumor.
(**d2**) Intraoperative view through a right pterional approach showing a tumor (t) fused (arrows) to
the inner surface of the infundibulum (If). *Critical CP adherence (Severity level V)*: (**e1**) Sagittal
section showing a suprasellar-secondary intraventricular CP (t) which has broken into the third
ventricle. The position of the hypothalamus relative to the tumor is around its mid-third portion
(red arrows). (**e2**) Intraoperative view through the lamina terminalis after radical removal of a CP
which had invaded the 3V. Notice the breached TVF allowing a direct view of the basilar artery (B)
and the right posterior cerebral artery (P1). *Ch* chiasm

hypothalamus associate a poor outcome in about one-tenth of the cases. Level IV of
adherence severity corresponds to CPs with tenacious and extensive adhesions
between the TVF/3V walls and the tumor. Release of these adhesions may lead to a
poor outcome in about a quarter of cases due to long-term disabling hypothalamic
damage. These tumors are either fused to or have replaced the TVF/3V walls, and
the area of tumor-brain contact may have a bowl-like morphology (the adhesion

covers the tumor's bottom portion), a ring-like shape (the adhesion encircles the tumor's middle portion like a band), or a circumferential morphology (the adhesion entirely covers the tumor surface like wrapping paper). The most severe, critical level of adherence (level V) occurs in aggressive CPs extending from the sella to the 3V roof that encroach upon all the structures that form the vertical pituitary–hypothalamic axis. The invasion or replacement of the TVF may lead to a rate of poor outcome/death as high as 40% in this group [39]. A breached TVF can typically be seen on postoperative MRI scans following radical removal of CPs presenting each of the two latter adherence levels [40, 48]. CP topography has been identified as the variable showing the strongest relation with the level of adherence severity [39]: the mild level adherence severity is typically associated with the sellar-suprasellar topography; the moderate level with the strictly intraventricular topography; the serious level with the suprasellar-pseudointraventricular group; the severe level of adherence severity is usually observed in the infundibulo-tuberal topography; lastly, the critical level is generally associated with the secondary intraventricular category. CP topography, however, only explains by itself the surgical risk derived from the degree of tumor-brain adherence in 73% of cases, as many other variables such as tumor size, presence of hydrocephalus, and clinical symptoms caused by hypothalamic dysfunction also contribute significantly to the surgical risk.

4.8 MRI Assessment of the Anatomical Compartments and Neural Structures Involved by the Tumor

The preoperative MRI evaluation of a CP should consider first the tumor's occupation of three different compartments: the sella turcica, the chiasmatic or suprasellar cistern, and the 3V. In a second step, the position and morphological appearance of the anatomical structures making up the pituitary–hypothalamic axis (PG, PS, TVF, and 3V walls) is assessed (Fig. 4.2). The systematic definition of the status of these compartments and anatomical structures on conventional T1 and T2 images has proven sufficient to establish the accurate CP topography and the relationships between the tumor and the surrounding neurovascular structures in most cases [38, 47]. The compartments whose occupation provide the most reliable information to define the CP-hypothalamus relationship are the 3V and the chiasmatic cistern. Lack of occupation of the 3V is only observed in the sellar-suprasellar topography, which comprises those CPs with a more favorable surgical outcome.

Differentiating among the four remaining topographical categories with 3V involvement is the most difficult task. One of the most valuable signs is the lack of occupation of the chiasmatic cistern, a sign which strongly indicates a strictly intraventricular position. In contrast, partial occupation of the chiasmatic cistern points to the infundibulo-tuberal topography. Finally, a cistern wholly obliterated by the tumor may occur in any of the three topographic categories that originate below the TVF (the sellar-suprasellar, pseudointraventricular, and secondary intraventricular varieties).

Regarding the anatomical distortions of the pituitary–hypothalamic axis caused by the tumor, the appearance of the PS and the relative anatomical position between the hypothalamus and the CP are the two most useful signs to accurately define the type of tumor-hypothalamus relationship [38, 47]. The appearance of the PS, best defined on midsagittal MRI sections, is the radiological sign showing the strongest correlation with CP topography. Four major patterns can be considered: (1) intact or wholly visible PS; (2) thickened PS due to macroscopic tumor infiltration; (3) amputated PS, whose upper portion is not visible due to tumor growth; and (4) not visible or unrecognizable PS due to tumor encroachment. Amputation of the PS's upper infundibular edge by the tumor and PS infiltration are two signs that strongly point to a not-strictly intraventricular or infundibulo-tuberal CP associating a severe (level IV) hypothalamic adhesion. On the contrary, a normal PS appearance points to a strictly intraventricular CPs with a moderate (level II) adherence to the 3V. Lastly, the lack of identification of the PS on preoperative MRI is a less specific sign, as it can occur in any of the three topographic categories that originate beneath the TVF and occupy the chiasmatic cistern.

Another fundamental MRI variable is the level of the hypothalamus relative to the tumor, a sign best assessed on transinfundibular-coronal MRI sections [47]. The hypothalamus may be found adjacent to the lower tumor pole, around its mid-third portion or above the top pole of the tumor. The position of the hypothalamus in relation to the tumor is the most informative MRI sign to estimate the severity of CP adherence. A position of the hypothalamus around the mid-third or central portion of the tumor strongly points to the presence of the most extensive and tenacious adhesions to the hypothalamus (severity levels IV and V). On the contrary, a position of the hypothalamus around the lower third of the tumor is typical of strictly intraventricular lesions, whereas its position above the upper third of the tumor is observed for the sellar-suprasellar and pseudointraventricular CP topographies, both associating a lower risk of hypothalamic injury [47].

Finally, some macroscopic CP features such as the tumor size, consistency, shape, or presence of calcifications should be defined. Among these features, the tumor's shape has proven particularly useful to predict the severity of CP-hypothalamus adhesion. A round or pear-like tumor shape points to the presence of loose, mild attachment to the TVF that associates the lowest risk of hypothalamic injury. A pear-like outline on midsagittal MRI scans is usually observed for intrasellar CPs that push the diaphragma sellae upward against the optic chiasm and are thus covered with a layer of dura mater which separates the tumor from the vital hypothalamic nuclei. Conversely, elliptical shapes are often observed for infundibulo-tuberal and secondarily intraventricular CPs showing severe degrees of hypothalamic attachment (levels IV and V).

4.9 Optic Chiasm Distortions Caused by Craniopharyngiomas: Their Relation to Visual Function and Postoperative Visual Outcome

A precise MRI definition of the anatomical distortion caused by CPs on the optic chiasm represents valuable information to predict not only the accurate CP topography, but more importantly, the reversibility of visual impairment and the long-term visual outcome [49]. The position and shape of the optic chiasm are best assessed on midsagittal MRI sections (Fig. 4.4). The close proximity of the optic chiasm to CPs makes their growth usually grossly distort this structure. A wholly normal chiasm is only observed in approximately 10% of CP cases, either in those which exclusively occupy the sella turcica or in small tumors within the 3V cavity. Two major types of pathological distortion of the optic chiasm may occur, compression and stretching; typically, the former occurs in CPs originated within the TVF, behind the chiasm, whereas the latter is often observed in tumors growing below the chiasm

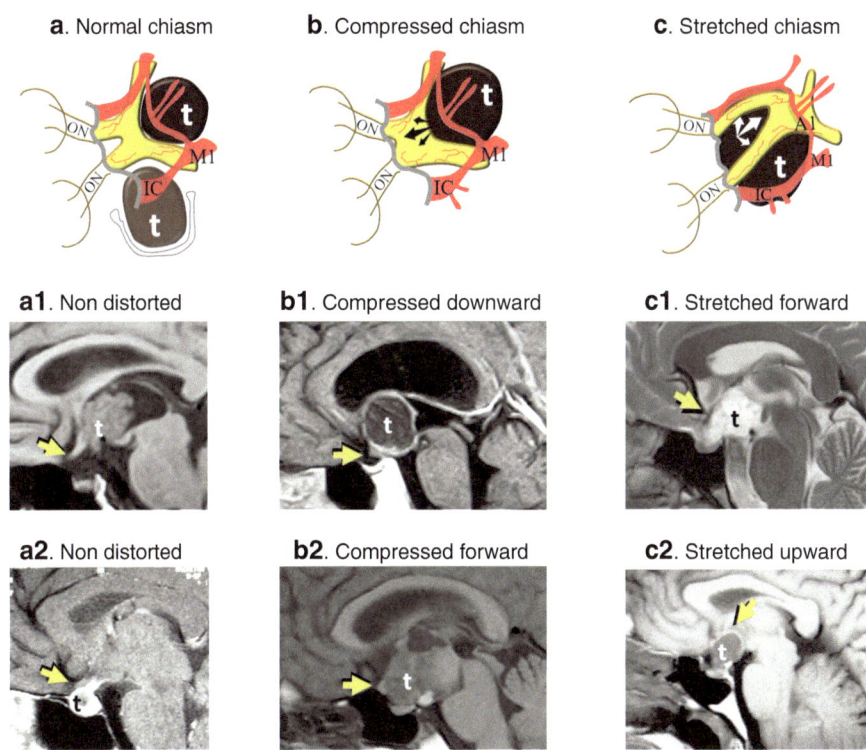

Fig. 4.4 MRI assessment of optic chiasm distortions caused by craniopharyngiomas and their relation with tumor topography. Yellow arrows point to the position of the optic chiasm in MRI midsagittal sections. (**a**) Illustrative scheme showing a chiasm with a normal position and shape. (**a1**) Normal or non-distorted chiasm as observed on T1-weighted MRI midsagittal scan from a patient with a strictly intraventricular CP (t). (**a2**) Normal or non-distorted chiasm in another case of a small sellar-suprasellar tumor CP (t). (**b**) Compressed distortions caused by intraventricular-retrochiasmatic CPs pushing on the chiasm and displacing it towards the tuberculum sellae. (**b1**) Compressed downward chiasm, placed beneath the anteroinferior margin of a pure intraventricular tumor (t) and flattened by its downward compressive force. (**b2**) Chiasm compressed forward against the bone of the planum sphenoidale by a not-strictly intraventricular CP (t). (**c**): Stretched distortions of the optic chiasm caused by suprasellar-subchiasmatic lesions pushing upwards on this structure, which becomes progressively elongated. (**c1**) Stretched forward chiasm along the anterior margin of a secondary intraventricular CP (t). (**c2**) Stretched upward chiasm along the superior surface of a sellar-suprasellar CP (t)

plane. Additional chiasm deformation subtypes can be defined depending on the direction the chiasm is displaced. A chiasm stretched upward strongly points to the suprasellar-pseudointraventricular topography; whereas a chiasm stretched and displaced forward, that is elongated along the anterior margin of the tumor, suggests a secondary intraventricular position. Among the compressed chiasms, those displaced forward and flattened against the tuberculum sellae (compressed forward) are typically associated with the not-strictly intraventricular topography, whereas the compressed chiasms downwardly displaced at the anteroinferior margin of the tumor point to the strictly intraventricular topography.

The type of chiasm distortion is related to the presence of visual disturbances and especially to the degree of visual impairment. Vision is usually spared in CP cases with either normal or downwardly compressed chiasms, whereas visual deficits occur in more than 80% of tumors associated with forward compression or forward/upward chiasm stretching [49]. The upward stretched pattern is the one associating the most severe visual disturbances, present in 75% of the cases. This is the result of irreversible axonal degeneration caused by stretching forces, indicated by the long-term thinned appearance of the chiasm on postoperative MRI midsagittal scans [49]. Accordingly, visual outcome after CP removal is significantly related to both the type of preoperative and postoperative chiasm distortion. The best visual outcome is found among CP patients whose optic chiasms show either a normal or downward compressed morphology on preoperative MRI. In contrast, the worst visual outcome is observed among patients with stretched chiasms. About one-third of the patients in these latter cases will not experience any improvement in their visual deficits following surgery, in particular when the postoperative MRI shows a chiasm with a thinned appearance [49].

4.10   Clinical-MRI Correlation for a Proper Assessment of Surgical Risks

Functional impairment of the hypothalamus represents one of the most feared complications of CP surgery, as Harvey Cushing wisely recognized towards the end of his career [1, 50]. The flood of information provided by current neuroradiological studies should not underestimate the value of preoperative clinical symptoms in predicting the type of hypothalamic involvement. For this reason, and despite this chapter being focused on MRI signs, we would like to briefly emphasize the importance of a proper preoperative assessment of clinical symptoms, in particular of those related to the impairment of hypothalamic functions. The *infundibulo-tuberal* syndrome is especially worth noting. It includes the symptoms of sexual infantilism, obesity, diabetes insipidus, and/or abnormal somnolence [40, 51]. The presence of this syndrome is highly predictive of a primary involvement of the basal hypothalamus (the region of the TVF, including the infundibulum and tuber cinereum) by the tumor. The arcuate, lower ventromedial, periventricular, and tubero-mammillary nuclei, as well as the supra-optic-hypophyseal and tubero-hypophyseal tracts included within this thin layer of neural tissue, are involved in the regulation of sexual functions, feeding behavior, water metabolism, and control of sleep cycles [51, 52]. Despite the surgeon's experience and skills, attempts to perform a radical

CP removal in patients with symptoms typical of the infundibulo-tuberal syndrome associate a high risk of hypothalamic injury and severe postoperative morbidity, even patient death [40, 51].

In addition, patients with CPs involving the 3V may present a wide set of alterations related to the loss of hypothalamic regulation of mental and/or vital bodily functions, caused by the damage of those hypothalamic nuclei and pathways situated above the TVF, within the 3V walls, as well as of the mammillary bodies. This *hypothalamic syndrome*, in contrast to the more restricted infundibulo-tuberal syndrome, includes psychiatric, behavioral and/or emotional alterations, severe impairment of memory and cognitive functions, abnormal changes in body temperature, loss of hemodynamic homeostasis, gait disturbances, and/or sphincter incontinence [51]. The presence of these alterations, usually associated with CPs developed within the 3V, should be thoroughly evaluated before surgery in order to avoid undue surgical maneuvers for the release of the CP-hypothalamic adhesions.

4.11 Accuracy of Conventional MRI to Predict CP Topography and the Severity of Hypothalamic Adherence

Accurate preoperative definition of CP topography and severity of CP adhesions to the hypothalamus can be achieved in 85–90% of cases with the use of conventional MRI sequences (T1- and T2-weighted) [38, 47]. For a proper assessment of CP topography, a multivariate analysis of MRI data investigated in a cohort of 200 surgically treated CPs selected seven fundamental radiological variables: (1) tumor occupation of the sella; (2) tumor occupation of the chiasmatic cistern; (3) PS appearance; (4) level of the hypothalamus relative to the CP; (5) value of the MBA; (6) CP shape; and (7) type of chiasm distortion [38] (Figs. 4.5, 4.6, 4.7,

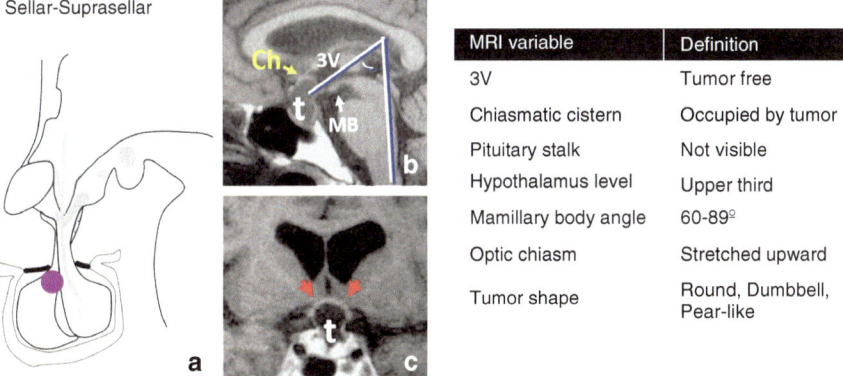

MRI variable	Definition
3V	Tumor free
Chiasmatic cistern	Occupied by tumor
Pituitary stalk	Not visible
Hypothalamus level	Upper third
Mamillary body angle	60-89º
Optic chiasm	Stretched upward
Tumor shape	Round, Dumbbell, Pear-like

Fig. 4.5 Sellar-suprasellar topography: MRI signs suggesting this category. (**a**) Illustrative scheme showing the origin of these CPs, at the junction between the pituitary stalk and the pituitary gland (purple circle). Midsagittal (**b**) and coronal-transinfundibular (**c**) MRI sections of a sellar-suprasellar craniopharyngioma (t). Red arrows point to the position of the hypothalamus, over the top of the tumor. *Ch* chiasm, *3V* third ventricle. *MB* mammillary body. The table summarizes the MRI signs typically observed in this group

Pseudointraventricular

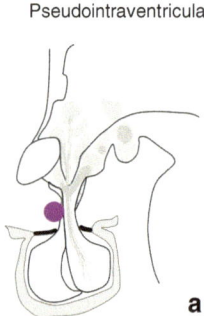
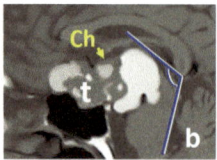
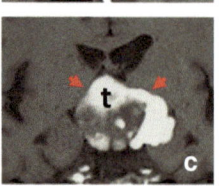

MRI variable	Definition
3V	Occupied by tumor
Chiasmatic cistern	Occupied by tumor
Pituitary stalk	Not visible
Hypothalamus level	Upper third
Mamillary body angle	>90º
Optic chiasm	Stretched upward
Tumor shape	Multiobulated

Fig. 4.6 Pseudointraventricular topography: MRI signs suggesting this category. (**a**) The origin of these CPs usually takes place at the pars tuberalis enveloping the anterior surface of the pituitary stalk (purple circle). Midsagittal (**b**) and coronal-transinfundibular (**c**) MRI sections of a craniopharyngioma (t) mimicking an intraventricular position. Red arrows point to the position of the hypothalamus, around the upper pole of the tumor. *Ch* chiasm. The table summarizes the MRI signs typically seen in this group

Secondary intraventricular

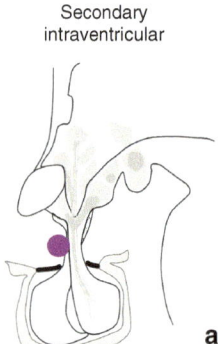
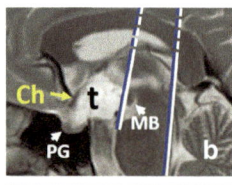
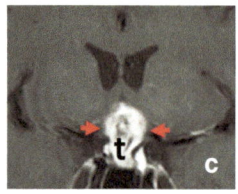

MRI variable	Definition
3V	Occupied by tumor
Chiasmatic cistern	Occupied by tumor
Pituitary stalk	Not visible
Hypothalamus level	Mid third
Mamillary body angle	30-59º
Optic chiasm	Stretched forward
Tumor shape	Multilobulated, Elliptical

Fig. 4.7 MRI predictors of the suprasellar-secondary intraventricular topographical category. (**a**) Illustrative scheme of the hypophyseal-hypothalamic region showing the origin of this group of CPs, at the suprasellar portion of the pituitary stalk (purple circle). Midsagittal (**b**) and coronal-transinfundibular (**c**) MRI sections of a craniopharyngioma (t) originated below the third ventricle floor which has broken through it into the third ventricle cavity. Red arrows point to the position of the hypothalamus, around the central portion of the tumor. *Ch* chiasm, *MB* mammillary body, *PG* pituitary gland. The table summarizes the MRI signs typically observed in this group

4.8, and 4.9). However, it should be noted that the accuracy of this model to predict CP topography is not homogeneous among the different categories. The best discrimination occurred for the sellar-suprasellar, pseudointraventricular, and strictly intraventricular topographies in which a correct diagnosis was made in up to 90% of the cases. On the contrary, the secondary intraventricular topography proved to be the most difficult to identify, being correctly predicted in less than 70% of cases. The difficulties in obtaining a correct preoperative diagnosis of the

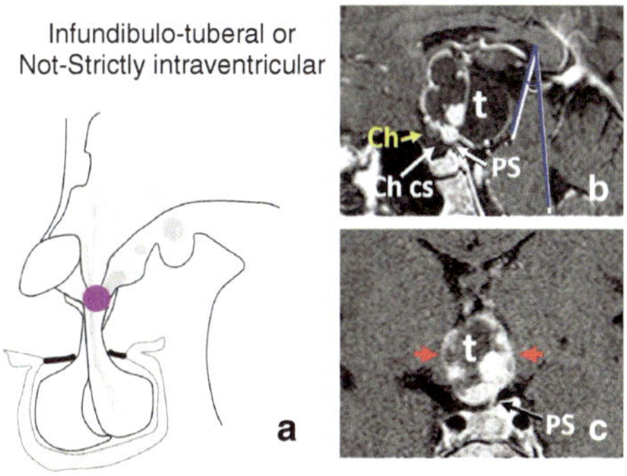

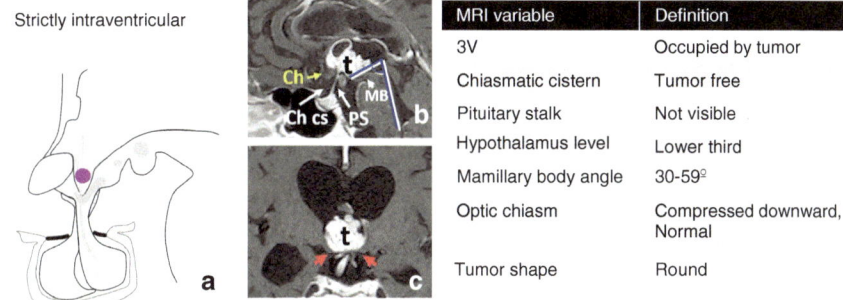

Fig. 4.8 MRI signs pointing to the infundibulo-tuberal or not-strictly intraventricular topographical category. (**a**) Hypothalamic-pituitary scheme showing the area of origin of this group of CPs, at a subpial position within the neural tissue of the third ventricle floor (purple circle). Midsagittal (**b**) and coronal-transinfundibular (**c**) MRI sections of a craniopharyngioma (t) largely growing within the third ventricle. Red arrows point to the position of the hypothalamus, around the central portion of the tumor. *Ch* chiasm, *Ch cs* chiasmatic cistern, *PS* pituitary stalk. The table summarizes the MRI signs typically found in this group

Fig. 4.9 MRI signs suggestive of the strictly intraventricular topographical category. (**a**) Illustrative scheme showing the origin of this group of CPs, from the ependymal (inner) layer of the third ventricle floor (purple circle). Midsagittal (**b**) and coronal-transinfundibular (**c**) MRI sections of a craniopharyngioma (t) purely located in the third ventricle. Red arrows point to the position of the hypothalamus. *Ch* chiasm, *Ch cs* chiasmatic cistern, *MB* mammillary body, *PS* pituitary stalk. The table summarizes the MRI signs typically found in this group

secondary intraventricular category (which invades the 3V from a suprasellar position) can be explained by the heterogenous anatomic distortions of the surrounding structures that this subtype of CPs may cause. Nevertheless, a high suspicion of the secondary intraventricular topography should be considered when the sella turcica, the chiasmatic cistern, and the 3V are occupied by the tumor and the PS is not visible, particularly if the hypothalamus is positioned around the mid-third portion of a multilobulated-shaped lesion [38, 46].

With regard to the severity of CP adherence, the multivariate model selected three basic MRI signs: (1) hypothalamus position relative to the tumor; (2) PS

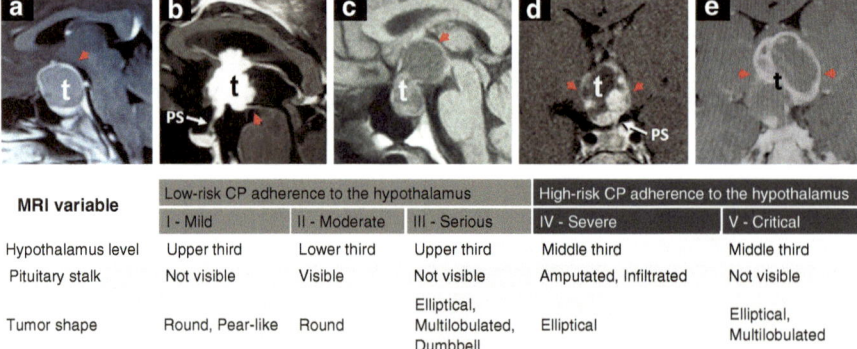

MRI variable	Low-risk CP adherence to the hypothalamus			High-risk CP adherence to the hypothalamus	
	I - Mild	II - Moderate	III - Serious	IV - Severe	V - Critical
Hypothalamus level	Upper third	Lower third	Upper third	Middle third	Middle third
Pituitary stalk	Not visible	Visible	Not visible	Amputated, Infiltrated	Not visible
Tumor shape	Round, Pear-like	Round	Elliptical, Multilobulated, Dumbbell	Elliptical	Elliptical, Multilobulated

Fig. 4.10 MRI predictors of the craniopharyngioma adherence severity level. The table below the row of MR images summarizes the specific signs associated with each level of CP adhesion severity. (**a**) Preoperative midsagittal MRI scan showing a pear-like craniopharyngioma (t) growing in the sellar and suprasellar compartments beneath the intact hypothalamus (red arrow). The tumor has encroached upon the pituitary stalk, no longer visible. (**b**) Midsagittal MRI showing a round papillary tumor (t) purely located within the third ventricle. The hypothalamus in located below the tumor (red arrow). Note the intact pituitary stalk (PS) and tumor-free chiasmatic cistern. (**c**) Midsagittal MRI scan showing a dumbbell craniopharyngioma (t) displacing upward the third ventricle floor (red arrow) (**d**) Coronal MRI scan showing an infundibulo-tuberal CP developed at the TVF. The hypothalamus is situated around the mid-third level. The PS is amputated. (**e**) Coronal MRI scan showing a large multilobulated CP growing in the sellar, suprasellar, and third ventricle compartments (secondary intraventricular tumor). The PS is not visible and the hypothalamus can be identified around the mid-third portion of the tumor (red arrows)

appearance; and (3) CP shape (Fig. 4.10). Distinction between high-risk adherence levels (IV-severe or V-critical) and low-risk adherence levels (I-mild, II-moderate, and III-serious) was correctly predicted in almost 90% of the cases by assessing only these three variables [47]. An incomplete tumor removal is strongly advocated when the position of the hypothalamus is around the mid-third of the lesion, the PS is amputated or infiltrated by the tumor, and the CP has an elliptical shape, as CPs showing severe or critical adhesions to the hypothalamus will be found in most cases with these MRI signs [16, 38, 40, 46, 47].

4.12 CP Topographical Diagnosis with New High-Resolution MRI Techniques: Future Perspectives

Recent MRI studies on sellar/parasellar lesions have demonstrated that high-resolution sequences such as the heavily T2-weighted and the fast-imaging employing steady state acquisition (FIESTA) MR imaging sequences offer a better definition of the tumor boundaries and the CP-brain relationships [53–56]. The 3D-FIESTA sequence has proven an invaluable tool to picture the exact position and status of the TVF in relation to the tumor [54], being particularly useful to measure the MBA [56]. These new methods are particularly promising to improve the topographical diagnosis of CPs of a large size and/or a secondary intraventricular position, which are currently the most difficult categories to define. In approximately 15% of cases, the MBA and the optic chiasm are unrecognizable with conventional T1- and T2-weighted MRI scans, a figure that very probably will be reduced with these new high-resolution sequences. We highly recommend including these new sequences in further studies on CPs.

4.13 MRI Assessment of Craniopharyngiomas: How It Can Guide the Optimal Surgical Approach and Degree of Tumor Resection

The optimal treatment of CPs remains controversial even today. A wide range of surgical approaches can be employed, such as the transcallosal, frontal-transventricular, pterional, subfrontal, interhemispheric, or transsphenoidal, and the use of one or another has been mostly based on the surgeon's preference. Regarding the degree of removal, some authors advocate a radical removal with the aim of preventing recurrences and the riskier procedures for recurrent tumors, whereas others propose limited resections followed by radiotherapy to avoid permanent invalidating sequelae. The heterogeneity of CPs in size, topography, and adherence, in addition to the high variability of patient age, makes it easy to understand that there is no generalized optimal treatment scheme for this complex type of tumor. Surgical planning for each individual case should take into consideration two aspects: where to begin; when to stop. The first question concerns the surgical route to be chosen, and the second the degree of removal to be attempted. Both matters should seriously take into account that the anatomical and functional preservation of the hypothalamus is paramount. With this premise in mind, the optimal surgical route would be the one that provides the best direct view of the lesion boundaries and the cleavage plane between the CP and the hypothalamus [39]. Moreover, CP surgery should pursue the maximum safe resection on the first attempt, to reduce the likelihood of CP recurrence, as recurrent lesions usually present the most severe adhesions to the hypothalamus [57].

As previously discussed, the detailed assessment of preoperative MRI studies provides enough clues to predict the accurate CP topography and the adherence level that will be found in the surgical procedure. The upper trans-ventricular routes can only be safely used in strictly intraventricular CPs in which the hypothalamus is situated below the tumor. These lesions usually present small attachments to the inner side of the TVF that can usually be released straightforwardly by employing an intraventricular approach. On the contrary, these routes associate a high risk of hypothalamic damage when used to remove any of the remaining topographical CP categories involving the 3V. The upper trans-ventricular routes do not offer a direct view of the wide and strong attachments to the hypothalamus shown by most not-strictly intraventricular and secondary intraventricular CPs. The presence of TVF remnants encircling the mid-third of the tumor makes it advisable to use the trans-lamina terminalis approach, either through a pterional, subfrontal, or interhemispheric route, in order to have a direct view of these delicate ring-like adhesions. The endoscopic transsphenoidal routes provide an even better view of the whole area of attachment of the not-strictly and secondary intraventricular categories, but at the expense of a high risk of cerebrospinal fluid fistula due to the direct connection left behind between the 3V and the nose.

4.14   Conclusions

A precise knowledge of the CP-hypothalamus relationships is essential to guide a proper, judicious decision regarding the optimal approach to the tumor and the degree of removal suitable for each case. The systematic assessment of a limited set of neuroradiological findings that can be easily identified on conventional MRI scans has proven highly reliable to accurately predict both CP topography and the level of CP adherence to the hypothalamus that will be found in surgery. Specifically, the position of the hypothalamus relative to the tumor, the appearance of the pituitary stalk, the occupation of the chiasmatic cistern and the 3V by the tumor, the MBA, the type of chiasm distortion, and the tumor shape are the most useful MRI signs to accurately define CP topography and adherence. An obtuse MBA strongly points to a pseudointraventricular topography, whereas a tumor-free chiasm cistern strongly indicates a strictly intraventricular tumor. The lowest risk of hypothalamic injury occurs in cases whose MRI shows a tumor-free 3V as they correspond to CPs developed below the TVF, in the sellar-suprasellar compartments. Radical tumor removal should be avoided in CPs presenting extensive and strong hypothalamic adhesions. CP adhesions to the hypothalamus associating high surgical risk should be suspected when the hypothalamus is positioned around the mid-third portion of the tumor, the upper infundibular portion of the PS is amputated and the tumor is elliptical.

References

1. Cushing H. Congenital tumors: the craniopharyngiomas. In: Intracranial tumors. Notes upon a series of two thousand verified cases with surgical-mortality percentages pertaining thereto. Springfield: Charles C Thomas; 1932. p. 93–104.
2. Prieto R, Pascual JM, Castro-Dufourny I, Carrasco R, Barrios L. Craniopharyngioma: surgical outcome as related to the degree of hypothalamic involvement. World Neurosurg. 2017;104:1006–10.
3. Fahlbusch R, Honegger J, Paulus W, Huk W, Buchfeledr M. Surgical treatment of craniopharyngiomas: experience with 168 patients. J Neurosurg. 1999;90:237–50.
4. Shi XE, Wu B, Fan T, Zhou ZQ, Zhang YL. Craniopharyngioma: surgical experience of 309 cases in China. Clin Neurol Neurosurg. 2008;110:151–9.
5. Pan J, Qi S, Lu Y, Fan J, Zhang X, Zhou J, Peng J. Intraventricular craniopharyngioma: morphological analysis and outcome evaluation of 17 cases. Acta Neurochir. 2011;153:773–84.
6. Rossi A, Cama A, Consales A, Gandolfo C, Garrè ML, Milanaccio C, Pavanello M, Piatelli G, Ravegnani M, Tortori-Donati P. Neuroimaging of pediatric craniopharyngiomas: a pictorial essay. J Ped. Endocrinol Metab. 2006;19:299–319.

7. Buslei R, Paulus W, Rushing EJ, Burger C, Giangaspero F, Santagata S. Craniopharyngioma. In: Louis DN, Ohgaki H, Wiestler OD, Cavenee WK, editors. WHO classification of tumors of the central nervous system. 4th ed. Lyon: IARC Press; 2016. p. 324–9.
8. Pascual JM, Prieto R. Harvey Cushing's craniopharyngioma treatment. Part 1: identification and clinicopathological characterization of this challenging pituitary tumor. J Neurosurg. 2018;131:949–63.
9. Pascual JM, Prieto R, Carrasco R, Castro-Dufourny I, Barrios L. Craniopharyngioma adherence to the hypothalamus. Neurosurg Focus. 2014;37:1–7.
10. Qi S, Lu Y, Pan J, Zhang X, Long H, Fan J. Anatomic relations of the arachnoidea around the pituitary stalk: relevance for surgical removal of craniopharyngiomas. Acta Neurochir. 2011;153:785–96.
11. Erdheim J. Über Hypophysengangsgeschwülste und Hirncholesteatome. Sitzungsb Kais Akad Wissen Math Naturw Klin. 1904;113:537–726.
12. Pascual JM, Rosdolsky M, Prieto R, Strau S, Winter E, Ulrich W. Jakob Erdheim (1874–1937): father of hypophyseal-duct tumors (craniopharyngiomas). Virchows Arch. 2015;467:459–69.
13. Cushing H. The pituitary body and its disorders. Philadelphia: JB Lippincott; 1912.
14. Fulton JF. Harvey Cushing. A biography. Springfield: Charles C. Thomas; 1946.
15. McKenzie KG, Sosman MC. The roentgenological diagnosis of craniopharyngeal pouch tumors. Am J Roentgenol. 1924;11:171–6.
16. Pascual JM, Prieto R, Castro-Dufourny I, Carrasco R, Strasuss S, Barrios L. Development of intracranial approaches for craniopharyngiomas: an analysis of the first 160 historical procedures. Neurosurg Focus. 2014;36:E13.
17. Pascual JM, Prieto R. Harvey Cushing and pituitary case number 3 (Mary D.): the origin of this most baffling problem in neurosurgery. Neurosurg Focus. 2016;41:E6.
18. Prieto R, Pascual JM. Harvey Cushing's craniopharyngioma treatment. Part 2: surgical strategies and results of his pioneering series. J Neurosurg. 2018;131:964–78.
19. Dandy WE. Ventriculography following the injection of air into the cerebral ventricles. Ann Surg. 1918;68:5–11.
20. Dandy WE. Benign tumors in the third ventricle of the brain: diagnosis and treatment. Springfield: Charles C. Thomas; 1933.
21. Pertuiset B, Janny P, Allegre G, Olivier L. Craniopharyngiomes simulant une tumeur antérieure du III ventricule. Presse Med. 1962;26:1846–8.
22. Pascual JM, González-Llanos F, Barrios L, Roda JM. Intraventricular craniopharyngiomas: topographical classification and surgical approach selection based on an extensive overview. Acta Neurochir. 2004;146:785–802.
23. Steno J, Malácek M, Bízik I. Tumor-third ventricular relationships in supradiaphragmatic craniopharyngiomas: correlation of morphological, magnetic resonance imaging, and operative findings. Neurosurgery. 2004;54:1051–60.
24. Pascual JM, Carrasco R, Prieto R, Gonzalez-Llanos F, Alvarez F, Roda JM. Craniopharyngioma classification. J Neurosurg. 2008;109:1180–3.
25. Banna M. Craniopharyngioma: based on 160 cases. Br J Radiol. 1976;49:206–23.
26. Pertuiset B. Craniopharyngiomas. In: Vinken PJ, Bruin GW, editors. Handbook of clinical neurology, vol. 19, Part II: tumors of the brain and skull. Amsterdam: North Holland Publishing Company; 1975. p. 531–72.
27. Rougerie J. What can be expected from surgical treatment of craniopharyngiomas in children. Childs Brain. 1979;5:433–49.
28. Hoffman JH, Hendrick EB, Humphreys RP, Buncic JR, Armstrong DL, Jenkin RD. Management of craniopharyngioma in children. J Neurosurg. 1977;47:218–27.
29. Raybaud C, Rabehanta P, Girard N. Aspects radiologiques des craniopharyngiomes. Neurochirurgie. 1991;37(Suppl 1):44–58.
30. Sartoretti-Schefer S, Wichmann W, Aguzzi A, Valavanis A. MR differentiation of adamantinomatous and squamous-papillary craniopharyngiomas. AJNR Am J Neuroradiol. 1997;18:77–87.

31. Adamson TE, Wiestler OD, Kleihues P, Yaşargil MG. Correlation of clinical and pathological features in surgically treated craniopharyngiomas. J Neurosurg. 1990;73:12–7.
32. Samii M, Tatagiba M. Surgical management of craniopharyngiomas: a review. Neurol Med Chir (Tokyo). 1997;37:141–9.
33. Steno J. Microsurgical topography of craniopharyngiomas. Acta Neurochir Suppl (Wien). 1985;35:94–100.
34. Apps JR, Martinez-Barbera JP. Molecular pathology of adamantinomatous craniopharyngioma: review and opportunities for practice. Neurosurg Focus. 2016;41:E4.
35. Prieto R, Pascual JM. Can tissue biomarkers reliably predict the biological behavior of craniopharyngiomas? A comprehensive overview. Pituitary. 2018;21:431–42.
36. Qi S, Pan J, Lu Y. Frontiers in neurosurgery, vol 4, craniopharyngiomas – classification and surgical treatment. Sharjah: Bentham Science Publishers; 2017.
37. Prieto R, Pascual JM. Craniopharyngiomas with a mixed histological pattern: the missing link to the intriguing pathogenesis of adamantinomatous and squamous-papillary varieties. Neuropathology. 2013;33:682–6.
38. Prieto R, Pascual JM, Barrios L. Topographic diagnosis of craniopharyngiomas: the accuracy of MRI findings observed on conventional T1 and T2 images. AJNR Am J Neuroradiol. 2017;38:2073–80.
39. Prieto R, Pascual JM, Rosdolsky M, Castro-Dufourny I, Carrasco R, Strauss S, Barrios L. Craniopharyngioma adherence: a comprehensive topographical categorization and outcome related risk stratification model based on the methodical examination of 500 tumors. Neurosurg Focus. 2016;41:E13.
40. Pascual JM, Prieto R, Carrasco R. Infundibulo-tuberal or not strictly intraventricular craniopharyngioma: evidence for a major topographical category. Acta Neurochir. 2011;153:2403–26.
41. Pascual JM, Prieto R, Carrasco R, Barrios L. Response to Craniopharyngiomas and the hypothalamus. J Neurosurg. 2013;119:1650–3.
42. Lubuulwa J, Lei T. Pathological and topographical classification of craniopharyngiomas: a literature review. J Neurol Surg Rep. 2016;77:e121–7.
43. Kassam AB, Gardner PA, Snyderman CH, Carrau RL, Mintz AH, Prevedello DM. Expanded endonasal approach, a fully endoscopic transnasal approach for the resection of midline suprasellar craniopharyngiomas: a new classification based on the infundibulum. J Neurosurg. 2008;108:715–28.
44. Sainte-Rose C, Puget S, Wray A, Zerah M, Grill J, Brauner R, Boddaert N, Pierre-Kahn A. Craniopharyngioma: the pendulum of surgical management. Childs Nerv Syst. 2005;21:691–5.
45. Puget S, Garnett M, Wray A, Grill J, Habrand JL, Bodaert N, Zerah M, Bezerra M, Renier D, Pierre-Kahn A, Sainte-Rose C. Pediatric classification and treatment according to the degree of hypothalamic involvement. J Neurosurg. 2007;106:3–12.
46. Pascual JM, Prieto R, Carrasco R, Barrios L. Displacement of mammillary bodies by craniopharyngiomas involving the third ventricle: surgical-MRI correlation and use in topographical diagnosis. J Neurosurg. 2013;119:381–405.
47. Prieto R, Pascual JM, Rosdolsky M, Barrios L. Preoperative assessment of craniopharyngioma adherence: magnetic resonance imaging findings correlated with the severity of tumor attachment to the hypothalamus. World Neurosurg. 2018;110:e404–26.
48. De Vile CJ, Grant DB, Hayward RD, Kendall BE, Neville BG, Stanhope R. Obesity in childhood craniopharyngioma: relation to post-operative hypothalamic damage shown by magnetic resonance imaging. J Clin Endocrinol Metab. 1996;81:2734–7.
49. Prieto R, Pascual JM, Barrios L. Optic chiasm distortions caused by craniopharyngiomas: clinical and magnetic resonance imaging correlation and influence on visual outcome. World Neurosurg. 2015;83:500–29.
50. Cushing H. Papers relating to the pituitary body, hypothalamus and parasympathetic nervous system. Springfield: Charles C. Thomas; 1932. p. 43–56.
51. Castro-Dufourny I, Carrasco R, Prieto R, Pascual JM. Infundibulo-tuberal syndrome: the origins of clinical neuroendocrinology in France. Pituitary. 2015;18:838–43.

52. Dudás B. The human hypothalamus: anatomy, functions and disorders. New York: Nova Science Publishers; 2013.
53. Saeki N, Murai H, Kubota M, Fujimoto N, Luichi T, Yamaura A, Sunami K. Heavily T2 weighted MR images of the anterior optic pathways in patients with sellar and parasellar tumors: prediction of surgical anatomy. Acta Neurochir. 2002;144:25–35.
54. Xie T, Zhang XB, Yun H, et al. 3D-FIESTA MR images are useful in the evaluation of endoscopic expanded endonasal approach for midline skull-base lesions. Acta Neurochir. 2011;153:12–8.
55. Watanabe K, Kakeda S, Yamamoto J, Watanabe R, Nishimura J, Ohnari N, Nishizawa S, Korogi Y. Delineation of optic nerves and chiasm in close proximity to large suprasellar tumors with contrast-enhanced FIESTA MR imaging. Radiology. 2012;264:852–8.
56. Gu Y, Zhang X. Mammillary body and craniopharyngioma. J Neurosurg. 2014;120:1243–5.
57. Prieto R, Pascual JM, Subhi-Issa I, Jorquera M, Yus M, Martinez R. Predictive factors for craniopharyngioma recurrence: a systematic review and illustrative case report of a rapid recurrence. World Neurosurg. 2013;79:733–49.

How Far with Surgery in the Modern Era of Endoscopy: Nasal Route

5

Matteo Zoli, Federica Guaraldi, Ernesto Pasquini, Marco Faustini-Fustini, and Diego Mazzatenta

5.1 Introduction

The hypothesis of resecting a craniopharyngioma (CP) through the transsphenoidal (TS) route has a long history [1–3]. Indeed, it was firstly proposed by Harvey Cushing at the beginning of the twentieth century, at the beginning of the neurosurgical era, but then progressively abandoned because of technical difficulties, mainly consistent in visualization issues [1–3]. The renaissance of TS surgery occurred in the 1960s, thanks to the experience of Guiot and Hardy, who suggested that such route could be suitable with good results for intrasellar subdiaphragmatic lesions [1–3]. Based on these results, in 1987 Weiss proposed a microscopic extended TS approach, enlarging the osteo-dural opening from the sella to the tuberculum sellae and planum region, to manage also selected cases of CP with supradiaphragmatic extensions [1–3]. This approach had the advantage to adopt a complete extra cranial corridor, therefore avoiding brain retraction or vasculo-nervous structures manipulation. However, due to the limitations given by the microscopic technique, for a long time this approach has been considered a route for "virtuosos," meaning for few highly trained surgeons, and was limited by the potential dramatic risk of CSF leak [4].

M. Zoli · F. Guaraldi · D. Mazzatenta (✉)
Center of Diagnosis and Treatment of Pituitary and Skull Base Tumors-Pituitary Unit, IRCCS Institute of Neurological Sciences of Bologna, Bologna, Italy

Department of Biomedical and Neuromotor Sciences, University of Bologna, Bologna, Italy
e-mail: matteo.zoli4@unibo.it; diego.mazzatenta@unibo.it, diego.mazzatenta@isnb.it

E. Pasquini
ENT Department, Bellaria Hospital, Bologna, Italy

M. Faustini-Fustini
Center of Diagnosis and Treatment of Pituitary and Skull Base Tumors-Pituitary Unit, IRCCS Institute of Neurological Sciences of Bologna, Bologna, Italy
e-mail: marco.faustini@isnb.it

© Springer Nature Switzerland AG 2020
E. Jouanneau, G. Raverot (eds.), *Adult Craniopharyngiomas*,
https://doi.org/10.1007/978-3-030-41176-3_5

79

A fundamental step forward in the routinely adoption of the TS approach for the treatment of CP was made with the introduction of the endoscope [5], firstly proposed for the treatment of pituitary adenomas by Jho and Carrau [5]. The authors suggested that the endoscope could improve the visualization of the surgical field, giving a more detailed and focused view, as well as a panoramic vision of the anatomical structures [5]. Moreover, for its versatility and maneuverability, it allows to tailor the surgical approach according to the lesion extension by combining different surgical corridors, and giving access to the vast majority of median and paramedian skull base regions [6, 7]. Therefore, thanks to the combination of the improved feasibility of extended approaches given by the endoscope and the advantages of the transsphenoidal route, the endoscopic endonasal approach (EEA) has progressively become the first choice approach for a large number of CPs [8–12]. In line with the trend reported by international literature, the number of procedures performed by EEA has continuously increased also at our center in the last 20 years (Fig. 5.1) [8]. Interestingly, the surgical outcome is similar among the different centers, demonstrating the reproducibility and standardization of this technique that can be, therefore, considered to be not for virtuosos only [8].

Although CSF leak still remains an important issue, requiring a meticulous plastic repair and a dedicate care and nursing in the post-operative time, the advantages of EEA in properly selected cases have been reported by many papers in the last years [8–12]. Indeed, EEA allows to resect the tumor following its own pattern of growth without trespassing the arachnoid plane and, therefore, avoid the manipulation of the optic nerves and chiasm, or of its vasculature. This is reflected by the good results in terms of visual outcome reported by many authors that represent one of the most relevant advantages for the patients [8–12].

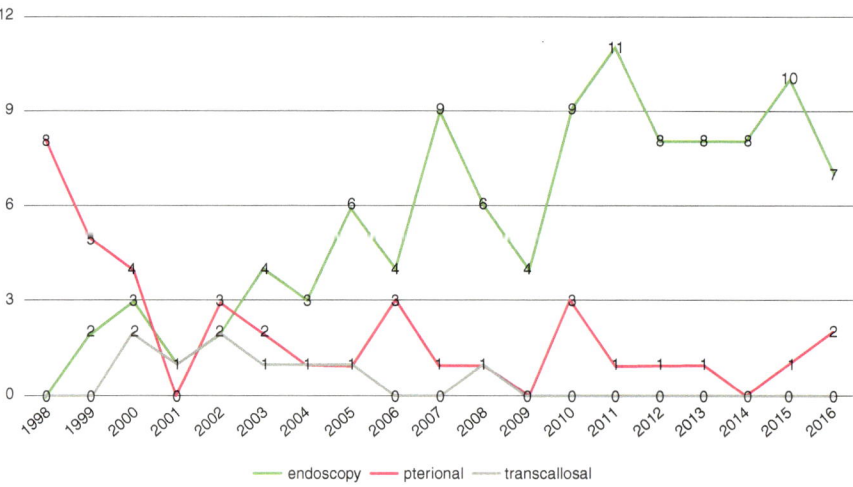

Fig. 5.1 The graph represents the increasing trend in adopting the endoscopic endonasal approach together with the concomitant reduction of transcranial approaches after the introduction of the endoscopic technique in 1998 at our center

However, despite the abovementioned advantages and positive outcome, it should be reminded that craniotomy still has some specific indications that should be well kept in mind by the surgeon while planning every treatment [13–16]. Indeed, a surgeon facing challenging tumors like CPs should master all the different types of approaches, including transcranial routes and endoscopic endoventricular technique, in order to choose the most appropriate one for every single case, sometimes also combining them, to improve the final outcome [13–16]. The recent advances in the knowledge of CP biology, pathology, and molecular patterns have led to the development of complementary treatments, i.e., radiotherapy—eventually with heavy particles—and medications [17–19]. Therefore, the surgeon should be able to tailor not only the surgical approach, but also to combine surgery with other treatments, in order to offer the most effective treatment strategy possible with the aim of controlling disease and preserving patient quality of life.

5.2   Endoscopic Endonasal Approach: Surgical Technique

Based on our experience, we prefer to place the patient in a semi-sitting position, with the thorax slightly elevated on the operating table [20], that helps in keeping the surgical field clean from blood. A supine position has also been proposed and is currently adopted by other groups.

Surgery is performed under general anesthesia with oro-tracheal intubation. The laryngopharynx is packed with gauzes to prevent blood and fluid passage in the upper airways rod lens endoscopes (model Hopkins II; Ø 4 mm, length 18 cm; 0° and 30° scopes; Karl Storz Endoscopy-America, Inc., Culver City, CA) with a high definition camera are adopted. The 4 mm endoscope is adopted also to treat pediatric patients because even if the diameter of the instrument reduces the working space—especially during the nasal phase—it allows a much better visualization, particularly during the more delicate phase of the intradural tumor resection. Neuronavigation (StealthStation S7 MEDTRONIC, Louisville, CO) is routinely adopted for extended approaches. It is mandatory in case of conchal or pre-sellar variant of the sphenoid sinus, typical of children. A CT-angiogram (CTA) merged with the pre-operative MRI of the patient, processed through StealthMerge Software (MEDTRONIC, Louisville, CO) is used as reference image. High-speed diamond drill is adopted in case of incomplete pneumatization, or to complete bony opening of the tuberculum/planum region. We recommend to use the drill under continuous irrigation, particularly when working close to the optic canal, to avoid heat-related damages to these structures. In general, it is difficult to adopt CUSA® (Integra LifeSciences Corporation, Plainsboro, NJ) in the transsphenoidal corridor, so it is of limited utility. Conversely, other non-coaxial but side-cutting instruments, such as NICO Myriad® (NICO Corporation Indianapolis, IN) can be useful for tumor debulking [21]. Intraoperative Eco-Doppler with a dedicated mini-probe for TS surgery (Mizuho America, Union City, CA) is routinely adopted to localize the carotid artery, after the bone drilling, or other major intradural vessels.

If the tumor is completely intrasellar, a simple midline TS approach, similar to the routine technique used for pituitary adenomas, is generally sufficient. This approach requires a posterior septostomy, followed by an anterior sphenoidotomy. After the identification of the common landmarks of the posterior wall of the sphenoidal sinus—represented by the sellar bulge, the clivus indentation, the optic nerves, the carotid arteries impressions, and by the medial and lateral optic-carotid recess between these structures, the sella is opened by a Kerrison rongeur. After dura incision, the tumor is removed, trying to avoid intraoperative CSF-leak due to the damage of the diaphragm. Otherwise, a plastic repair with abdominal fat, and a graft or flap of mucoperiosteum from the middle turbinate, or from the septum, is necessary to prevent post-operative leak potentially complicated by meningitis.

When the tumor extends suprasellar in the supradiaphragmatic region, as for the majority of CPs, an extended transplanum/transtuberculum approach is needed to gain access to the intradural space. The landmarks of the nasal phase are the same adopted for the standard approach, mainly constituted by the middle and superior turbinate, which points with its tail to the sphenoid ostium. Normally, we prefer to resect the middle turbinate of the narrowest nasal fossa, while the contralateral is displaced laterally. Recently, for selected cases with a good pneumatization of paranasal sinuses, and a wide working room in the nasal fossae and in the sphenoid sinus, we have avoided turbinectomy. Then, a posterior septostomy is performed to work through both nostrils. When necessary, unilateral (anterior and/or posterior) ethmoidectomy is performed to expose the posterior wall of the sphenoid, followed by wide anterior sphenoidotomy. Indeed, in selected cases with wide sphenoid pneumatization, the ethmoidectomy can be avoided with a drastic reduction of the risk of post-operative anosmia. Based on intraoperative anatomical landmarks (i.e., optic-carotid recess) the bony floor of the sella is identified and progressively removed with a high-speed diamond drill or a Kerrison rongeur (Fig. 5.2). Bone removal is extended superiorly to the tuberculum sellae and planum sphenoidalis. The intercavernous sinus is coagulated and then the dura is opened superiorly to expose the suprasellar cistern (Fig. 5.3). For the intradural phase of the surgery, we prefer to fix the endoscope with a holder, so to proceed with a "four hands-two surgeons" technique.

The tumor removal is performed according to the principles of the microsurgical technique. Briefly, the tumor is initially debulked centrally, then it is dissected following the surrounding arachnoidal layer (Fig. 5.4), that allows to preserve the arachnoid covering the optic nerves and their tiny feeding vessels, and the superior hypophyseal artery. Then the tumor is progressively dissected by the hypothalamus. In case of intrapial infiltration, this maneuver is arrested to avoid permanent neurological sequelae (Fig. 5.4). Once the tumor removal has been completed, an exploration of the surgical cavity is usually performed through angled scopes (Fig. 5.4).

A watertight plastic repair is performed with free-flaps multilayer technique, in which three layers are usually adopted for closure (Fig. 5.5). The first layer is placed intracranially and intradurally and is made with fascia lata or heterologous dural substitute, such as Biodesign® (Cook Medical, Bloomington, IN). It is fundamental that the covering tissue is larger than the osteo-dural defect to be

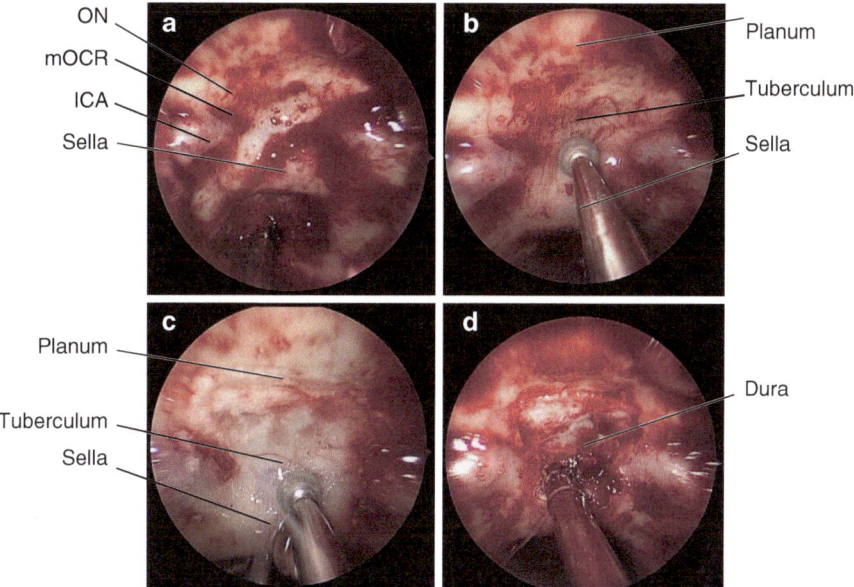

Fig. 5.2 Intraoperative images obtained using a 0° scope during endoscopic endonasal approach (EEA). Approach phase. (**a**) The anatomical landmarks in the posterior wall of the sphenoidal sinus are visible. (**b**) After the identification of the sellar bulge and of the medial optic-carotid recess, it is possible to open the bone from the sella toward the tuberculum region. (**c**) The bone is progressively removed by high speed diamond drill and Kerrison rongeur in a trapezoidal shape. (**d**) The dura covering the sella and the tuberculum region is exposed after bone removal. Lateral limits of this opening are represented by the medial border of the medial optic-carotid recess to avoid vascular injury

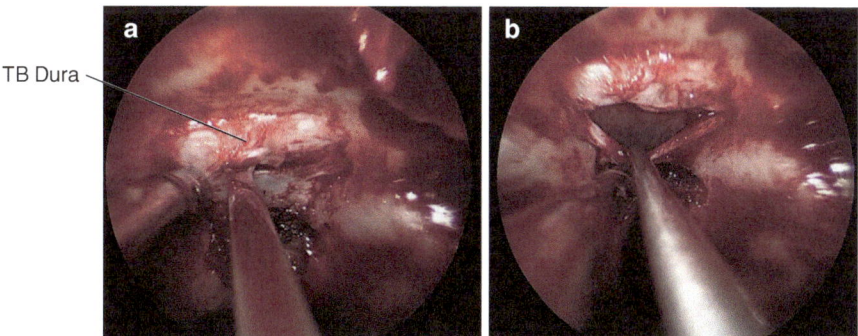

Fig. 5.3 Intraoperative images obtained using a 0° scope during endoscopic endonasal approach (EEA). Approach phase. (**a**) Dura is cut in an inverted H shape. (**b**) After the first cut, the dura is dissected from the other surgical planes, such as arachnoid. (**c**, **d**) Superior intercavernous sinus is coagulated and then cut to gain access to the suprasellar space

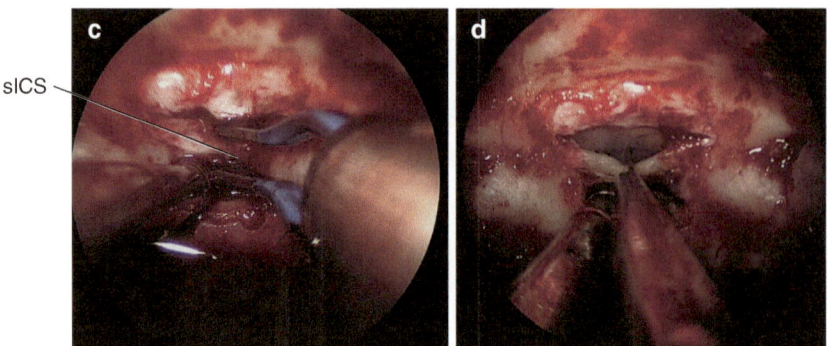

Fig. 5.3 (continued)

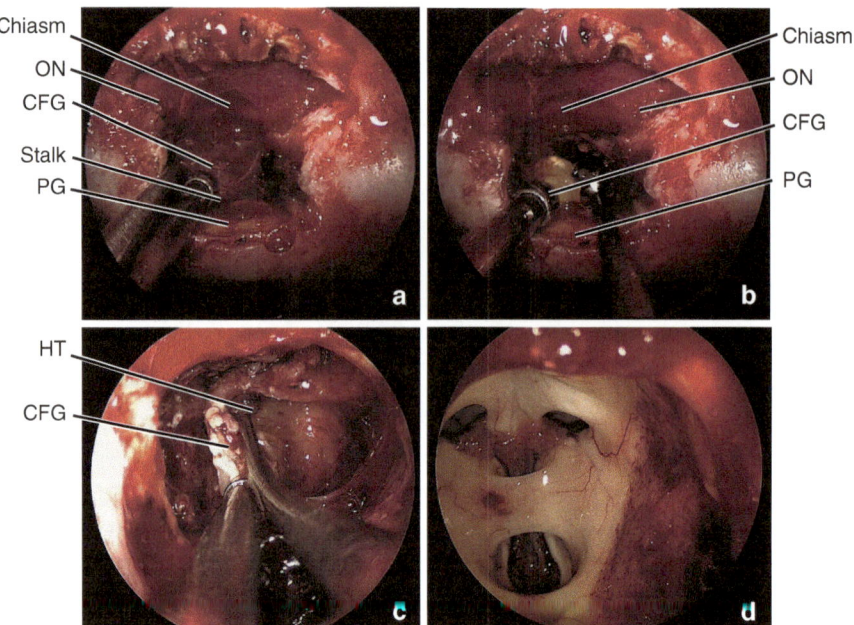

Fig. 5.4 Intraoperative images obtained using the endoscopic endonasal approach (EEA). Tumor removal phase. (**a**) The suprasellar anatomical structures, such as optic nerves and chiasm and pituitary stalk, are visible after dura opening. (**b**) Tumor is removed with bimanual microsurgical technique. Initially, it is centrally debulked to reduce the mass volume. (**c**) Afterwards, it can be dissected by the surrounding structures with optimal visualization of the tumor–hypothalamus interface. (**d**) At the end of the tumor removal, the third ventricle is visible, demonstrating the complete tumor removal. Images (**a–c**) are obtained using a 0° scope, while (**d**) is obtained by a 30° scope

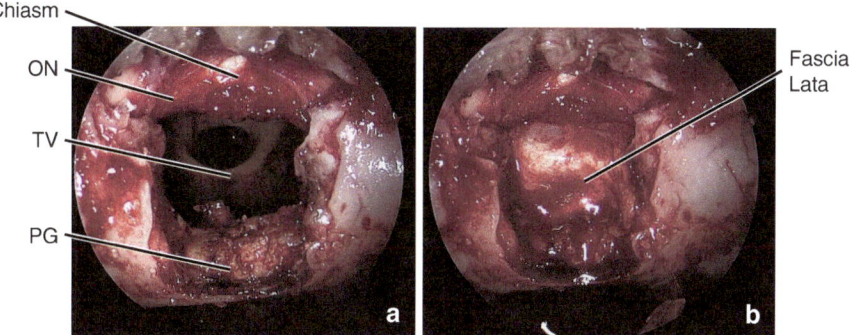

Fig. 5.5 Intraoperative images obtained using a 0° and a 30° scope during endoscopic endonasal approach (EEA). Closure phase. (**a**) The osteo-dural opening, representing the working window toward the suprasellar space, can be detected. (**b**) A first layer of fascia lata (or of other heterologous substitutes) is placed intracranially intradurally

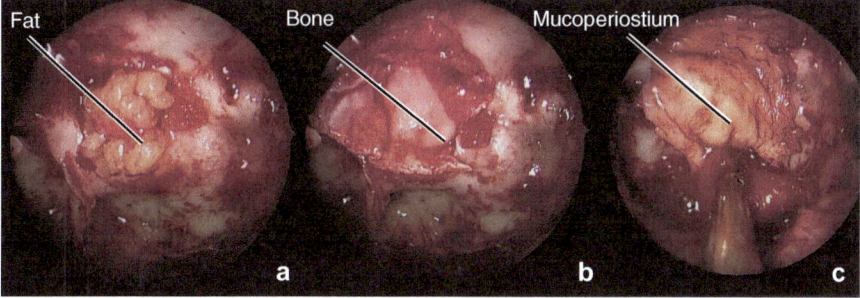

Fig. 5.6 Intraoperative images obtained using a 0° and a 30° scope during endoscopic endonasal approach (EEA). Closure phase. (**a**) After a second layer placed intracranially extradurally, a piece of abdominal fat is added to fill the space between the layers. (**b**) A rigid bony scaffold is placed to sustain the closure. (**c**) An outer layer of graft or flap of mucoperiosteum covers the closure

sure to cover it entirely and properly. Then, a further intracranial extradural layer of the same materials is placed to sustain the previous closure. Whenever possible, a rigid scaffold, such as a bony or a cartilage fragment, can be applied to increase the mechanic support to the closure (Fig. 5.6). Afterwards, an extracranial layer of mucoperiosteum, usually with a naso-septal flap or with a turbinate or septal graft, is applied to cover the osteo-dural defect (Fig. 5.6). A single 8-cm Merocel® (Merocel Corp., Mystic, CT) swab is placed in both nostrils for the following 72 h to prevent epistaxis.

5.3   Endoscopic Endonasal Approach: Indications and Contraindication

Tumor location and its relationship with the most relevant suprasellar structures (i.e., the optic chiasm, the pituitary stalk, and the hypothalamus) have to be analyzed to define the indication to EEA. As suggested by Ciric, CPs may arise from different locations, from the nasopharynx to the third ventricle [22, 23], since they take origin from the ectodermal remnants of Rathke's pouch or of the craniopharyngeal duct that have remained entrapped during their migration from the embryonic stomodeum toward the infundibulum [4]. Intracranial tumors can be classified, depending on their origin, into subdiaphragmatic, supradiaphragmatic extrapial, and supradiaphragmatic intrapial [3]. This classification has a relevant prognostic value, since the chances of radical resection and, therefore, the risk of recurrence vary according to the anatomic site of origin.

Conversely, as proposed by Hoffman, CPs may be classified, according to their location in relation with the optic chiasm, into intrasellar or pre-chiasmatic, and post-chiasmatic [24]. Although this scheme was initially proposed to help the surgeon in choosing between an anterior (i.e., sub-frontal) or lateral (i.e., pterional) approach for craniotomy, it keeps a determinant role also for endoscopic surgery. Indeed, as showed in Fig. 5.11, in case of a suprasellar CP, EEA can be chosen only in the absence of relevant structures along the surgical corridor given by the extended approach. In case the chiasm is pushed anteriorly and inferiorly by the tumor at the level of the tuberculum, the EEA could be hampered by this structure, that is, at major risk of damage, and could significantly reduce the chance to achieve a satisfactory tumor resection [25]. On the other hand, a postero-superior displacement of the chiasm by the tumor represents the more favorable condition for EEA [25].

In 2008, Kassam et al. have proposed a further classification of CPs based on their relationship with the pituitary stalk [26]. Five grades were considered: intrasellar, pre-infundibular, trans-infundibular, retro-infundibular, and intraventricular [26] (Figs. 5.7, 5.8, 5.9, and 5.10). The authors strongly advised to adopt the EEA for the first three categories and in selected cases of retro-infundibular CPs [26], but not for intraventricular forms [26]. In the last decade, several studies have investigated the outcome of EEA for the treatment of CPs to optimize the criteria applied for case selection [27–33]. In 2016, Marisako et al. proposed a management algorithm and suggested the EEA for intrasellar, pre-infundibular, and trans-infundibular CPs [34]. Conversely, they suggested the transcranial approach for retro-peduncular tumor larger than 30 mm and with calcifications [34]. Indubitably, tumor size and location, as well as the presence of calcifications are very important features to be considered while planning surgical approach, especially if the lesion is close to major vessels, for the consistent risk of a direct damage of these structures. Based on our experience, we consider the most appropriate surgical approach the one that allows the largest working room and the most direct angle possible to reach the tumor [20]. The extended EEA gives both these advantages for most retropeduncular forms [20]. Furthermore, if needed, additional space can be obtained by partially

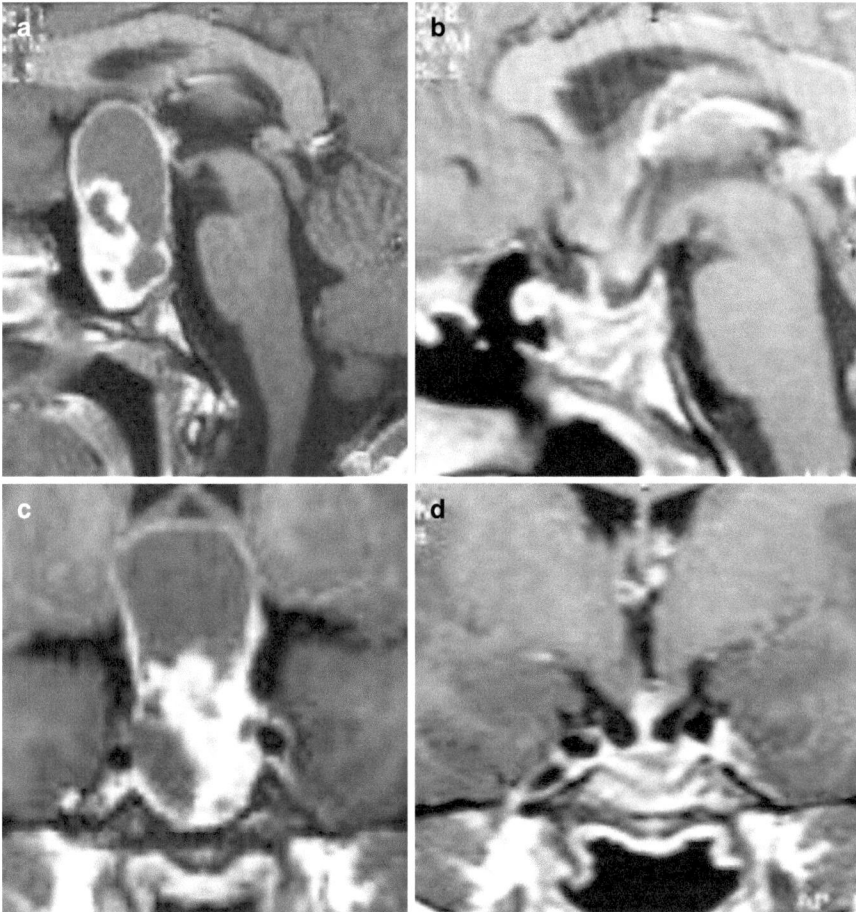

Fig. 5.7 Sagittal and coronal MRI T1 weighted images obtained after gadolinium injection. (**a, c**) A pre-peduncular craniopharyngioma is presented in the pre-operative MRI. (**b, d**) The radical tumor removal obtained by endoscopic endonasal approach (EEA) can be appreciated at the post-operative MRI

resecting the dorsum sellae to gain access to the interpeduncular cistern [35]. In our opinion, the most relevant features to be considered in the pre-surgical planning are the tumor location in relation with the chiasm that determines the possibility of having a satisfactory surgical corridor from the planum/tuberculum region to the tumor, and the lateral extension [25]. Indeed, the ventral route does not represent the best option in case of insufficient working space to resect the tumor, as for the cases in which the chiasm is displaced toward the tuberculum, or if the CP has a relevant lateral extension and, therefore, the angle for surgical approach is not coaxial to the tumor (Fig. 5.11). An issue associated with the ventral approach in retrochiasmatic CPs is represented by the anterior displacement of the stalk [33]. If this structure is

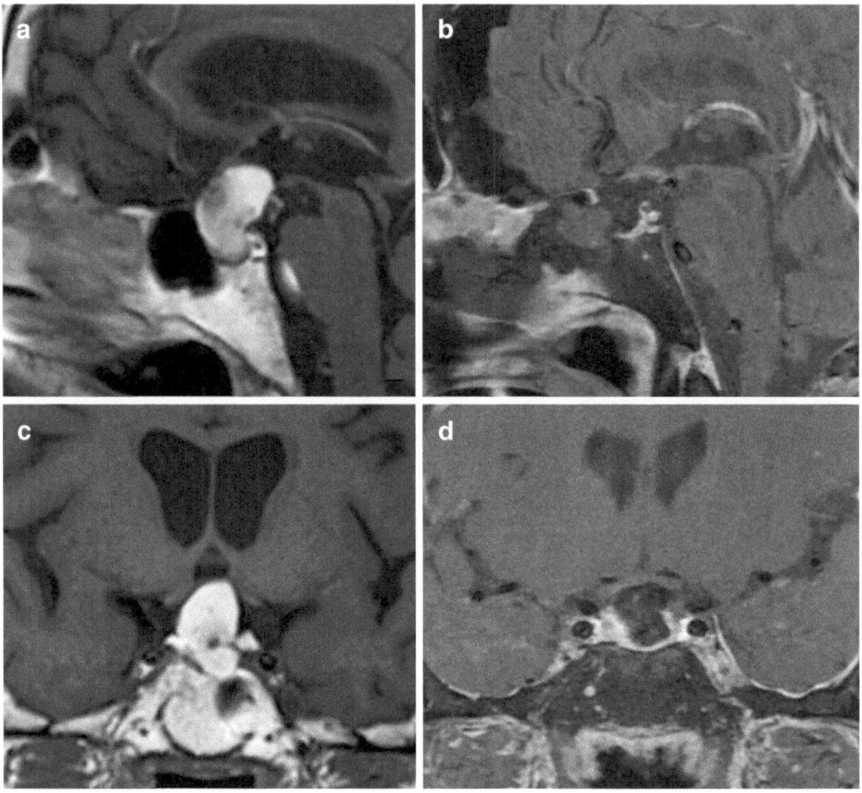

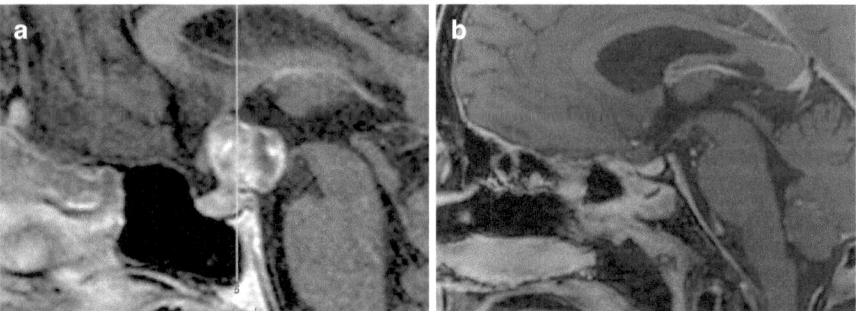

Fig. 5.8 Sagittal and coronal MRI T1 weighted images obtained after gadolinium injection. (**a, c**) Transpeduncular craniopharyngioma. (**b, d**) The radical tumor resection obtained by endoscopic endonasal approach (EEA) can be appreciated at the follow-up MRI

Fig. 5.9 Sagittal and coronal MRI T1-weighted images obtained after gadolinium injection. (**a, c**) A retropeduncular craniopharyngioma compressing and superiorly displacing the third ventricle floor. (**b, d**) Complete tumor removal with preservation of hypothalamic structures was obtained by endoscopic endonasal approach (EEA) and can be appreciated at the follow-up MRI

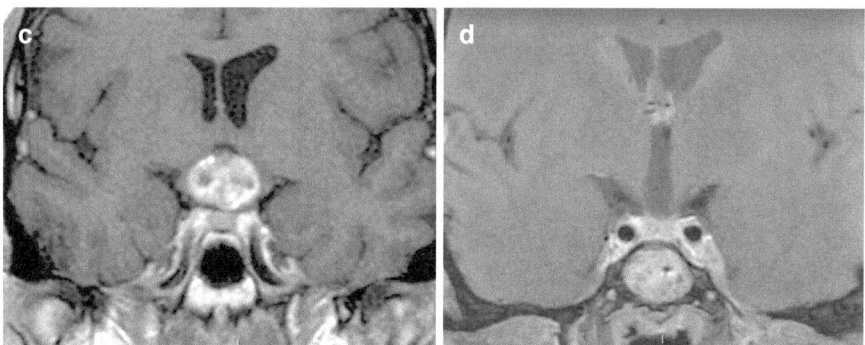

Fig. 5.9 (continued)

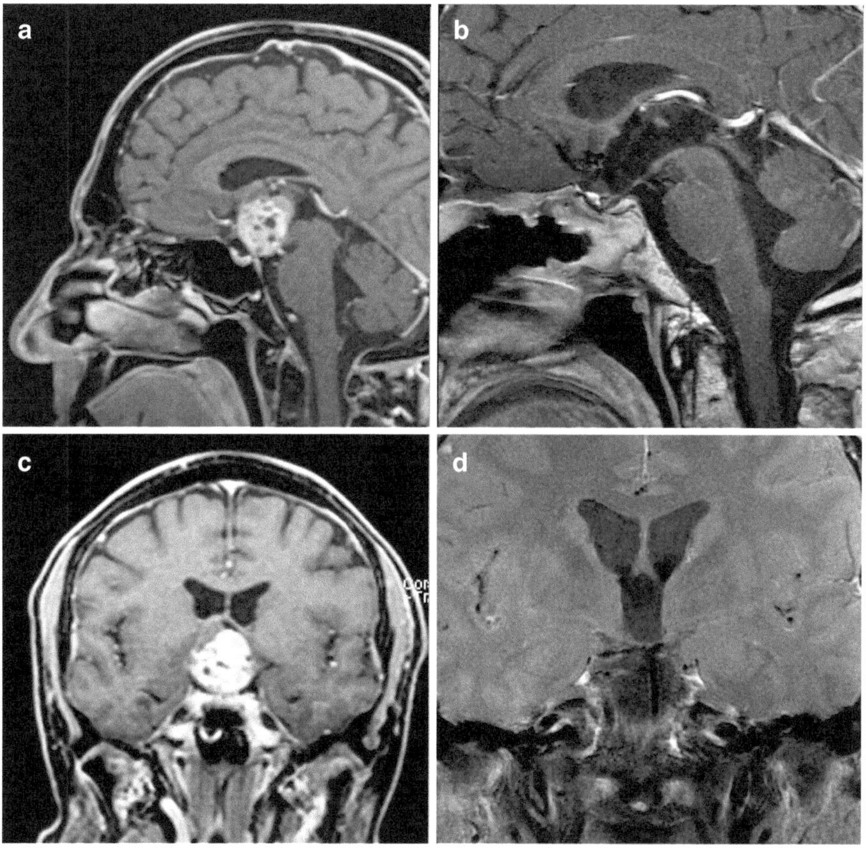

Fig. 5.10 Sagittal and coronal T1-weighted images obtained after gadolinium injection. (**a, c**) A third ventricle craniopharyngioma is presented. Considering the favorable mammillary body angle and the superior displacement of the chiasm, an endoscopic endonasal approach (EEA) was chosen. (**b, d**) Post-operative MRI demonstrating the radical resection of this tubers-infundibular craniopharyngioma together with hypothalamic anatomical sparing

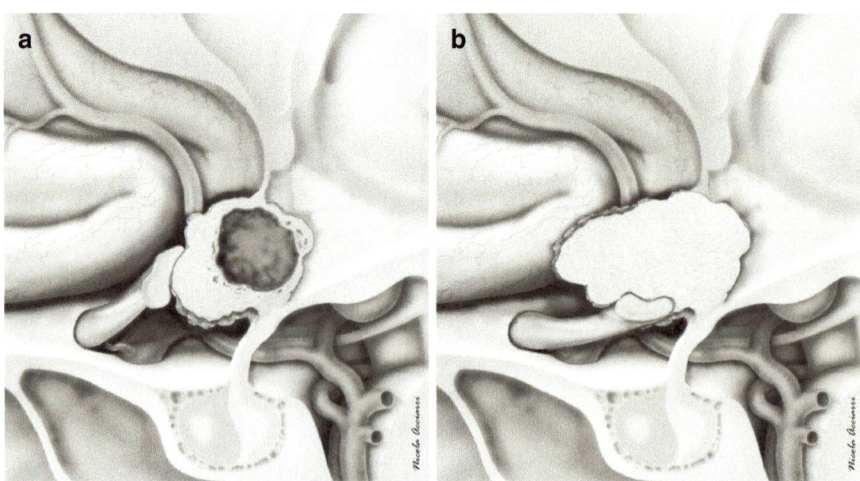

Fig. 5.11 Schematic drawing representing the relevancy of the optic chiasm displacement in the choice of endoscopic endonasal approach (EEA) for the treatment of retropeduncular or tubero-infundibular craniopharyngiomas. (**a**) The chiasm is displaced superiorly, giving a straight angle to approach the lesion, and sufficient working room using the ventral approach. (**b**) On the contrary, the antero-inferior displacement of the chiasm represents an obstacle along the surgical trajectory that impairs the endoscopic endonasal approach (EEA)

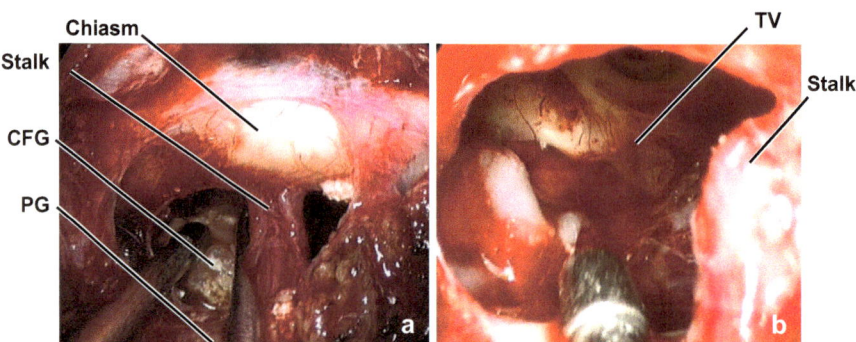

Fig. 5.12 Intraoperative images obtained using a 0° during endoscopic endonasal approach (EEA). (**a**, **b**) Tumor removal through a progressive dissection lateral to the pituitary stalk that allows its transection. Unfortunately, anatomical stalk preservation does not correspond to its functional integrity and could increase the risk of tumor recurrence

recognizable, the surgeon should try to spare it by working on both sides (Fig. 5.12). However, in the vast majority of published CP series, the endocrinological outcome is usually poor independently from stalk sparing [27–33] and some authors suggest that its preservation may only increase the risk of tumor recurrence without leading to real advantages [27–33]. Therefore, to date, the best management of the pituitary stalk in these cases remains debated.

The EEA for the treatment of endoventricular CPs remains controversial and some points have to be considered to give an updated and honest evaluation about the chances of success associated with this technique. According to Pascual, these tumors may be divided into infundibulo-tuberal or not strictly intraventricular, arising from the pituitary stalk at its upper part, and thus extending suprasellar primary and involving the third ventricle floor during their growth; and purely endoventricular, characterized by a complete intraventricular extension [36, 37]. According to Steno et al., in the first case the hypothalamus is circumferentially displaced around the tumor, which creates a straight and direct corridor to get access from the suprasellar region into the third ventricle, favorable for the endoscopic endonasal approach [38]. Conversely, in the second case the floor of the third ventricle is displaced inferiorly by the tumor toward the suprasellar region, thus preventing a ventral approach to spare the intact hypothalamus [38]. Therefore, for these cases the precise pre-operative consideration about the relationship between the tumor and the hypothalamus is relevant. Some authors have recently proposed a method based on the measurement of the so-called mammillary body angle, comprised between a plane tangential to the base of the mammillary bodies and a plane parallel to the floor of the fourth ventricle in midsagittal plane [39]. If the angle is <60°, it is highly probable that the tumor is intraventricular, so it cannot be resected through the EEA [39]. Conversely, if the angle is >90°, it could be a tubero-infundibular or a suprasellar CP with intraventricular expansion, thus suitable for ventral approach [3]. In conclusion, EEA can be chosen to treat CPs of the third ventricle when the tumor has already displaced laterally the hypothalamus, creating a straight corridor that reaches the ventricle following the mass (Fig. 5.13). Other approaches, such as transcallosal or trans-lamina terminalis, should be preferred in the other cases.

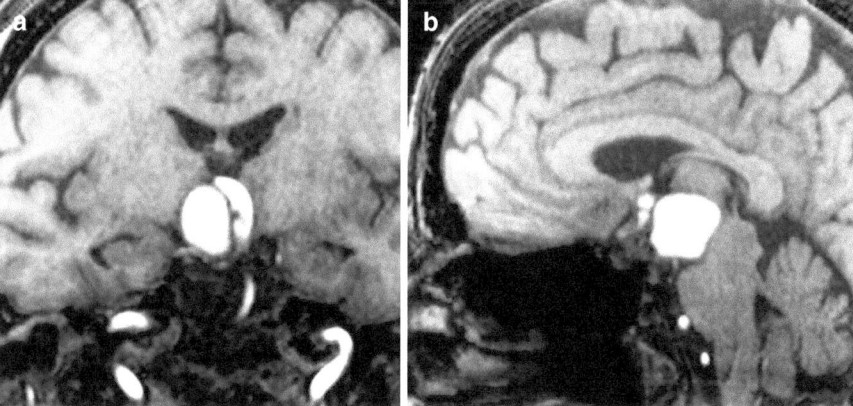

Fig. 5.13 Sagittal and coronal MRI T1-weighted images with gadolinium. Two cases of third ventricle craniopharyngioma are presented. (**a**, **b**) The tumor is completely endoventricular, displacing the floor of the ventricle and the chiasm inferiorly. For this purely ventricular case, a transcranial approach is preferable. (**b**) The tubero-infundibular craniopharyngioma displaces circumferentially the hypothalamus, creating a direct path to reach the ventricle from the ventral route that can be suitable for such cases

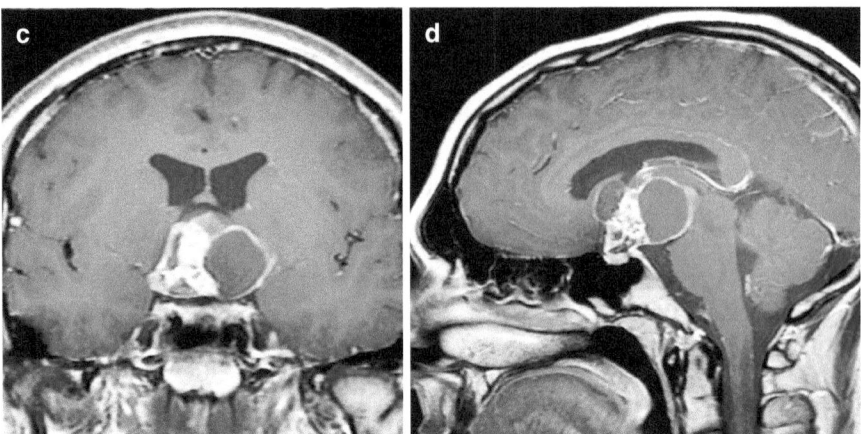

Fig. 5.13 (continued)

Finally, in adults, the nasal and paranasal sinuses anatomy does not represent an absolute contraindication to the EEA [40], since the lack of pneumatization or the conchal variant of the sphenoidal sinus, can be managed thanks to advanced operative technologies, i.e., the neuronavigation, and the collaboration with an expert ENT surgeon [40].

A further limit given by suprasellar CPs is their adherence to the hypothalamus [41]. As originally observed by Ciric, prognosis of supradiaphragmatic forms in terms of tumor removal, risk of hypothalamic damages, and recurrence or tumor progression is very different between intra- and extrapial tumors [4]. In the latter case, despite tumor adhesion, a cleavage plane given by the arachnoid is usually present, allowing a complete tumor resection with no brain damage. If absent, tumor removal should be arrested to avoid hypothalamic injury. This crucial limit in the therapeutic role of surgery for CPs does not dependent on the selected approach, but is associated with intrinsic tumor features [31].

5.4   Outcome of Endoscopic Endonasal Approach

Traditionally, the outcome of CP surgery has always been considered not fully satisfactory since tumor removal is often limited by the adherence to the surrounding structures, the endocrinological function is hampered, and complications leading to the reduction of patients quality of life are not rare [1–3]. In his historical paper published at the beginning of the 1990s, Yasargil et al. reported a mortality rate of 8.6%, a poor outcome in 5.3%, and a moderate worsening in patient quality of life in 17% of cases after radical tumor resection [42].

Considering these results, the pendulum of the goal of treatment for CPs has moved from the widest possible resection to a less extensive resection characterized by a reduced rate of complications and post-operative sequelae and, therefore, the preservation of patient quality of life [43]. This concept has led surgeons to prefer minimally invasive surgical approaches and subtotal resection, when the radical was not possible or very risky, combined with complementary treatments, mainly radiotherapy [43]. The advent of innovative complementary therapeutic strategies allowing satisfactory outcomes for both the surgeons and the patients has further encouraged the adoption of extracranial, minimally invasive approaches, like EEA. In their meta-analysis, Komotar et al. have observed that radical resection was achieved in a significantly higher percentage of the cases by EEA with respect to the trans-cranial approach (66.9 vs. 48.3%, respectively) [44]. Although a selection bias may be present in this analysis, the results support the validity of EEA in the treatment of CPs. In our experience, based on 111 adults with CPs, the rate of gross total resection was similar between the craniotomic and the EEA (94 cases, 80%). The main advantage associated with EEA was the better visual outcome [44], in agreement with Komotar et al. who had reported an improvement of visual function in 56.2% of the cases after a ventral approach vs. 33.1% after a transcranial surgery [44]. With the limits of the possible selection bias, the better visual outcome associated with the EEA could be absence of traction or manipulation of the nerve, particularly during the early surgical stages, when the optic pathways are stretched and distorted by the tumor and may be more susceptible to a direct damage [45]. Moreover, the tumor may be cleaved by the surrounding arachnoid plane that protects the arterial feeders of the chiasm coming from the carotid [45], thus reducing the risk of vascular indirect damage of the nerves [45].

On the other hand, the ventral approach is characterized by a significantly higher risk of CSF leak [27–33], whose prevalence is approximately 18% in major series, although only few cases were complicated by meningitis [44]. In our experience, CSF leak led to meningitis only in 2.6% of the patients treated for CP via EEA [46]. Therefore, if properly treated, CSF leak does not usually have any significant consequences on patient quality of life and functional outcome [46]. Conversely, the morbidity rate associated with trans-cranial approaches is certainly lower, but surgical complications, such as seizures or hydrocephalus, reported by Komotar et al. in 8.5 and 10.1% of cases, respectively, may have a permanent negative impact on patient quality of life, requiring long-life medications or the placement of devices, such as a ventriculo-peritoneal shunt, with a nonnegligible rate of malfunctions or infections [44]. In our experience, the key point to properly manage the CSF leak is represented by the collaboration with a trained ENT surgeon [47]. Indeed, the intraoperative closure phase is a crucial step, like tumor approach and removal, considering that its failure may compromise the entire surgery. Moreover, the post-operative care and nursing with bed rest for 72 h, gradual awakening from anesthesia, and the avoidance of coughing, sneezing, or violent Valsalva maneuvers are crucial to reduce the risk of post-operative CSF leak [47]. However, whenever it occurs, a quick and proper management is needed. In our experience, we prefer to avoid lumbar drainage, for the potential associated tensive pneumocephalus, limiting its adoption in selected cases with uncertain CSF leak and irrelevant presence of intracranial air demonstrated by the CT-scan [47]. In these cases, we prefer to control the drainage output by keeping a constant outflow of 20 cc every 6 h. For all the other cases, an urgent endoscopic endonasal plastic revision is performed to arrest the CSF leak.

Unfortunately, the endocrinological outcome is usually very poor, with the development of panhypopituitarism in almost all patients, independently from the type of surgical approach [44]. It should be reminded that CP arises from the pituitary stalk; therefore, its functional preservation is difficult, even in case of anatomical preservation of this structure. Such complication has a stronger impact in children for the associated arrest of statuary growth and pubertal maturation due to GH and gonadotropins deficiency [48]. Like for other cases of iatrogenic hypopituitarism, replacement treatment for anterior and/or posterior pituitary deficiency is mandatory in both children and adults, and is primarily aimed at replacing adrenal and thyroid function and diabetes insipidus (in case of posterior pituitary damage), followed by estradiol and progesterone replacement in women of fertile age, and testosterone replacement in all men with suggestive symptoms of testosterone deficiency, independently from age [49, 50]. Several large studies have demonstrated the need and safety of GH replacement in children affected by CP, whereas replacement therapy in adults, especially in those with residual tumor, is still debated [50, 51]. Treatment type, timing, and follow-up controls have to be performed according to international guidelines [49].

An often neglected aspect of CP, particularly for suprasellar and intraventricular forms, is presented by the hypothalamic function damages [49–51]. These disturbances, often misinterpreted by physician and sometimes by the patient him/herself, may significantly affect patient quality of life [52–53]. The most scaring hypothalamic disorder induced by the disease itself and/or surgery is the rapid and massive weight gain that can lead to morbid obesity. Other hypothalamic functions that can be potentially impaired are sleep-wake rhythm, body temperature homeostasis, memory, and behavior [55–59]. Therefore, special care should be paid during tumor removal in identifying the brain–tumor interface, thus avoiding hypothalamic damage, but also in instructing patients and care givers adequately to recognize and manage these disorders. As previously mentioned, the EEA provides an excellent view of the crucial relationship between the tumor and the surrounding structures, thus allowing to stop tumor removal if they appear infiltrated, and, therefore, surgery becomes risky. Anyhow, pre- and post-operative dietary counseling is highly suggested to control weight gain; in selected cases of iatrogenic morbid obesity bariatric surgery becomes necessary [54–59]. At the same time, particular attention has to be given to patient neurocognitive assessment since hypothalamic injuries may lead to mild to severe behavioral and neurocognitive alterations that may strongly reduce patient quality of life [60].

5.5   Conclusions

Indications to endoscopic endonasal approach (EEA) for craniopharyngioma (CP) treatment have progressively increased, thanks to technological innovation and advancement in the endoscopic technique skills. To date, EEA is considered the first choice for a large number of midline CPs in different centers worldwide, for the advantages associated with the wide view, and ability in detection of anatomical reference points and vulnerable structures, thus avoiding their damage. At the same time, tumor and patient anatomy have to be carefully evaluated before choosing the approach. Despite the surgeon's abilities and technical advantages, EEA, as all surgical approaches, is still burdened by high rates of post-operative hypopituitarism and, to a lesser extent, hypothalamic dysfunction and CSF leak that require prompt and multidisciplinary management.

References

 1. Barkhoudarian G, Laws ER. Craniopharyngioma: history. Pituitary. 2013;16(1):1–8.
 2. Lindholm J, Nielsen EH. Craniopharyngioma: historical notes. Pituitary. 2009;12(4):352–9.
 3. Roderick E, Karavitaki N, Wass JA. Craniopharyngiomas. Historical aspects of their management. Hormones. 2008;7(3):271–4.
 4. Ciric IS, Cozzens JW. Craniopharyngiomas: transsphenoidal method of approach--for the virtuoso only? Clin Neurosurg. 1980;27:169–87.
 5. Jho HD, Carrau RL. Endoscopic endonasal transsphenoidal surgery: experience with 50 patients. J Neurosurg. 1997;87(1):44–51.
 6. Kassam A, Snyderman CH, Mintz A, Gardner P, Carrau RL. Expanded endonasal approach: the rostrocaudal axis. Part I. Crista galli to the sella turcica. Neurosurg Focus. 2005;19(1):E3.
 7. Kassam A, Snyderman CH, Mintz A, Gardner P, Carrau RL. Expanded endonasal approach: the rostrocaudal axis. Part II. Posterior clinoids to the foramen magnum. Neurosurg Focus. 2005;19(1):E4.
 8. Schwartz TH, Morgenstern PF, Anand VK. Lessons learned in the evolution of endoscopic skull base surgery. J Neurosurg. 2019;130(2):337–46.
 9. Nishioka H, Nagata Y, Fukuhara N, Yamaguchi-Okada M, Yamada S. Endoscopic endonasal surgery for subdiaphragmatic type craniopharyngiomas. Neurol Med Chir. 2018;58(6):260–5.
10. Mangussi-Gomes J, Vellutini EA, Truong HQ, Pahl FH, Stamm AC. Endoscopic endonasal transplanum transtuberculum approach for the resection of a large suprasellar craniopharyngioma. J Neurol Surg B Skull Base. 2018;79(Suppl 3):S249–50.
11. Zenonos GA, Snyderman CH, Gardner PA. Endoscopic endonasal approach for a suprasellar craniopharyngioma. J Neurol Surg B Skull Base. 2018;79(Suppl 3):S241–2.
12. Todeschini AB, Montaser AS, Shahein M, Revuelta JM, Otto BA, Carrau RL, Prevedello DM. Endoscopic endonasal approach to a suprasellar craniopharyngioma. J Neurol Surg B Skull Base. 2018;79(Suppl 3):S237–8.
13. Jean WC. Transcallosal, transchoroidal resection of a recurrent craniopharyngioma. J Neurol Surg B Skull Base. 2018;79(Suppl 3):S259–60.
14. Patel NJ, Dunn I. Resection of a retrochiasmatic craniopharyngioma by combined modified orbital craniotomy and transnasal endoscopic techniques. J Neurol Surg B Skull Base. 2018;79(Suppl 3):S243–4.
15. Lin YJ, Chen KT, Lee CC, Toh CH, Wu TE, Huang YC, Hsu PW, Lu YJ, Chuang CC, Chen PY, Wei KC. Anterior skull base tumor resection by transciliary supraorbital keyhole craniotomy: a single institutional experience. World Neurosurg. 2018;111:e863–70.
16. Jeswani S, Nuño M, Wu A, Bonert V, Carmichael JD, Black KL, Chu R, King W, Mamelak AN. Comparative analysis of outcomes following craniotomy and expanded endoscopic endonasal transsphenoidal resection of craniopharyngioma and related tumors: a single-institution study. J Neurosurg. 2016;124(3):627–38.
17. Brastianos PK, Shankar GM, Gill CM, Taylor-Weiner A, Nayyar N, Panka DJ, Sullivan RJ, Frederick DT, Abedalthagafi M, Jones PS, Dunn IF, Nahed BV, Romero JM, Louis DN, Getz G, Cahill DP, Santagata S, Curry WT Jr, Barker FG. Dramatic response of BRAF V600E mutant papillary craniopharyngioma to targeted therapy. J Natl Cancer Inst. 2015;108(2):djv310.

18. Lesueur P, Calugaru V, Nauraye C, Stefan D, Cao K, Emery E, Reznik Y, Habrand JL, Tessonnier T, Chaikh A, Balosso J, Thariat J. Proton therapy for treatment of intracranial benign tumors in adults: a systematic review. Cancer Treat Rev. 2019;72:56–64.
19. Ajithkumar T, Mazhari AL, Stickan-Verfürth M, Kramer PH, Fuentes CS, Lambert J, Thomas H, Müller H, Fleischhack G, Timmermann B. Proton therapy for craniopharyngioma - an early report from a single European Centre. Clin Oncol. 2018;30(5):307–16.
20. Frank G, Pasquini E, Doglietto F, Mazzatenta D, Sciarretta V, Farneti G, Calbucci F. The endoscopic extended transsphenoidal approach for craniopharyngiomas. Neurosurgery. 2006;59(1 Suppl 1):75–83.
21. McLaughlin N, Ditzel Filho LF, Prevedello DM, Kelly DF, Carrau RL, Kassam AB. Side-cutting aspiration device for endoscopic and microscopic tumor removal. J Neurol Surg Skull Base. 2012;73:11.
22. de Lara D, Ditzel Filho LF, Muto J, Otto BA, Carrau RL, Prevedello DM. Surgical management of craniopharyngioma with third ventricle involvement. Neurosurg Focus. 2013;34(1 Suppl):5.
23. Magill JC, Ferguson MS, Sandison A, Clarke PM. Nasal craniopharyngioma: case report and literature review. J Laryngol Otol. 2011;125(5):517–9.
24. Hoffman HJ. Craniopharyngiomas. Can J Neurol Sci. 1985;12(4):348–52.
25. Zoli M, Mazzatenta D, Valluzzi A, Marucci G, Acciarri N, Pasquini E, Frank G. Expanding indications for the extended endoscopic endonasal approach to hypothalamic gliomas: preliminary report. Neurosurg Focus. 2014;37(4):E11.
26. Kassam AB, Gardner PA, Snyderman CH, Carrau RL, Mintz AH, Prevedello DM. Expanded endonasal approach, a fully endoscopic transnasal approach for the resection of midline suprasellar craniopharyngiomas: a new classification based on the infundibulum. J Neurosurg. 2008;108(4):715–28.
27. Radovanovic I, Dehdashti AR, Turel MK, Almeida JP, Godoy BL, Doglietto F, Vescan AD, Zadeh G, Gentili F. Expanded endonasal endoscopic surgery in suprasellar craniopharyngiomas: a retrospective analysis of 43 surgeries including recurrent cases. Oper Neurosurg. 2019;17(2):132–42. https://doi.org/10.1093/ons/opy356.
28. Forbes JA, Ordóñez-Rubiano EG, Tomasiewicz HC, Banu MA, Younus I, Dobri GA, Phillips CD, Kacker A, Cisse B, Anand VK, Schwartz TH. Endonasal endoscopic transsphenoidal resection of intrinsic third ventricular craniopharyngioma: surgical results. J Neurosurg. 2018;1:1–11.
29. Jamshidi AO, Beer-Furlan A, Prevedello DM, Sahyouni R, Elzoghby MA, Safain MG, Carrau RL, Jane JA. Laws ER. A modern series of subdiaphragmatic craniopharyngiomas. J Neurosurg. 2018;1:1–6.
30. Koutourousiou M, Fernandez-Miranda JC, Wang EW, Snyderman CH, Gardner PA. The limits of transsellar/transtuberculum surgery for craniopharyngioma. J Neurosurg Sci. 2018;62(3):301–9.
31. Hardesty DA, Montaser AS, Beer-Furlan A, Carrau RL, Prevedello DM. Limits of endoscopic endonasal surgery for III ventricle craniopharyngiomas. J Neurosurg Sci. 2018;62(3):310–21.
32. Ottenhausen M, Rumalla K, La Corte E, Alalade A, Nair P, Forbes J, Ben Nsir A, Schwartz TH. Treatment strategies for craniopharyngiomas. J Neurosurg Sci. 2019;63(1):83–7.
33. Dho YS, Kim YH, Se YB, Han DH, Kim JH, Park CK, Wang KC, Kim DG. Endoscopic endonasal approach for craniopharyngioma: the importance of the relationship between pituitary stalk and tumor. J Neurosurg. 2018;129(3):611–9.
34. Morisako H, Goto T, Goto H, Bohoun CA, Tamrakar S, Ohata K. Aggressive surgery based on an anatomical subclassification of craniopharyngiomas. Neurosurg Focus. 2016;41(6):E10.
35. Kassam AB, Prevedello DM, Thomas A, Gardner P, Mintz A, Snyderman C, Carrau R. Endoscopic endonasal pituitary transposition for a transdorsum sellae approach to the interpeduncular cistern. Neurosurgery. 2008;62(3 Suppl 1):57–72.
36. Prieto R, Pascual JM, Rosdolsky M, Castro-Dufourny I, Carrasco R, Strauss S, Barrios L. Craniopharyngioma adherence: a comprehensive topographical categorization and outcome-related risk stratification model based on the methodical examination of 500 tumors. Neurosurg Focus. 2016;41(6):E13.

37. Pascual JM, Prieto R, Dufourny IC, Simoes RG, Carrasco R. Hypothalamus-referenced classification for craniopharyngiomas: evidence provided by the endoscopic endonasal approach. Neurosurg Rev. 2013;36(2):337–9.
38. Steno J, Malácek M, Bízik I. Tumor-third ventricular relationships in supradiaphragmatic craniopharyngiomas: correlation of morphological, magnetic resonance imaging, and operative findings. Neurosurgery. 2004;54(5):1051–8.
39. Pascual JM, Prieto R, Carrasco R, Barrios L. Displacement of mammillary bodies by craniopharyngiomas involving the third ventricle: surgical-MRI correlation and use in topographical diagnosis. J Neurosurg. 2013;119(2):381–405.
40. Kuan EC, Kaufman AC, Lerner D, Kohanski MA, Tong CCL, Tajudeen BA, Parasher AK, Lee JYK, Storm PB, Palmer JN, Adappa ND. Lack of sphenoid pneumatization does not affect endoscopic endonasal pediatric skull base surgery outcomes. Laryngoscope. 2018;129(4):832–6. https://doi.org/10.1002/lary.27600.
41. Prieto R, Pascual JM, Castro-Dufourny I, Carrasco R, Barrios L. Craniopharyngioma: surgical outcome as related to the degree of hypothalamic involvement. World Neurosurg. 2017;104:1006–10.
42. Yaşargil MG, Curcic M, Kis M, Siegenthaler G, Teddy PJ, Roth P. Total removal of craniopharyngiomas. Approaches and long-term results in 144 patients. J Neurosurg. 1990;73(1):3–11.
43. Sainte-Rose C, Puget S, Wray A, Zerah M, Grill J, Brauner R, Boddaert N, Pierre-Kahn A. Craniopharyngioma: the pendulum of surgical management. Childs Nerv Syst. 2005;21(8-9):691–5.
44. Komotar RJ, Starke RM, Raper DM, Anand VK, Schwartz TH. Endoscopic endonasal compared with microscopic transsphenoidal and open transcranial resection of craniopharyngiomas. World Neurosurg. 2012;77(2):329–41.
45. Cavallo LM, Frank G, Cappabianca P, Solari D, Mazzatenta D, Villa A, Zoli M, D'Enza AI, Esposito F, Pasquini E. The endoscopic endonasal approach for the management of craniopharyngiomas: a series of 103 patients. J Neurosurg. 2014;121(1):100–13.
46. Milanese L, Zoli M, Sollini G, Martone C, Zenesini C, Sturiale C, Farneti P, Frank G, Pasquini E, Mazzatenta D. Antibiotic prophylaxis in endoscopic endonasal pituitary and skull base surgery. World Neurosurg. 2017;106:912–8.
47. Pasquini E, Frank G. Complications of endoscopic skull base surgery. In: Kennedy DW, Hwang PH, editors. Rhinology: diseases of the nose, sinus and skull base. 1st ed. New York: Thieme; 2012.
48. Patel VS, Thamboo A, Quon J, Nayak JV, Hwang PH, Edwards M, Patel ZM. Outcomes after endoscopic endonasal resection of craniopharyngiomas in the pediatric population. World Neurosurg. 2017;108:6–14.
49. Fleseriu M, Hashim IA, Karavitaki N, Melmed S, Murad MH, Salvatori R, Samuels MH. Hormonal replacement in hypopituitarism in adults: an Endocrine Society clinical practice guideline. J Clin Endocrinol Metab. 2016;101(11):3888–921.
50. Karavitaki N. Hypopituitarism oddities: craniopharyngiomas. Horm Res. 2007;68(Suppl 5):151–3.
51. Alotaibi NM, Noormohamed N, Cote DJ, Alharthi S, Doucette J, Zaidi HA, Mekary RA, Smith TR. Physiologic growth hormone-replacement therapy and craniopharyngioma recurrence in pediatric patients: a meta-analysis. World Neurosurg. 2018;109:487–496.e1.
52. Pekic S, Stojanovic M, Popovic V. Controversies in the risk of neoplasia in GH deficiency. Best Pract Res Clin Endocrinol Metab. 2017;31(1):35–47.
53. Zada G, Kintz N, Pulido M, Amezcua L. Prevalence of neurobehavioral, social, and emotional dysfunction in patients treated for childhood craniopharyngioma: a systematic literature review. PLoS One. 2013;8(11):e76562.
54. Foschi M, Sambati L, Zoli M, Pierangeli G, Cecere A, Mignani F, Barletta G, Sturiale C, Faustini-Fustini M, Milanese L, Cortelli P, Mazzatenta D, Provini F. Site and type of craniopharyngiomas impact differently on 24-hour circadian rhythms and surgical outcome. A neurophysiological evaluation. Auton Neurosci. 2017;208:126–30.

55. Zoli M, Sambati L, Milanese L, Foschi M, Faustini-Fustini M, Marucci G, de Biase D, Tallini G, Cecere A, Mignani F, Sturiale C, Frank G, Pasquini E, Cortelli P, Mazzatenta D, Provini F. Postoperative outcome of body core temperature rhythm and sleep-wake cycle in third ventricle craniopharyngiomas. Neurosurg Focus. 2016;41(6):E12.

56. van Iersel L, Brokke KE, Adan RAH, Bulthuis LCM, van den Akker ELT, van Santen HM. Pathophysiology and individualized treatment of hypothalamic obesity following craniopharyngioma and other suprasellar tumors: a systematic review. Endocr Rev. 2019;40(1):193–235.

57. Thompson CJ, Costello RW, Crowley RK. Management of hypothalamic disease in patients with craniopharyngioma. Clin Endocrinol. 2019;90(4):506–16. https://doi.org/10.1111/cen.13929.

58. Ni W, Shi X. Interventions for the treatment of craniopharyngioma-related hypothalamic obesity: a systematic review. World Neurosurg. 2018;118:e59–71.

59. van Iersel L, Meijneke RWH, Schouten-van Meeteren AYN, Reneman L, de Win MM, van Trotsenburg ASP, Bisschop PH, Finken MJJ, Vandertop WP, van Furth WR, van Santen HM. The development of hypothalamic obesity in craniopharyngioma patients: A risk factor analysis in a well-defined cohort. Pediatr Blood Cancer. 2018;65(5):e26911.

60. Heinks K, Boekhoff S, Hoffmann A, Warmuth-Metz M, Eveslage M, Peng J, Calaminus G, Müller HL. Quality of life and growth after childhood craniopharyngioma: results of the multinational trial KRANIOPHARYNGEOM 2007. Endocrine. 2018;59(2):364–72.

Cranial Surgery for Adult Craniopharyngiomas: Techniques and Indications

6

E. Jouanneau, H. Dufour, and R. Manet

Abbreviations

AC V	Anterior choroidal vein
ACA1	First segment of the cerebral artery
AChA	Anterior choroidal artery
ACoA	Anterior communicating artery
AO-CP	Adult onset craniopharyngiomas
CCPs	Cystic craniopharyngiomas
Ch	Chiasm
ChP	Choroid plexus
FL	Frontal lobe
GTR	Gross total removal
hS V	Thalamostriate vein
HW	Hypothalamic walls
IC V	Internal cerebral vein
ICA	Internal carotid
III V	Third ventricle

E. Jouanneau (✉)
Pituitary and Skull Base Neurosurgical Department,
Neurological Hospital, Hospices Civils de Lyon, Lyon, France

Claude Bernard University Lyon 1, Lyon, France
e-mail: emmanuel.jouanneau@chu-lyon.fr

H. Dufour
Neurosurgical Department, La Timone Hospital,
Marseille, France

R. Manet
Pituitary and Skull Base Neurosurgical Department,
Neurological Hospital, Hospices Civils de Lyon, Lyon, France

© Springer Nature Switzerland AG 2020
E. Jouanneau, G. Raverot (eds.), *Adult Craniopharyngiomas*,
https://doi.org/10.1007/978-3-030-41176-3_6

LT	Lamina terminalis
MBA	Mammillary body angle
MF	Foramen of Monro
ON	Optic nerve
PG	Pituitary gland
PS	Pituitary stalk
RXT	Radiotherapy
SF	Sylvian fissure
STR	Subtotal removal
TC	Trans-callosal approach
TF	Trans-frontal approach
Th	Thalamus
TL	Temporal lobe
TLT	Trans-lamina terminalis approach

6.1   Indications and Principles of the Surgery

Surgical excision remains the accepted first-line treatment for the large majority of AO-CP and should be systematically considered in the absence of major co-morbidities.

However, the optimal surgical modalities used for AO-CPs remain uncertain. The extension of resection remains controversial and it is still unclear if GTR leads to a better prognosis than STR associated with RXT in AO-CPs even though the rates of recurrence are clearly lower for the first of these options [1]. AO-CPs cohorts are too small for a definitive conclusion to be drawn. Pituitary stalk conservation, whenever possible, can be recommended but not at the expense of a GTR. Indeed, hormonal substitution is quite easy to manage (see chapter by G Raverot in this book). The challenge is at the level of the infundibulum and the hypothalamus. Recent data has shown that the hypothalamic part of the tumor can be removed whenever possible with an acceptable morbidity [2]. However, the authors would not recommend a GTR for all cases and a universal approach. Surgeons need to study all pre-operative parameters, especially the MRI results (outlined in the chapter by R. Prieto). Pre-operative hypothalamic syndrome indicates a lesion from the tumor but does not mean that a pseudo-gliosis cleavage plane cannot be found. It is therefore of paramount importance to have the best vision of such a plane.

The surgical approach is therefore designed to expose the tumor, in the best possible way, with minimal morbidity.

Endoscopic transnasal techniques have benefited from an impressive development over the last two decades [3–5] and have become the best option, especially in AO-CP. Indeed, sellar-suprasellar spaces are in the axis of the endonasal route and the endoscopic approach offers a great benefit for controlling the retrochiasmatic part of the tumor and the third ventricle floor exposure (Fig. 6.1) [2, 6]. Moreover, a posterior extension toward the posterior perforating space or behind the clivus can be managed through an extended trans-clival approach [7].

Fig. 6.1 Better exposure of the third ventricle floor using the extended endonasal endoscopic technique. (**a**) Operative view of a suprasellar craniopharyngioma operated on using a sub-fronto-pterional approach. The sub- and retrochiasmatic spaces are difficult or impossible to expose without pushing on the optic nerve. The surgeon is gently pushing away the optic nerve to work in between the internal carotid and the optic nerve (arrow). The third ventricle floor, behind and below the chiasm, cannot be directly exposed and the tumor will be removed by a piece-meal technique without being able to see the hypothalamus floor. (**b, c**) Operative views of the same type of craniopharyngioma. Using an extended trans-tubercular route, the surgeon has good exposure of third ventricle floor after tumoral debulking when approaching the endoscope. The dissection, under direct visualization, can be softer and safer to preserve, as much as possible, the hypothalamus while doing radical removal of the tumor. *ON* optic nerve, *ICA* internal carotid artery, *Ch* Chiasm, *PS* pituitary stalk, *PG* pituitary gland, *HW* hypothalamic walls, *III V* third ventricle

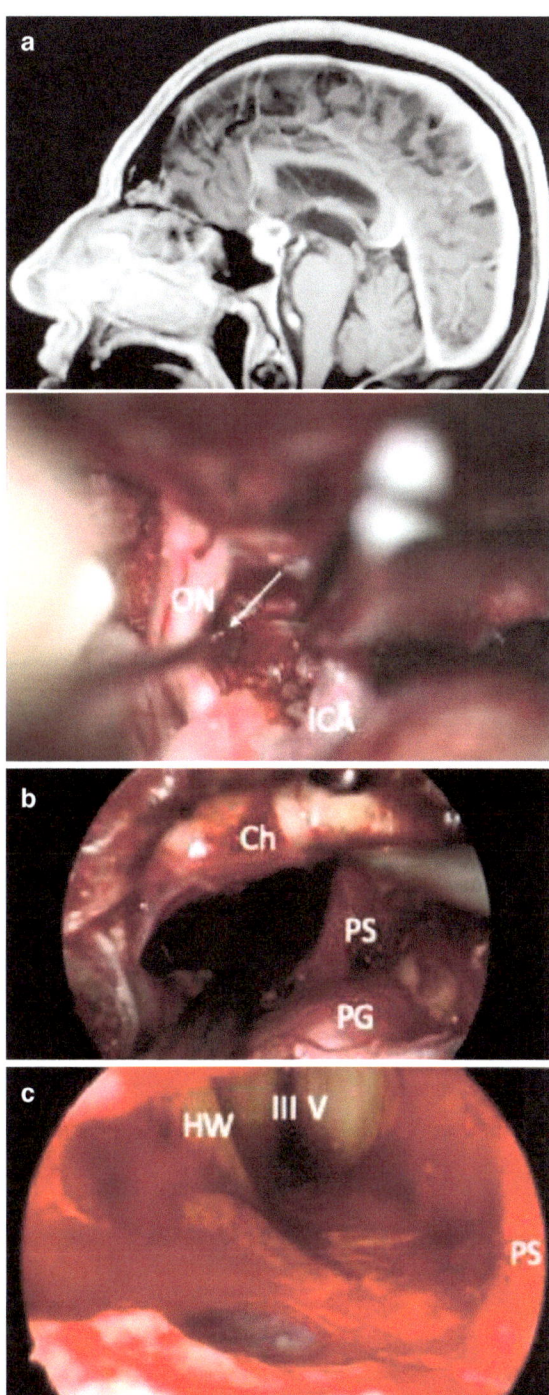

6.2   Trans-Cranial Approaches

Cranial routes are therefore less frequently used in adults. This approach is considered when the tumor extends towards the anterior skull base or the Sylvian fissure (Fig. 6.2) [6].

When using pterional subfrontal approaches, microsurgical techniques must be used without any specificity for the cisternal part of the tumor: debulking, and after extracapsular dissection, working through the usual inter-optic, inter-opticocarotid, and retro-carotid spaces, and paying close attention to the small perforating arteries [8]. The surgical steps are described in Fig. 6.3.

The specificity comes from the management of the ventricular extension of the tumor, where this is present, especially in case of a pre-fixed chiasma. Conversely to a nasal approach (see Fig. 6.1), the exposure of the third ventricle floor from a transcranial approach is far more complicated and can lead to unsatisfactory control of the intraventricular portion of the tumor (and thus to an incomplete removal).

A trans-lamina terminalis route can be used in two ways: the first is to use a cottonoid to push down the third ventricle and the tumor and thus expose it in the infrachiasmatic space; the second is to actually remove the tumor through the small window. More detail of this approach is given below.

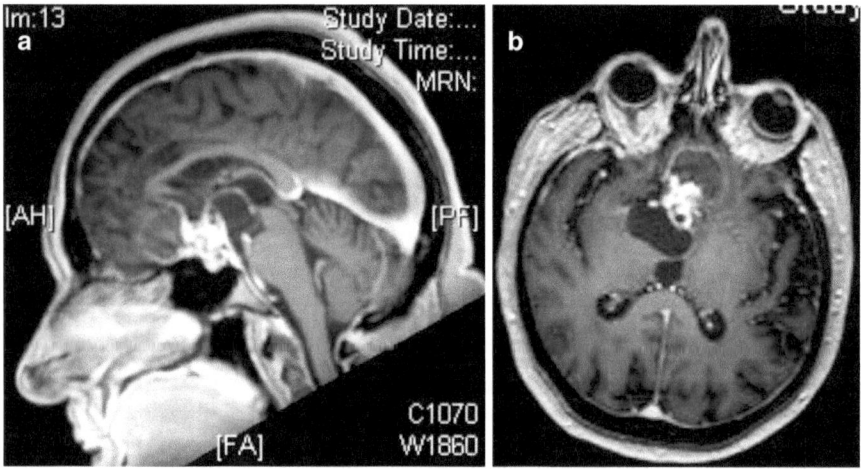

Fig. 6.2 A typical indication for cranial surgery in an AO-CP because of multiples cysts that extend anteriorly and laterally

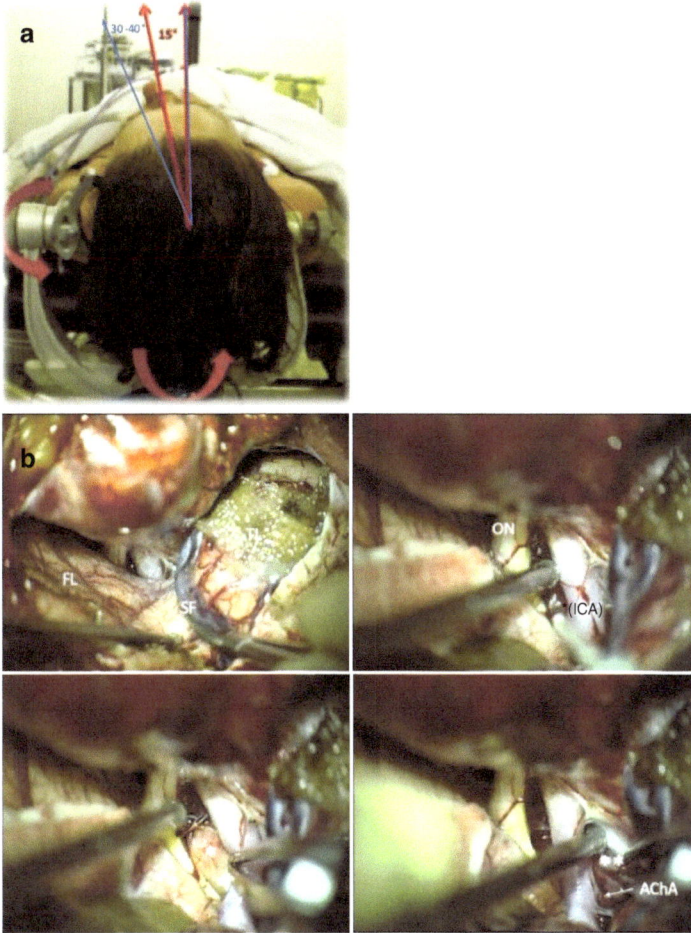

Fig. 6.3 Surgical steps for a pterional sub-frontal approach. (**a**) The patient is supine, the head slightly extended and turned, depending on the tumor extension. To work in the inter-optic space, 15° lateral tilt is required but for retro-carotid space, the head should be tilted around 30–40°. (**b**) The suprasellar cistern and Sylvian fissure are opened up largely for CSF drainage and to expose all of the crucial landmarks, the optic Nerve (ON), internal carotid (ICA), and the inter-optico-carotid space (*). Working behind the ICA is dangerous because of the perforating arteries (anterior choroidian artery, AChA, and other small hypothalamic vessels coming from the posterior communicating artery).

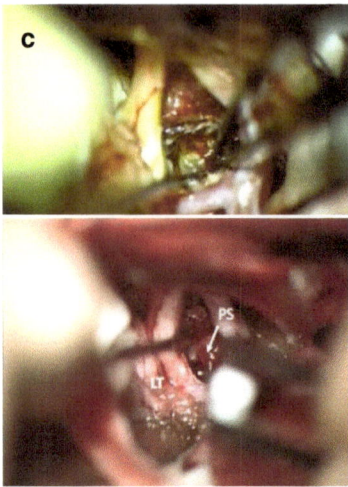

Fig. 6.3 (continued) (**c**) The surgical technique is similar to that used for other extra-cerebral tumors, piece-meal first followed by dissection. The particularity in this case is the hypothalamus dissection. The lamina terminalis (LT) can be opened up to expose the ventricular part of the tumor or left alone in case of a pure intraventricular CP. In that case, after an intratumoral debulking, the pituitary stalk (PS) has been located and kept intact. Unfortunately, the patient's condition worsened, with a pan-hypopituitarism post-surgery. *FL* frontal lobe, *TL* temporal lobe, *SF* sylvian fissure, *LT* lamina terminalis, *ICA* internal carotid, *AChA* anterior choroidal artery, *PS* pituitary stalk

6.3   Specific Situations

6.3.1   Combined Approaches for Giant CPs

Combined approaches form part of the history of surgery for CPs. From a sub-frontal route, in the 1930s, Dott proposed to intentionally cut and sacrifice the blind optic nerve to control the retrochiasmatic extension, with a second surgical step using a trans-frontal trans-ventricular approach for the ventricular extension (see the chapter on Epidemiology in this book [9]). Using this ventricular approach, he was the first to recognize the role of the hypothalamus, observing that in the case of a sharp dissection, the patient's state worsened with an increased hypothalamic syndrome.

In our era, combined approaches can be considered for management of huge CPs. The transcranial route allows the management of anterior and lateral extensions and the transnasal route allows the management of the retrochiasmatic and ventricular extensions. In these cases of giant tumors, achieving a GTR without major neurological damage is illusory. Thus, the goal of this strategy must be to achieve STR combined with RXT. The goal is to decompress the brain and optic pathway, reducing the size of the tumor so that it can be efficiently treated by RXT. The optimal sequence—transcranial approach followed by transnasal versus transnasal followed by transcranial—is dictated as for giant pituitary adenomas by the question: which route is best for decompression of the optic apparatus? This strategy is easier to use in CPs. Indeed, contrary to giant pituitary adenomas, the risk of apoplexia of the residual tumoral portion that is left is far lower in CPs.

This strategy was used in the case illustrated in Fig. 6.7. This patient was referred to our center after sub-frontal surgery where a simple biopsy was done. The patient was almost blind and had total pituitary insufficiency. Surprisingly, no hypothalamic syndrome was present. The tumor was then approached using a trans-frontal trans-ventricular approach to remove the upper part. We left in place a piece of tumor that was too strongly adhered to the optic chiasm and the ventricle. The proposal was thereafter for upfront radiotherapy. Unfortunately, the patient postponed treatment and returned 9 months later with a recurrence, which was treated using a nasal approach. The small piece of remaining tumor was treated using conformal radiotherapy and the patient was free of recurrence after 4 years. The clinical status of the patient was unchanged with an optic atrophy, as was observed pre-operatively, and with no hypothalamic syndrome.

Lastly, considering the issue of CSF leak when two surgical steps (nasal and cranial) are scheduled, the two approaches should be performed as separate surgeries.

6.3.2   Management of Intraventricular Tumor

It is sometimes very difficult to determine if the CP is located inside the 3rd ventricle or if it is a suprasellar tumor that has secondarily extended to the ventricle. This is a key point in selecting the best approach. Using the wrong route, in particular reaching the tumor through the third ventricle floor by a transnasal approach may lead to dramatic damage to the hypothalamus.

In our experience, MRI T2 sequences, especially the mid-sagittal view, are the best option to determine this anatomical situation. The position of the mammillary bodies and the mammillary body angle (MBA) must be carefully studied. An MBA inferior to 50° indicates an intraventricular CP (Fig. 6.4). This rule is, however, not absolute as can be seen in Fig. 6.5, where despite an MA inferior to 50°, the tumor appeared to pass through the third ventricle, therefore, being accessible using an endonasal approach. Readers can also refer to the chapter by Prieto in this book for more details.

The 3rd ventricle can be accessed by a number of routes: a trans-lamina terminalis approach (TLT), a trans-frontal approach (TF), or a trans-callosal (TC) approach.

The choice should be made by considering the following parameters:

- the size of the tumor and its height: small- or medium-sized tumors that do not extend too greatly superiorly or inferiorly are good candidates for a TLT approach;
- The presence of hydrocephalus: For a large tumor with ventricle dilatation, a TF route may be adequate; while for a large tumor without ventricle dilatation, a TC route may be more appropriate including its variants (inter-forniceal; inter thalamo-trigonal);
- The surgeon's own previous experience.

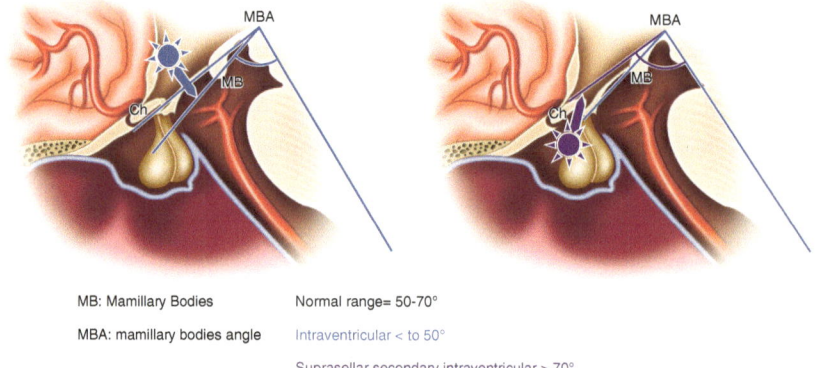

MB: Mamillary Bodies   Normal range= 50-70°

MBA: mamillary bodies angle   Intraventricular < to 50°

                                        Suprasellar secondary intraventricular > 70°

Fig. 6.4 Mamillary bodies angle (MBA) for intra- or extra-ventricular CPs (modified from R Prieto)

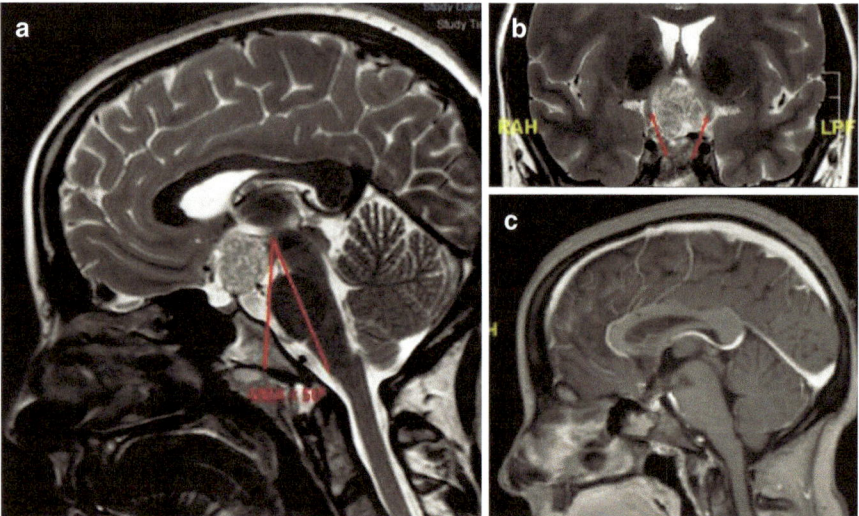

Fig. 6.5 One example of CP with an MA < 50° that was, however, approached using an endonasal route. The CP passing through the 3rd ventricle floor can be approached from below with few additional morbidity than the tumor already creates. (**a**) MA < 50° suggesting an intraventricular CP and a transventricular approach. (**b**) In the coronal view the tumor passes through the ventricle floor to point into the suprasellar space (ventricle walls with the optic pathway on both sides [arrowed]). (**c**) An endonasal endoscopic extended approach has been employed therefore to completely remove the tumor. The visual outcome was good, but the patient's endocrine state worsened, which was expected as the tumor originated from the infundibulum. Pre-operatively, the patient was overweight, and this increased slightly after surgery and was controlled by diet and exercise

6.3.2.1 Trans-Lamina Terminalis Route (Fig. 6.6)

Considering the role of the extended endonasal approach, the trans-lamina terminalis window may be considered useful in two different situations:

– As a complement during a sub-frontal approach to reach the retrochiasmatic or intraventricular part of a CPs
– For a pure intraventricular CPs, as in the case presented in Fig. 6.6

This technique, which has been used for many years, is outlined in numerous publications [10–14].

For a pure TLT approach, an interhemispheric approach may be preferable to a pterional sub-frontal in order to obtain a perfect exposure of the ventricle walls on both sides. Though, as shown in Fig. 6.6, with a sub-frontal approach, the hypothalamic wall on the same side as the approach can be difficult to expose. A trans-sinus approach (or a midline bi-frontal craniotomy in case of small sinuses) can therefore be performed with the patient placed supine, the head neutral and strictly midline in a three-pin head holder.

Once the lamina terminalis has been exposed, it can be opened up to directly access the tumor. This strategy is therefore a piece-meal technique and as usual, the critical point is the dissection of the tumor from the hypothalamic walls where the

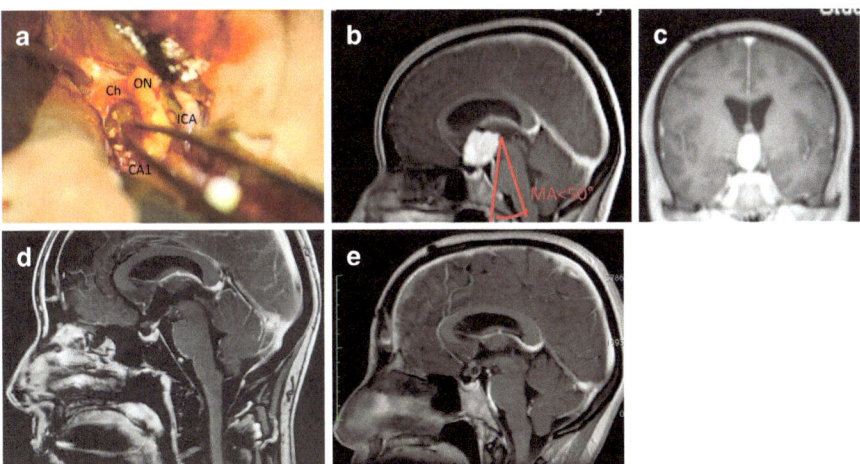

Fig. 6.6 A case of a pure intraventricular CPs removed through a pterional sub-frontal TLT approach. (**a**) Operative view showing a sub-frontal TLT approach. The ipsilateral hypothalamic wall may be difficult to expose without pushing on the optic nerve. (**b, c**) The mammillary body angle (MBA) is inferior to 50° indicating an intraventricular tumor. (**d**) Post-operative MRI at 3 months. The result was classified as a GTR without endocrine and visual symptoms. (**e**) At 6 months, a small cystic recurrence at the level of the pituitary stalk appeared, which was treated by conformational radiotherapy. The patient is disease free at 4 years. *ON* optic nerve, *ICA* internal carotid, *Ch* chiasm, *CA1* anterior cerebral artery first segment

surgeon must decide between a pseudo-gliosis plan, where a GTR can be attempted, and an invasion where a STR would be advised. The same formula can be used whichever approach is used: when the tumor can be easily and gently mobilized (soft dissection), it can be removed. In other situations, in case of a sharp dissection, the tumor should be kept in place.

Pros:

– Direct ventricle vision is obtained without crossing any neurological structures, allowing tumor removal without causing endocrine deficit, as in the case presented in Fig. 6.6 and as has been reported in the literature [14]
– Such an approach is independent of the length of the optic nerves

Cons:

– Provides a narrow window, especially in case of short ACA1 or fenestrated ACoA, and sometimes difficult to mobilize. Splicing the ACoA can be used when the artery length is sufficient with, however, the sacrifice of an anastomosis that may be useful in where there are stroke issues with age
– Vascular risks for the ACoA and the perforating arteries of the anterior complex
– Limited exposure of the upper part and the third ventricle floor that can lead to STR, as illustrated in the Fig. 6.6. An endoscopic-assisted technique can be used, however, this requires caution as the window is quite narrow and there can be issues with warming if approaching too close to the endoscope tip.

6.3.2.2 Trans-Frontal Trans-ventricular Route (Fig. 6.7)

When the tumor is located in the 3rd ventricle and results in an hydrocephalus, the surgeon can choose a transcortical trans-frontal approach.

The craniotomy is performed one-third behind the coronal suture, two-thirds in front, without crossing the midline. A 3 cm antero-posterior cortical incision is made and the frontal horn of the ventricle reached at a depth of about 4 cm. Usually, the tumor is approached through the dilated Monro foramen which can be enlarged posteriorly using a interthalamic forniceal approach through the choroidal fissure and the superior tela after coagulation and section of the septal vein. Great care should be taken for the fornix and of the other veins.

Pros:

– An easy approach with less complicated structures involved than the transcallosal approach

Cons

– Only possible when there is hydrocephalus
– Transcortical approach can result in sequelae seizure

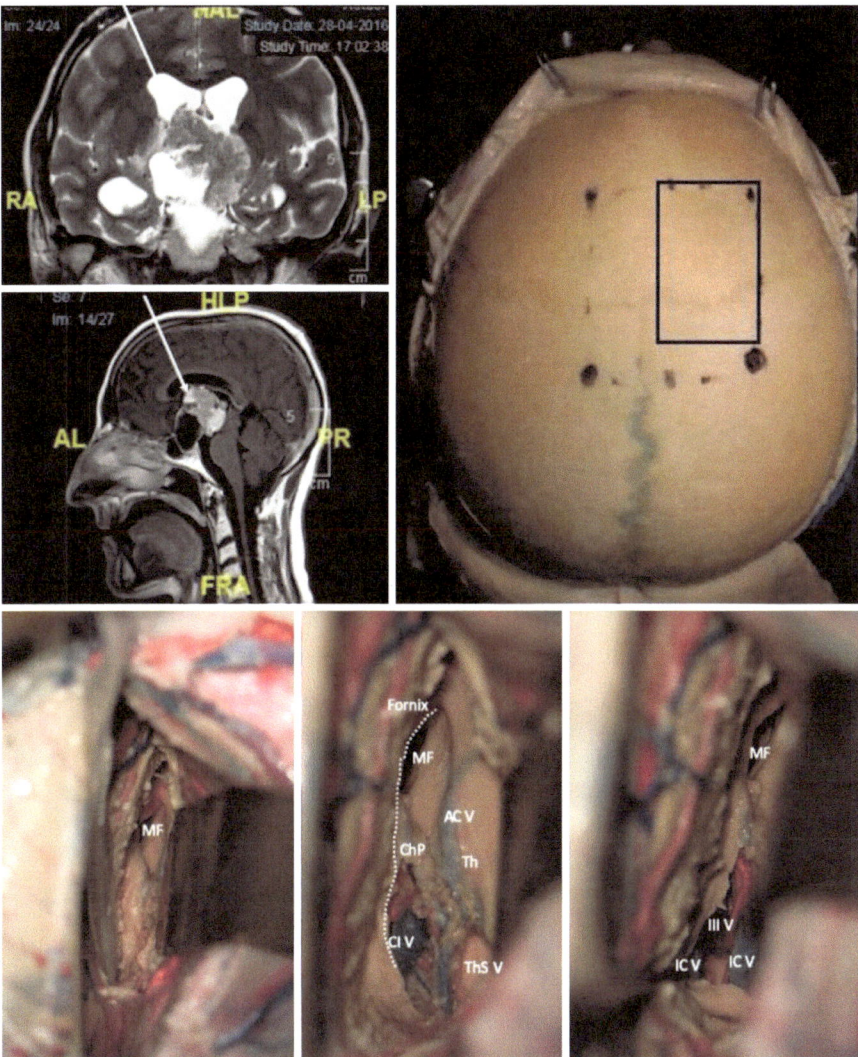

Fig. 6.7 A case of a huge CP which was first operated in another center using a sub-frontal approach without satisfactory removal. A second step using a trans-frontal approach was possible to performed because of the hydrocephalus. After a linear incision, a frontal craniotomy is carried out one-third behind the coronal suture—two-thirds in front. *Cadaveric study*: The foramen of Monro (MF) is exposed after entering the frontal horn. Tumor exposure can be improved using a transchoroidal approach, separating the fornix (dotted line) and the thalamus medially to the choroid plexus (ChP) to get inside the third ventricle. *MF* foramen of Monro, *AC V* anterior choroidal vein, *ThS V* thalamostriate vein, *Th* thalamus, *ChP* choroid plexus, *IC V* internal cerebral vein, *III V* third ventricle. *The different surgical steps for the patient*:

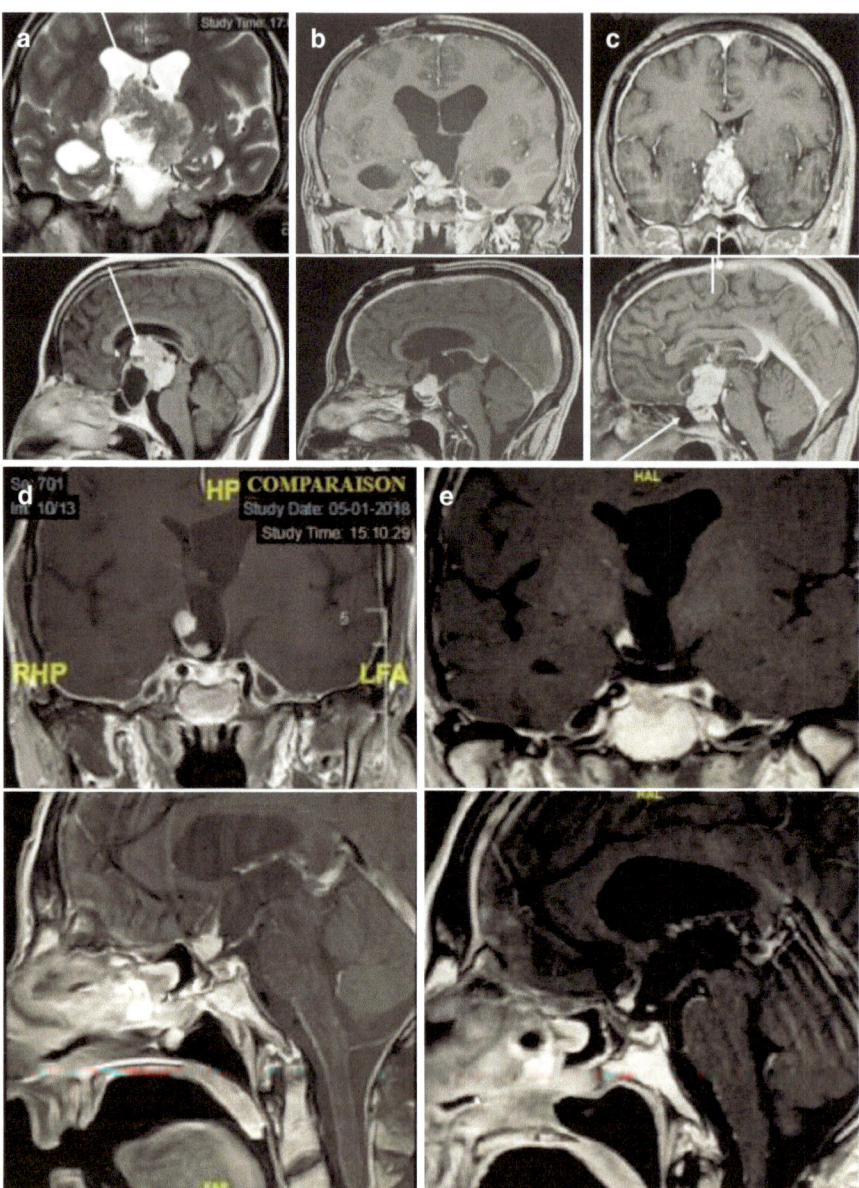

Fig. 6.7 (continued) (**a**) Pre-operative MRI; (**b**) After the trans-frontal approach with a deep tumor remnant at the level of the ventricle floor. (**c**) Radiotherapy was delayed due to the patient and 9 months later a recurrence in the ventricle was observed. The patient was operated on using an endonasal approach. (**d**) Post-operative result with a piece of tumor left in place because of strong adhesions. Radiotherapy was performed at 4 months. (**e**) At last follow-up, after 3 years, there was still perfect control of the tumor

- Not a midline approach
- Deepest part of the tumor is difficult to expose at the level of the posterior perforating space

6.3.2.3 Trans-Callosal Route (Fig. 6.8)

In the absence of hydrocephalus (or when a shunt has been placed before), an interhemispheric trans-callosal approach can be used, including its three variants: interforniceal (between the fornix bodies), and the inter thalamo-trigonal approaches with its trans- and subchoroidal variants (opening the choroidal fissure on the fornix and on the thalamic side, respectively) [15, 16].

The patient positioning is the same as that used for a transcortical trans-frontal approach, with a craniotomy crossing the midline in order to achieve an interhemispheric approach.

The dura mater is opened in a U shape and great care is taken of the afferent veins to the sagittal longitudinal sinus.

Once the corpus callosum is reached, a short 2 cm antero-posterior incision is made in between the pericallosal arteries.

A strictly midline approach can also be used, separating the fornix bodies to reach the third ventricle through the superior tela in between the internal cerebral veins.

Another option is to enter the frontal horn of the lateral ventricle. The third ventricle is therefore reached using the same approach as using the trans-frontal one, using a transchoroidal or a subchoroidal variant. The difference between the two latter approaches is minor, with perhaps a more direct and larger view obtained with the transchoroidal approach. To increase the antero-posterior exposure, the septal vein can be cut at the level of the Monro foramen. From that point, exactly the same principles as with the trans-frontal approach are followed.

Pros:

- Avoids the transcortical route and any brain lesion

Cons:

- Difficult management of veins
- Involves manipulation of the Fornix with possible sequelae memory impairments
- The deepest part of the tumor is difficult to expose at the level of the posterior perforating space

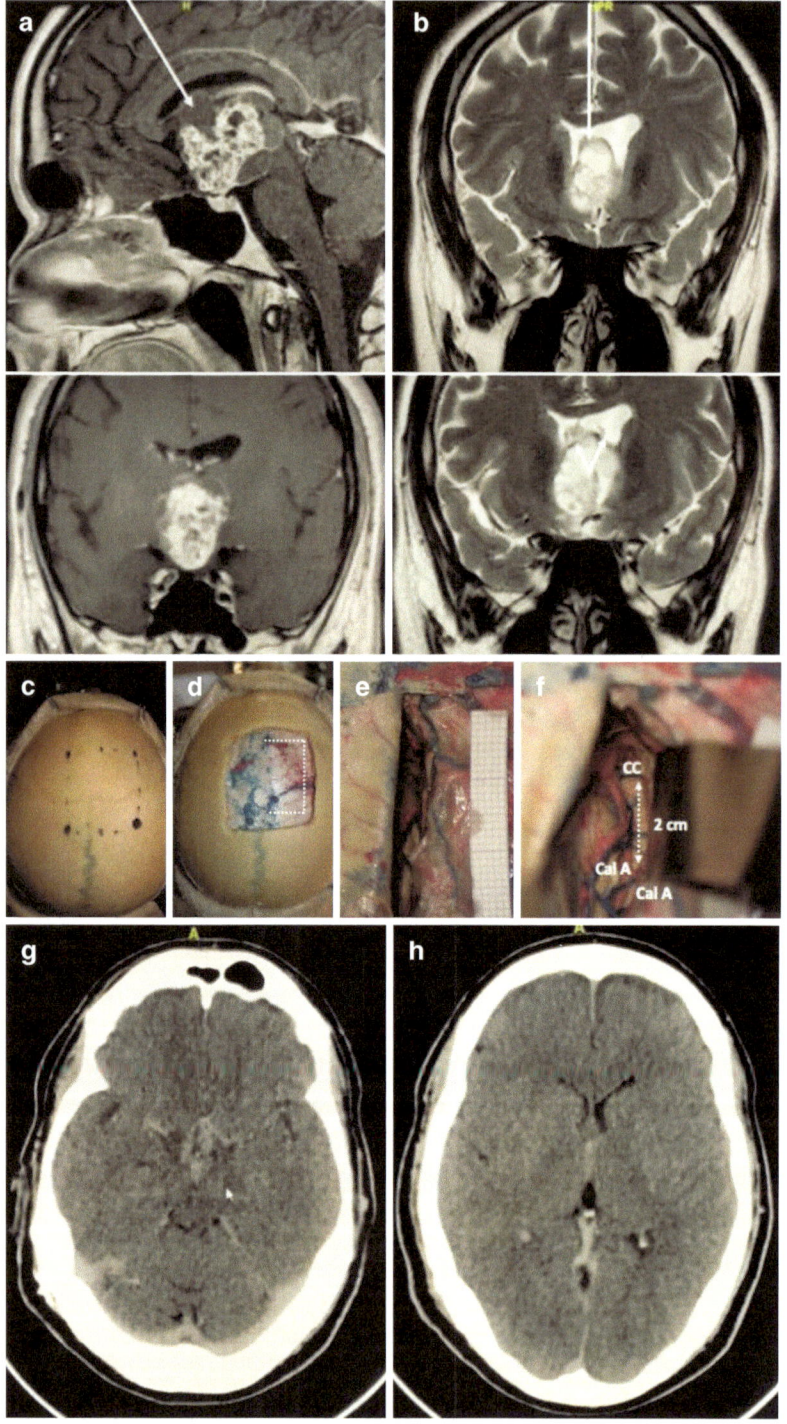

6.3.3   Management of Cystic Craniopharyngiomas (CCPs)

There is a considerable number of publications regarding pediatric-onset Cystic Craniopharyngiomas (cCP). In huge cCP in children, where total excision may be impossible and when radiotherapy may have to be postponed for developmental reasons, drainage and local therapies may be the best options. Intracystic therapies are based on the inflammatory theory of the tumoral walls at the origin of the cyst, recently validated by molecular studies (see chapter by Martinez-Barbera in this book [17]).

To date, Bleomycin and IFN-α have been the most tried therapies, either at initial diagnosis or after recurrence.

The first step is to insert a catheter inside the cyst, connected to a sub-cutaneous Ommaya reservoir. A few days after confirming that the system is "watertight" (especially for Bleomycin), the treatment can be started.

Bleomycin has been generally used three times per week with a median dose of 0.43 mg/kg/week for a total dose of between 8 and 75 mg (mean 36 mg). The treatment duration is several weeks [18].

For IFN-α, 3 MIU/day is injected inside the cyst, after withdrawing as much of the liquid as possible, on occasion up to a total of 36 MIU over several courses in cases where the cyst did not respond well [19].

Bleomycin treatment appeared to be effective (with close to 100% of cyst response and a shrinkage superior to 90% in one quarter of cases), but the severe side effects observed have led to a loss of interest in Bleomycin. In addition, the shrinkage was also found to be transitory: less than 1 year for half of the population and with sustained benefit seen in the other half of the population, with a mean follow-up of 34 months [20].

Since the pioneering work of Cavalheiro in 2005, IFN-α has proven to be effective with less side effects than Bleomycin. A recent multicenter assessment concluded that IFN-α therapy was useful in delaying more invasive treatment in children [21, 22].

For adult onset cCP, data are scarce due to pure or predominantly cystic CP being uncommon. We recently reviewed our own data (11 cases) focusing on a single point: is drainage sufficient to manage cystic CP? Interestingly, with a mean follow-up of 40 months, only 27% of patients had recurrence, 2 in a cystic manner, one

---

Fig. 6.8 Trans-callosal approach. Huge intraventricular CPs without hydrocephalus. A trans-callosal approach was chosen. (**a**) A trans-callosal approach was chosen to remove this intraventricular CP, revealed by an ICP, with hydrocephalus. The patient has been firstly operated on to insert a shunt and was then referred to our center. (**b**) The variant used here was an inter-forniceal route because the CP had itself created the route. On the T2 coronal view, we can clearly see a cyst pointing in between the two fornix (arrows) and the internal cerebral veins. (**c**–**f**) Anatomical studies: the different steps for the interhemispheric trans-callosal approach are shown. A craniotomy crossing the midline is performed to prepare the interhemispheric approach (**c**). A U-shaped opening is made in the Dura-mater (**d**). A 2 cm incision of the corpus callosum (CC) is made between the peri-callosal arteries (Cal A) (**f**). (**g** and **h**) Post-operative contrast CT showing a sub-total removal. The inferior infiltration at the level of the third ventricle floor has been left in place. The outcome was uneventful with a total recovery of the patient's mnesic issues, without any endocrine or visual deficits

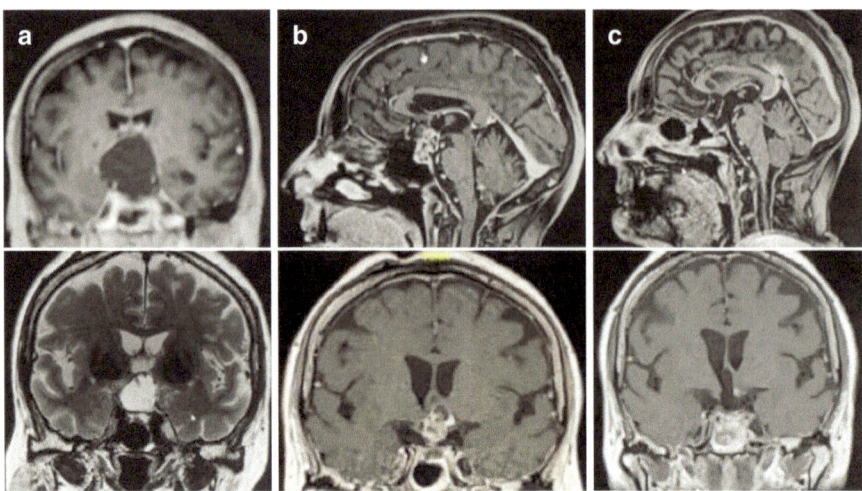

Fig. 6.9 Unpredictable evolution of a cystic CP after drainage. (**a**) Cystic CP diagnosed in a 68-year-old woman with pseudo-dementia syndrome which was completely resolved after drainage. (**b**) The cyst disappeared after 1 year and the solid part of the tumor started growing 3 years later. An endonasal approach has been performed. (**c**) Post-operative MRI after a STR via the nose

from a solid part of the tumor (Fig. 6.9). Only one patient required secondary drainage (using the Ommaya) and one patient in whom the catheter had been removed due to infection showed no recurrence after 5 years (Fig. 6.10). The high rate of tumor control produced by a simple drainage has been confirmed by other authors, as well as the low rate of repeated aspiration [23]. This observation can be explained by the continuous drainage of the cyst following the insertion of the catheter in the ventricle or CSF spaces. Thus, some authors advocate a large opening of the cyst in the ventricle, rather than a simple insertion of a catheter using the endoscopic technique [24, 25].

The role of IFN-α instillation in adult CCP remains unclear, and perhaps it may preferably be used in recurrence.

There is also very little data available on immediate post-drainage management, meaning a wait and see approach or upfront radiotherapy both need to be considered.

Considering the low recurrence rate after a simple drainage the unpredictable evolution of the tumor (recurrence may arise from the solid part rather than the cystic part of the tumor (Fig. 6.9) or the cyst disappearing after a single drainage (Fig. 6.10)), the possible enlargement of the cyst after radiotherapy, and similar recurrence after upfront radiotherapy versus a wait and see approach, palliative management of cCP only by drainage, may represent an interesting option ([23, 24], personal data). This allows not only good tumor control but also good clinical outcomes, including preservation of pituitary function, and preservation of good visual and cognitive function.

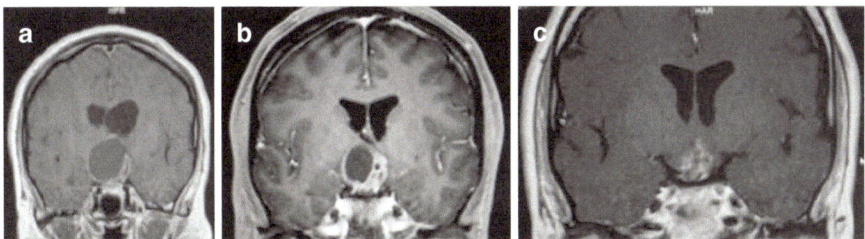

Fig. 6.10 One example of spontaneous regression of a cyst after a single drainage. (**a**) At diagnosis a predominant cystic CP was observed. A catheter was inserted using a stereotactic technique which was then removed at 3 months because of an infection. (**b**) The cyst remained stable at 1 year and the patient was free of symptoms. (**c**) Two years later, the cyst disappeared and the solid tumoral part remains stable 4 years after the initial diagnosis

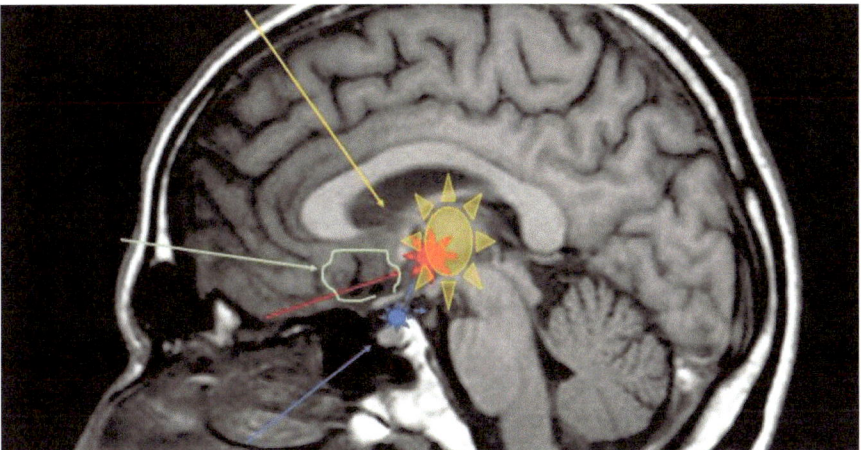

Fig. 6.11 Surgical choices according to CP anatomy. ──────➤ Sellar-suprasellar, retrochiasmatic CPs: nasal route; ──────➤ Anterior and lateral extensions: cranial route; ──────➤ Intraventricular small CPS: trans-lamina terminalis route; ──────➤ Intraventricular huge CPS: trans-frontal (if hydrocephalus present) or trans-callosal (without hydrocephalus) route

6.3.4   Key Points for Beginners: Fig. 6.11

- There are two routes to operate AO-CPs: the nasal route through the skull base and the historical cranial approach.
- There is no randomized study comparing the outcome of both routes, but all experts currently consider that the third ventricle floor is better exposed in the endoscopic endonasal approach with an expected improvement of the GTR.
- Therefore, AO-CPs which are mainly sellar-suprasellar tumors are operated on using the endoscopic endonasal techniques despite the issue of a higher rate of CSF leak not being completely solved.

Table 6.1 Respective indications and drawbacks

Surgical approach		Indications	Pros	Cons
Transnasal		Sellar-Suprasellar-retrochiasmatic-retroclival tumors	• Direct access to the tumor • Better exposure of the hypothalamus and pituitary stalk • Better GTR rate • Avoids optic nerve and chiasm mobilization	• Cannot control lateral extensions • Not adequate for pure intraventricular tumor • CSF Leaks • Meningitis • Rhino-sinusitis
Transcranial		Tumors with anterior and lateral extensions	Less issue of CSF leaks	• Worse exposure of the ventricle, the third ventricle floor and retrochiasmatic space • Mobilization of nerves and vessels • Issue of seizures • Worse visual outcome
Combined nasal and cranial		Huge tumors with intraventricular extensions		
Specific 3rd ventricle approaches	*TLT*	Medium- and small-sized intraventricular tumors	Easy access without nerve mobilization	• Narrow window • Vascular risks • Poor exposure of the third ventricle floor
	TF	Intraventricular tumor with hydrocephalus		• Vein and fornix risks • Seizure issues • Poor exposure of the deepest part of the tumor
	TC	Intraventricular tumor without hydrocephalus		• Vein and fornix risks • Poor exposure of the deepest part of the tumor

TC trans-callosal, *TF* trans-frontal approach, *TLT* trans-lamina terminalis approach

- Rare indications for cranial approaches still remain for AO-CPs, in particular when the CPs has developed away from the midline with lateral or anterior extension(s). When the tumors are located inside the third ventricle, the surgeon has three choices: reaching the tumor through the *lamina terminalis* just above the optic chiasm (small or middle size tumor), through the frontal cortex (possible when there is hydrocephalus), or through the corpus callosum (in the absence of a ventricle dilatation) (Fig. 6.11).
- Evolution of Cystic CPs is unpredictable and minimally invasive management with a simple drainage through a catheter and then a wait and see policy may be advisable. Around two-thirds of cystic CPs are controlled by a simple drainage after more than 3 years of follow-up. Continuous drainage of the cyst in the ventricle may contribute to better control. Thus, an endoscopic fenestration should be preferred rather than a simple catheter stereotactic insertion.

- The role of intracystic therapies, mainly using IFN-α, remains unclear for AO-CPs.
- The surgical treatment of these rare tumors is difficult and impacts directly on the outcomes, in particular the management of the ventricular portion of the tumor, requiring highly specific skills. Thus, these patients should preferably be managed in dedicated referral centers (Table 6.1).

References

1. Dandurand C, Sepehry AA, Asadi Lari MH, Akagami R, Gooderham P. Adult craniopharyngioma: case series, systematic review, and meta-analysis. Neurosurgery. 2018;83(4):631–41. https://doi.org/10.1093/neuros/nyx570.
2. Apra C, Enasceschu C, Lapras V, Raverot G, Jouanneau E. Is gross total resection reasonable in adults with craniopharyngiomas with hypothalamic involvement ? World Neurosurg. 2019; https://doi.org/10.1016/j.wneu.2019.06.037.
3. de Divitiis E, Cappabianca P, Cavallo LM, Esposito F, de Divitiis O, Messina A. Extended endoscopic transsphenoidal approach for extrasellar craniopharyngiomas. Neurosurgery. 2007;61(5 Suppl 2):219–27; discussion 228. https://doi.org/10.1227/01.neu.0000303220.55393.73.
4. Kassam AB, Gardner PA, Snyderman CH, Carrau RL, Mintz AH, Prevedello DM. Expanded endonasal approach, a fully endoscopic transnasal approach for the resection of midline suprasellar craniopharyngiomas: a new classification based on the infundibulum. J Neurosurg. 2008;108(4):715–28. https://doi.org/10.3171/JNS/2008/108/4/0715.
5. Cappabianca P, Cavallo LM, Colao A, et al. Endoscopic endonasal transsphenoidal approach: outcome analysis of 100 consecutive procedures. Minim Invasive Neurosurg. 2002;45(4):193–200. https://doi.org/10.1055/s-2002-36197.
6. Komotar RJ, Starke RM, Raper DMS, Anand VK, Schwartz TH. Endoscopic endonasal compared with microscopic transsphenoidal and open transcranial resection of craniopharyngiomas. World Neurosurg. 2012;77(2):329–41. https://doi.org/10.1016/j.wneu.2011.07.011.
7. Kassam AB, Prevedello DM, Thomas A, et al. Endoscopic endonasal pituitary transposition for a transdorsum sellae approach to the interpeduncular cistern. Neurosurgery. 2008;62(3 Suppl 1):57–72; discussion 72-74. https://doi.org/10.1227/01.neu.0000317374.30443.23.
8. Nanda A, Narayan V, Mohammed N, Savardekar AR, Patra DP. Microsurgical resection of suprasellar craniopharyngioma-technical purview. J Neurol Surg Part B Skull Base. 2018;79(Suppl 3):S247–8. https://doi.org/10.1055/s-0038-1625941.
9. Prieto R, Pascual JM. Norman M. Dott, master of hypothalamic craniopharyngioma surgery: the decisive mentoring of Harvey Cushing and Percival Bailey at Peter Bent Brigham Hospital. J Neurosurg. 2017;127(4):927–40. https://doi.org/10.3171/2016.9.JNS16702.
10. Dehdashti AR, de Tribolet N. Frontobasal interhemispheric trans-lamina terminalis approach for suprasellar lesions. Neurosurgery. 2005;56(2 Suppl):418–24.; discussion 418-424. https://doi.org/10.1227/01.neu.0000157027.80293.c7.
11. Choudhri O, Chang SD. Subfrontal trans-lamina terminalis approach to a third ventricular craniopharyngioma. Neurosurg Focus. 2016;40 Video Suppl 1:2016.1.FocusVid.15416. https://doi.org/10.3171/2016.1.FocusVid.15416
12. Silva PS, Cerejo A, Polónia P, Pereira J, Vaz R. Trans-lamina terminalis approach for third ventricle and suprasellar tumours. Clin Neurol Neurosurg. 2013;115(9):1745–52. https://doi.org/10.1016/j.clineuro.2013.04.010.
13. Weil AG, Robert T, Alsaiari S, Obaid S, Bojanowski MW. Using the trans-lamina terminalis route via a pterional approach to resect a retrochiasmatic craniopharyngioma involving the

third ventricle. *Neurosurg Focus*. 2016;40 Video Suppl 1:2016.1.FocusVid.15440. https://doi.org/10.3171/2016.1.FocusVid.15440

14. Maira G, Anile C, Colosimo C, Cabezas D. Craniopharyngiomas of the third ventricle: translamina terminalis approach. Neurosurgery. 2000;47(4):857–63.; discussion 863–865. https://doi.org/10.1097/00006123-200010000-00014.

15. Bozkurt B, Yağmurlu K, Belykh E, et al. Quantitative anatomic analysis of the transcallosal-transchoroidal approach and the transcallosal-subchoroidal approach to the floor of the third ventricle: an anatomic study. World Neurosurg. 2018;118:219–29. https://doi.org/10.1016/j.wneu.2018.05.126.

16. Rosenfeld JV, Freeman JL, Harvey AS. Operative technique: the anterior transcallosal transseptal interforniceal approach to the third ventricle and resection of hypothalamic hamartomas. J Clin Neurosci Off J Neurosurg Soc Australas. 2004;11(7):738–44. https://doi.org/10.1016/j.jocn.2004.03.008.

17. Apps JR, Carreno G, Gonzalez-Meljem JM, et al. Tumour compartment transcriptomics demonstrates the activation of inflammatory and odontogenic programmes in human adamantinomatous craniopharyngioma and identifies the MAPK/ERK pathway as a novel therapeutic target. Acta Neuropathol (Berl). 2018;135(5):757–77. https://doi.org/10.1007/s00401-018-1830-2.

18. Hukin J, Steinbok P, Lafay-Cousin L, et al. Intracystic bleomycin therapy for craniopharyngioma in children: the Canadian experience. Cancer. 2007;109(10):2124–31. https://doi.org/10.1002/cncr.22633.

19. Kilday J-P, Caldarelli M, Massimi L, et al. Intracystic interferon-alpha in pediatric craniopharyngioma patients: an international multicenter assessment on behalf of SIOPE and ISPN. Neuro-Oncology. 2017;19(10):1398–407. https://doi.org/10.1093/neuonc/nox056.

20. Steinbok P, Hukin J. Intracystic treatments for craniopharyngioma. Neurosurg Focus. 2010;28(4):E13. https://doi.org/10.3171/2010.1.FOCUS09315.

21. Cavalheiro S, Dastoli PA, Silva NS, Toledo S, Lederman H, da Silva MC. Use of interferon alpha in intratumoral chemotherapy for cystic craniopharyngioma. Childs Nerv Syst ChNS Off J Int Soc Pediatr Neurosurg. 2005;21(8–9):719–24. https://doi.org/10.1007/s00381-005-1226-1.

22. Cavalheiro S. Intracystic interferon-alpha in pediatric craniopharyngioma patients. Neuro-Oncology. 2017;19(10):1419. https://doi.org/10.1093/neuonc/nox123.

23. Moussa AH, Kerasha AA, Mahmoud ME. Surprising outcome of Ommaya reservoir in treating cystic craniopharyngioma: a retrospective study. Br J Neurosurg. 2013;27(3):370–3. https://doi.org/10.3109/02688697.2012.741732.

24. Spaziante R, De Divitiis E, Irace C, Cappabianca P, Caputi F. Management of primary or recurring grossly cystic craniopharyngiomas by means of draining systems. Topic review and 6 case reports. Acta Neurochir (Wien). 1989;97(3–4):95–106.

25. Lauretti L, Legninda Sop FY, Pallini R, Fernandez E, D'Alessandris QG. Neuroendoscopic treatment of cystic craniopharyngiomas: a case series with systematic review of the literature. World Neurosurg. 2018;110:e367–73. https://doi.org/10.1016/j.wneu.2017.11.004.

Definitive Radiotherapy in Adult Population Craniopharyngiomas

Loïc Feuvret, Julian Jacob, François Georges Riet, Kevin Cristina, Marguerite Cuttat, and Valentin Calugaru

7.1 Introduction

The craniopharyngioma (CP) is a rare, slow growing benign tumor, making up between 2% to 5% of all primary intracranial tumors [1]. The incidence is bimodal with peaks occurring from 5 to 15 and from 45 to 60 years old. About half of cases occur in adults according to data from a Danish study [2, 3]. Despite high proportion of CP in adult population, data are scarce and limited compared to those of childhood patients in literature. Consequently, main therapeutic strategies have mimicked those of pediatrics approaches in terms of surgery and radiation therapy to establish recommendations in adulthood patients.

Radical resection has been recommended for several decades as the gold standard of treatment. As a consequence of their infiltrative growth behavior and their high trend to relapse as a malignant disease, the treatment appears as a major neurosurgical challenge. Indeed, CP infiltrates adjacent organs like the neuroendocrine structures as pituitary gland, hypothalamus, optic pathways, blood vessels, and the 3rd ventricle causing significant morbidity and mortality due to a lack of clear line

L. Feuvret (✉)
Department of Radiation Oncology, Hospital Pitié-Salpêtrière Charles Foix, APHP, Paris, France

Proton Therapy Centre, Institut Curie, Orsay, France
e-mail: loic.feuvret@aphp.fr

J. Jacob · F. G. Riet · K. Cristina · M. Cuttat
Department of Radiation Oncology, Hospital Pitié-Salpêtrière Charles Foix, APHP, Paris, France
e-mail: julian.jacob@aphp.fr; francoisgeorges.riet@aphp.fr; kevin.cristina@aphp.fr

V. Calugaru
Proton Therapy Center, Institute Curie, Orsay, France
e-mail: valentin.calugaru@curie.fr

© Springer Nature Switzerland AG 2020   119
E. Jouanneau, G. Raverot (eds.), *Adult Craniopharyngiomas*,
https://doi.org/10.1007/978-3-030-41176-3_7

of cleavage between tumor and normal tissue. Hence, all of these make complete resection challenging. Currently that is why subtotal resection (STR) and complementary treatment hold a main role, although the optimal therapeutic approach remains controversial.

In 2018, two meta-analyses with more than 700 adult patients analyzed the role of two competing paradigms, either gross total resection (GTR) with minimal morbidity or safe STR associated with complementary radiation therapy (STR+RT). Both of them drew the same conclusions that safe STR and RT may have similar outcomes as GTR in pediatrics and in adult population. The rates of recurrence were 17% in the GTR group and 27% in the STR+RT group [4, 5]. Unfortunately, the incidence of relapse remains high for a benign disease. However, in the Dandurand's study, some limitations should be mentioned: 7 studies with only 22 patients treated from 1946 to 2016; subjectivity of variables (histological grade, extent of resection, appropriateness of RT); lack of analyze treatment-related morbidity and mortality. From the Surveillance, Epidemiology, and End Results (SEER) database from 2004 to 2012, multivariable analysis demonstrated that age (>65 years old) was considered as a negative prognostic factor of overall survival ($p < 0.001$), whereas treatment modality (RT/GTR/STR+RT) was not ($p = 0.2$) [2]. To understand the therapeutic potential of radiation therapy, it is worth mentioning two studies highlighting the potential efficacy of RT. Elowe-Gruau *et al.* published the results of a single institution study showing that a hypothalamus-sparing surgical strategy combined with adjuvant radiotherapy decreased the rate of serious long-term obesity in childhood patients without increasing their risk for local relapses [6]. In a prognostic univariate analysis of 122 patients, Schoenfeld *et al.* showed similarly that there was no significant difference in progression-free survival and overall survival between patients treated with GTR or STR+RT. Moreover, the authors reported the combination of STR and RT demonstrated a significantly lower risk of developing diabetes insipidus and panhypopituitarism in an adult and child population [7].

An interesting issue is which results could be expected by immediate post-operative RT to avoid relapse. The tumor relapse is considered as a surgical challenge worse than the first treatment. Morbidity and mortality rates of this surgery are higher than those observed after primary surgery. Furthermore, the rate of total removal is significantly limited. Moreover, Bishop *et al.* showed irradiation performed in childhood patients as salvage therapy rather than immediate post-operative treatment exposed to higher rates of visual and endocrine dysfunctions [8].

Thus, currently the main treatment option consists of surgical resection followed by radiation therapy in case of residual tumor in adult and pediatric patients [9]. In the literature, prospective studies assessing different treatment strategies and role of different RT techniques in adult patients are missing. Because this disease is quite rare, many studies combine adult and childhood onset. There are no evidence-based guidelines for the optimal RT of primary or recurrent CP in adults. In this chapter, first, we propose to define some concepts of radiation techniques used to treat CP patients, and second to report clinical results in terms of tumor control and side effects for different RT techniques applied to adult population.

7.2 Radiation Techniques

7.2.1 Generalities

New radiation technologies have the potential to transform how tumor is treated through precise tumor targeting and adaptive treatment at the delivery time. They are currently under investigation to reach an optimal balance between local control and the long-term effects for surrounding eloquent structures at risk such as a pituitary gland, hypothalamus, optic apparatus, arteries at the base to the skull, normal brain tissues. Technologic improvements in imaging, radiation planning, and dose delivery have improved the accuracy of radiation doses to target volumes and reduced the doses to nearby normal tissues to shallow the aforementioned concept. In clinical practice, the dose per fraction, the total dose, the radiation technique, the volume of normal structures irradiated, and the dose delivered to the healthy tissues define a course of radiation and influence the effectiveness and tolerance in CP treatment. In order to understand, we propose to define the fundamental principles governing the radiation therapy.

7.2.2 Dose Delivery

7.2.2.1 Fractionation

The multi-fraction radiotherapy was based on experiments performed in Paris in the 1920s. The radiation delivered in daily fractions over a period of time made antitumoral effect possible with minimal normal tissue damage compared to a single X-rays dose. Hence, classical radiation schedules using once daily (five per week) fractionation of 1.8–2 Gy over a period of 5–7 weeks and a total dose of 50.4–59.4 Gy for CPs have become the most applied ones.

Mono- and hypo-fractionation schedules use reduced number of fractions of larger size (1–5 fractions to a marginal dose of 13–25 Gy) in small target volumes over a period of 1–5 days.

7.2.2.2 Applications

Photon Beams
Most types of tumor radiotherapy use ionizing photon (X-rays or gamma rays) beams for the local or regional treatment of disease. Apart from conventional three-dimensional conformal radiation therapy, several modalities have been developed for radiotherapy delivery. The most advanced method for the delivery of high radiation doses with photon beams is intensity modulated radiation therapy (IMRT).

Three-Dimensional Conformal Radiation Therapy
Three-dimensional conformal radiation therapy (3DCRT) is a cancer treatment that refers to the radiation beams to match the shape of the tumor. 3DCRT has been the standard of practice for many decades in CP radiation therapy.

Treatment plans use several radiation beams, shaped to conform to the target volume and to optimize the conformality of the dose distribution. In the literature focused on CP, the most frequently used systems for delivering a conventional 3DCRT are linear accelerators. Consequently, the main presented results are extracted from 3DCRT series. It is worth mentioning that new RT techniques such as intensity modulated radiation therapy and stereotactic radiation therapy should over time replace 3DCRT.

Intensity Modulated Radiation Therapy

Intensity modulated radiation therapy (IMRT) is a form of 3DCRT, using multiple intensity modulated beams, and a computer-assisted iterative optimization. It delivers conformal radiation to the target tumor, by "crossing" multiple shaped beams of various intensities through ways that spare radiosensitive and critical adjacent tissues, as shown in Fig. 7.1. IMRT utilizes ionizing radiation in the form of X-rays generated by linear accelerators.

Stereotactic Radiation Therapy

Stereotactic radiation therapy (SRT) is a modality combining the precise focal delivery of total high dose with the radiobiological advantages of high dose per fraction. This technique applies the fact that the radiation tolerance of normal tissue is volume dependent. Thus, SRT reduces side effects in minimizing normal tissue margins. The term stereotactic radiosurgery (SRS) is used when all of the irradiation is done in one session, whereas the term hypofractionated stereotactic radiotherapy (HFSRT) is appropriate with 2 or more radiation fractions. SRT refers to using an accurate three-dimensional mapping technique to guide a procedure and requires a sophisticated treatment planning system and stereotactic mobilization devices. There are two basic kinds of equipment, each of which uses different tools and radiation sources: the Gamma Knife® (gamma rays) and Linear accelerator (LINAC) (X-rays) machines. Multiple manufacturers as Varian®, Elekta®, and Accuray® make LINAC, which have brand names such as Novalis Tx™, Elekta Synergy™, and CyberKnife®. In the literature focused on CP, the most frequently used device to deliver a single dose is the Gamma Knife®. This machine was made to administrate a single, large dose of highly conformal radiation (γ-rays) precisely to a number of intracranial sites using multiple fixed 60 Co sources aimed at a center point using a stereotactic fixed invasive frame (Fig. 7.2). The CyberKnife® is a dedicated frameless system used for SRT. It uses non-invasive image-guided localization, a lightweight photon-beam accelerator, and a robotic delivery system to deliver stereotactic radiation therapy. For treatment tracking, the 6D skull tracking mode allows to correct any residual offset between the patient's simulation position and that at the time of treatment. Hence, frameless technology as CyberKnife® and classical LINACs offer the opportunity to perform SRS or HFSRT (usually 1–5 fractions over 1–5 days).

Patients treated with SRT get a small tumor size, mainly solid tumors well circumscribed and located several millimeters away from organs at risk (optic pathways, brainstem).

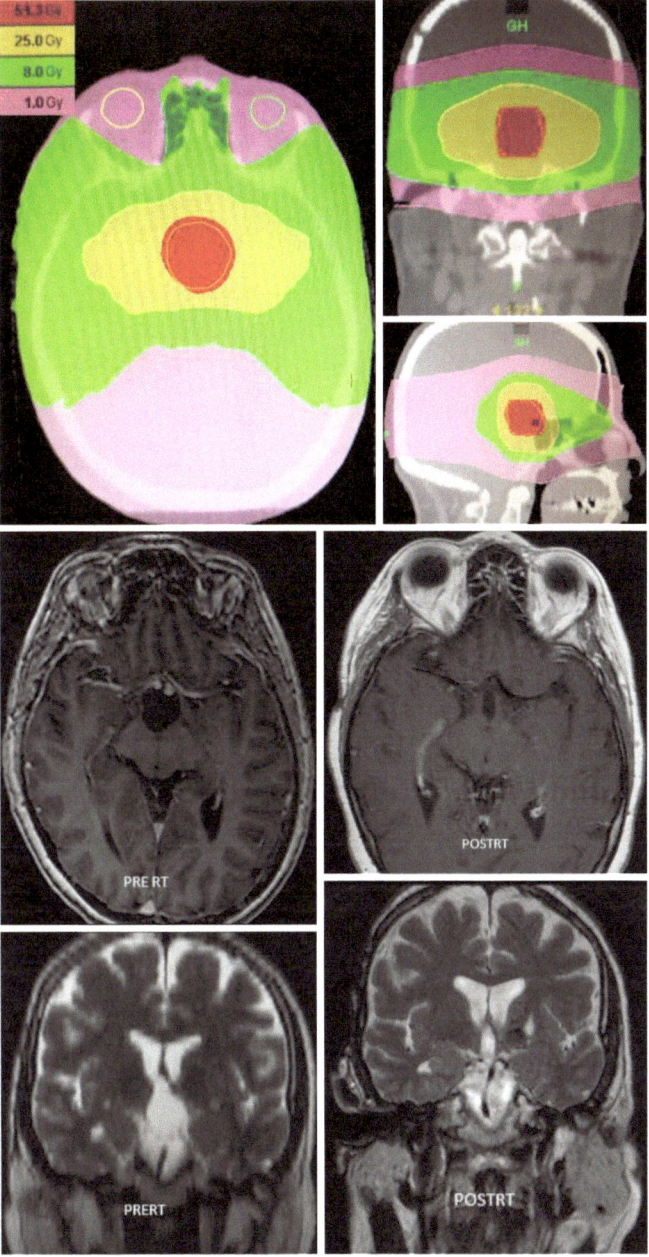

Fig. 7.1 Sample images (top) of the intensity modulated radiation therapy, helical tomotherapy treatment plan for a recurrent adult craniopharyngioma (54 Gy in 30 fractions, five per week). It demonstrates an optimal target coverage (Clinical Target Volume: orange line; red wash color: prescribed dose) with a sharp dose fall-off, but owing to helical tomotherapy arrangement with both entry and exit dose, a low dose is deposited diffusely in the region of the normal brain surrounding the central tumor (Yellow wash color: V25 Gy; Green wash color: V8 Gy; Rose wash color: V1 Gy). Follow-up MRI (bottom) showing a remarkable shrinkage of the cystic tumor

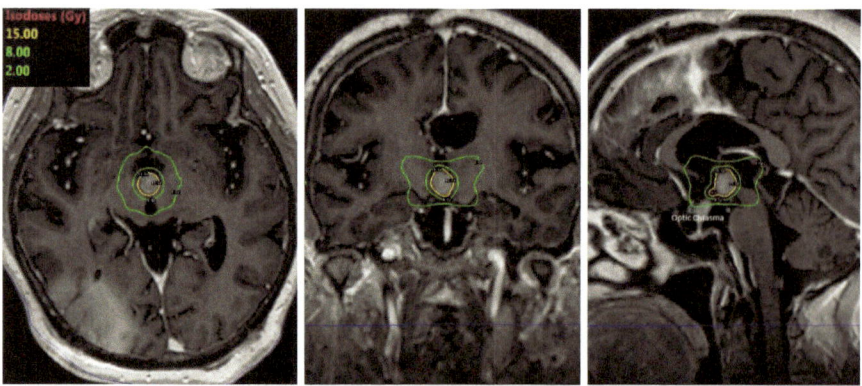

Fig. 7.2 An example of the dose distribution for Gamma Knife radiosurgery (15 Gy on 50% iso-dose—yellow line). Thanks a sharp dose fall-off, a low dose is deposited in the region of the normal brain surrounding the tumor (Green lines: V2 Gy and V8 Gy). The optic chiasma maximal dose is 2 Gy (Blue structure on sagittal MRI view)

Proton Beams

An alternative treatment modality is charged particle radiotherapy, which uses beams of protons. American physicist Robert R. Wilson was the first to suggest using protons for radiation therapy in a paper published in 1946. The first people to receive proton beam therapy were treated with pituitary irradiation to control metastatic breast cancer in 1954. Nowadays, proton radiation has been used to treat more than 160,000 people worldwide. Even with the rapid growth of proton treatment centers, proton therapy has been relatively inaccessible for most patients. Proton therapy has become the most accurate and advanced form of radiation treatment. It has been used to improve local control rates by increasing the dose delivered to the tumor, while sparing OARs. Indeed, this technique is an efficient way to improve the dose gradient between the gross tumor and surrounding structures due to the unique distribution in matter by the narrow lateral penumbra and the Bragg peak (point where all of the energy of the incident beam is delivered very sharply before dropping to zero). The Bragg peak must be modulated in proton beam therapy using an energy degrader and also shaped to deliver high conformal irradiation. As physic characteristics, protons offer dose distribution resulting in a significantly reduced integral dose of radiation to the surrounding normal tissues as compared to 3DCRT, as shown in Fig. 7.3. The experimental in vivo and clinical data indicate that continued employment of a generic relative biological effectiveness (RBE) value of 1.1 is reasonable for proton beams. Thus, proton therapy is considered as the best radiation technique for pediatric patients but its role should be assessed in adult population.

7.2.3 Organs at Risk

Most craniopharyngiomas are located in the sellar/parasellar region with suprasellar tumor mass extension. Its location places the temporal lobes, hippocampi,

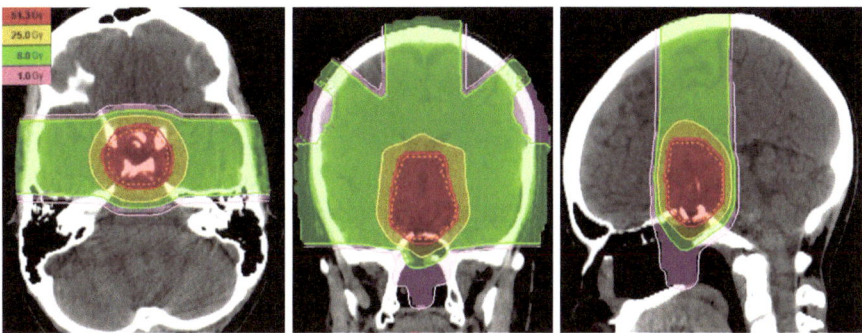

Fig. 7.3 An example of the dose distribution for passive-scatter proton therapy in a patient with craniopharyngioma demonstrates a homogenous target dose plan. Three-dimensional conformal proton therapy offers a sharp dose fall-off and, with a five-beam arrangement with no exit dose, offers less dose deposition in the normal brain tissue. This plan offers an optimal sparing of the supratentorial brain, cochleas, and orbits

hypothalamus, brainstem, cochleae, optic chiasm, and optic nerves at risk for radiation injury. About CP RT, late complications of RT could include visual defect, endocrine dysfunction, and cognitive impairment. New RT innovations aim at maintaining or increasing the tumor control rate while maintaining or reducing the normal tissue complications. Recently, publications reported the set of intracranial organs at risk delineation and dose constraints to the organs at risk in order to provide assistance in the difficult task of reaching the optimal plan for each patient. These guidelines might be a tool for daily practice and to decrease the risk of long-term side effects after RT in patients treated for CPs [10–12].

7.3 Clinical Results

7.3.1 Efficacy

7.3.1.1 Classical Fractionation

Photons
Satisfying long-term results of photon beams conventional conformal radiotherapy were reported in many retrospective series representing the most important data of CP radiation therapy in the literature. In 2018, a large systematic review focusing on adult population reported local recurrence rates recurrence of 27% in a group after STR+RT and 45% in a group after STR [5]. The mean times to recurrence for STR+RT and STR only were 81.3 and 23 months, respectively. In a mixed population, the 10- and 20-year, the actuarial local control rates were 89.1% and 54%, respectively (Fig. 7.1). The median follow-up was 12.1 years [13].

Protons
In adult population, proton beam series are very limited. The single series reporting results for adult patients was published by the Massachusetts General Hospital,

Harvard Medical School, Boston in 2006 [14]. The median dose delivered was 62.7 GyE (equivalent dose) in 10 adults of a pediatric and adult population. Actuarial 5- and 10-year local control rates were 93% and 85% without distinction between children and adults. The functional status of the living adult patients is unaltered from their baseline status; all of them continued leading normal or near normal working lives. Globally, classical fractionation radiotherapy, radiation total dose, and clinical tumor results were identical to these reported in photon radiation therapy series. As data are very scarce, studies combined adult and childhood onset. A final conclusion on the impact of proton therapy in adult patients can therefore not be clearly assessed particularly in terms of long-term side effects. Boehling et al. reported a dosimetric comparison of three-dimensional conformal proton radiotherapy, intensity modulated proton therapy, and intensity modulated radiotherapy for treatment of pediatric CP [15]. They showed that proton therapy was able to avoid excess integral radiation dose to a variety of normal structures at all dose levels while maintaining equal target volume coverage. Recently, a dosimetric comparison between proton radiation therapy and different photon techniques [16] concluded the effectiveness and safety of proton beam dose compared to photon radiation therapy depending on the intracranial tumor features, i.e., the size, the lateralization. These data should refine selection of radiation techniques and assess cost-effectiveness and clinical toxicity in adult population. Only prospective trials should examine the clinical benefits of these dosimetric advantages in adult patients. Currently, the website "clinicaltrials.gov" reports only two studies about proton therapy in pediatric patients treated for CP.

7.3.1.2 Hypo- and Monofractionation Stereotactic Radiation Therapy

Stereotactic radiation therapy (SRT) is an option at initial post-operative treatment or relapse for tumors selected according to the criteria mentioned below. Because it allows the accurate delivery of very high-dose radiation to the tumor, while minimizing irradiation of critical structures, SRT should reduce the risks of long-term side effects. Treatment using Gamma Knife is considered as an efficient strategy with low side effect risks [17]. However, although the targeting accuracy and dose fall-off of SRS treatment are great, it appears as not relevant for tumors closed to optic pathways or large (diameter >3 cm) due to the dose limitation to normal structures in a single session. The sparing of normal tissues, especially late-responding tissues such as the optic structures, should be more optimal by using lower daily doses with stereotactic fractionated radiation than with SRS.

Radiosurgery

SRS is the most frequently used technique as SRT and is considered as an alternative to fractionated radiotherapy in patients with small size CP. Series reported local control rates between 67 and 86% with a median follow-up of 64 months [62–75] [17–20]. One out of four series reported results for only adult patients. No significant difference appeared between adult and child patients. Despite promising outcomes, further prospective studies are needed to precise the role of SRS in terms of local control and potential long-term adverse effects.

Hypofractionated Stereotactic Radiation Therapy
Data about HFSRT are very poor. Only two series reported clinical results in a limited population (16–43 patients) with a short follow-up (15–40 months) [21, 22]. Different radiation delivery schedules were used: (18.0–38.0 Gy/3–10 fractions) in the Lee *et al.*'s series; 16.0 Gy/2 fractions, 21.0 Gy/3 fractions, and 25.0 Gy/5 fractions according to Iwata *et al.* Two-, 3-year local control rates were 85 and 91%, respectively. No comparison between SRS and HFSRT has been published.

7.3.2 Toxicity

Pituitary impairments are common at the time of diagnosis and after surgery due to the tumor proximity or involvement of the endocrine system. It is worth mentioning that there is no significant difference in terms of incidence of endocrine injury between GTR and STR+RT [6]. In a 1990s series, Regine *et al.* reported 46% of radiation complications in 39 adults [23]. The mean delivered dose was 62.43 Gy (43.2–70) with 2D RT. Radiation-related endocrine, neurologic, vascular, and/or visual sequelae appeared in all patients exposed to maximum doses upper to 61 Gy. It is worth mentioning RT was applied with ancient techniques and a delivered total dose was considered as very high compared to current guidelines. Thus, no conclusion could be drawn from this paper. Using pediatrics series to describe late side effects in adult population should be confounding and not relevant because data are scarce and normal tissues radiation sensitivity to radiation seems different between both populations. However, one series reported no significant difference in the probabilities of major visual field defects, hyperphagia/obesity, hemi/monoparesis, or epilepsy between childhood- and adult-onset disease [24]. In 2002, in one of the most illustrative series of adult patients ($n = 22$) treated by conventional RT (classical fractionation median dose 59.75 Gy) with long-term follow-up (12 years), Varlotto *et al.* reported complication-free survival rates at 10 and 20 years of 80.1% and 69.5%, respectively. The complications and interval after RT for the patients were as follows: infarction of the left side of the pons (12 years 1 month), optic neuropathy (2 years) and left-sided hemiparesis (3 years 4 months), visual field defect (3 years 2 months), mental status changes and thalamic infarct (4 years 9 months), memory loss (2 years 5 months), and left-sided visual field defect (5 years). Despite a variety of different treatment techniques, no complications occurred at a dose of 55 Gy (equivalent dose in 2-Gy fractions) [13]. In a recent series of patients treated with Gamma Knife, only one case (2%) of worsening of a preexistent visual defect 12 months after RT was reported. Long-term follow-up is recommended to assess long-term side effects rates, misjudged due to a retrospective design of studies and a low statistical power.

7.4 Conclusion

Currently standard radiation therapy for adult CP is fractionated radiotherapy. Numerous publications have clearly showed that RT after STR is associated with decreased risk of relapse as demonstrated in pediatric series. Long-term side effects are described in patients irradiated for CP. Thanks to RT innovations, adverse effects incidences are expected to decrease while maintaining a high local control rate. Although the integral dose in normal tissues decreases drastically, the benefit of IMRT, proton therapy, and SRT remains uncertain in adult patients. Currently, IMRT should appear, at least, as the optimal RT technique, which is highly spread throughout the world. Due to the rarity and cost of proton therapy, prospective studies are mandatory before declaring proton as the optimal RT method. SRT remains a standard option for suitable tumors. Finally, despite adjuvant RT efficacy, local control rate seems relatively low for a benign tumor (27% of recurrence), meaning the relative weakness of global therapeutic strategy. Only prospective trials in adult population should define the role of RT in terms of techniques, prescribed doses, fractionation, sparing organs at risk. In clinicaltrial.gov website, only one study is reported out of 26 occurrences (keywords: craniopharyngioma, adult) about radiation therapy of CP. It assesses the role of proton therapy. Notwithstanding these trials, progress towards guidelines publications would be slow.

References

1. Clark AJ, Cage TA, Aranda D, Parsa AT, Sun PP, Auguste KI, et al. A systematic review of the results of surgery and radiotherapy on tumor control for pediatric craniopharyngioma. Childs Nerv Syst. 2013;29(2):231–8.
2. Zhang C, Verma V, Lyden ER, Horowitz DP, Zacharia BE, Lin C, et al. The role of definitive radiotherapy in craniopharyngioma: a SEER analysis. Am J Clin Oncol. 2018;41(8):807–12.
3. Nielsen EH, Feldt-Rasmussen U, Poulsgaard L, Kristensen LØ, Astrup J, Jørgensen JO, et al. Incidence of craniopharyngioma in Denmark (n = 189) and estimated world incidence of craniopharyngioma in children and adults. J Neurooncol. 2011;104(3):755–63.
4. Wang G, Zhang X, Feng M, Guo F. Comparing survival outcomes of gross total resection and subtotal resection with radiotherapy for craniopharyngioma: a meta-analysis. J Surg Res. 2018;226:131–9.
5. Dandurand C, Sepehry AA, Asadi Lari MH, Akagami R, Gooderham P. Adult craniopharyngioma: case series, systematic review, and meta-analysis. Neurosurgery. 2018;83(4):631–41.
6. Elowe-Gruau E, Beltrand J, Brauner R, Pinto G, Samara-Boustani D, Thalassinos C, et al. Childhood craniopharyngioma: hypothalamus-sparing surgery decreases the risk of obesity. J Clin Endocrinol Metab. 2013;98(6):2376–82.
7. Schoenfeld A, Pekmezci M, Barnes MJ, Tihan T, Gupta N, Lamborn KR, et al. The superiority of conservative resection and adjuvant radiation for craniopharyngiomas. J Neurooncol. 2012;108(1):133–9.
8. Bishop AJ, Greenfield B, Mahajan A, Paulino AC, Okcu MF, Allen PK, et al. Proton beam therapy versus conformal photon radiation therapy for childhood craniopharyngioma: multi-institutional analysis of outcomes, cyst dynamics, and toxicity. Int J Radiat Oncol. 2014;90(2):354–61.
9. Zoicas F, Schöfl C. Craniopharyngioma in adults. Front Endocrinol [Internet]. 2012 [cited 2018 Nov 27];3. Available from: http://journal.frontiersin.org/article/10.3389/fendo.2012.00046/abstract
10. Lambrecht M, Eekers DBP, Alapetite C, Burnet NG, Calugaru V, Coremans IEM, et al. Radiation dose constraints for organs at risk in neuro-oncology; the European particle therapy network consensus. Radiother Oncol. 2018;128(1):26–36.

11. Milano MT, Grimm J, Soltys SG, Yorke E, Moiseenko V, Tomé WA, et al. Single- and multi-fraction stereotactic radiosurgery dose tolerances of the optic pathways. Int J Radiat Oncol [Internet]. 2018 Jan [cited 2018 Nov 27]; Available from: https://linkinghub.elsevier.com/retrieve/pii/S0360301618301251

12. Scoccianti S, Detti B, Gadda D, Greto D, Furfaro I, Meacci F, et al. Organs at risk in the brain and their dose-constraints in adults and in children: a radiation oncologist's guide for delineation in everyday practice. Radiother Oncol. 2015;114(2):230–8.

13. Varlotto JM, Flickinger JC, Kondziolka D, Lunsford LD, Deutsch M. External beam irradiation of craniopharyngiomas: long-term analysis of tumor control and morbidity. Int J Radiat Oncol. 2002;54(2):492–9.

14. Fitzek MM, Linggood RM, Adams J, Munzenrider JE. Combined proton and photon irradiation for craniopharyngioma: long-term results of the early cohort of patients treated at Harvard Cyclotron Laboratory and Massachusetts General Hospital. Int J Radiat Oncol. 2006;64(5):1348–54.

15. Boehling NS, Grosshans DR, Bluett JB, Palmer MT, Song X, Amos RA, et al. Dosimetric comparison of three-dimensional conformal proton radiotherapy, intensity-modulated proton therapy, and intensity-modulated radiotherapy for treatment of pediatric craniopharyngiomas. Int J Radiat Oncol. 2012;82(2):643–52.

16. Adeberg S, Harrabi S, Bougatf N, Verma V, Windisch P, Bernhardt D, et al. Dosimetric comparison of proton radiation therapy, volumetric modulated arc therapy, and three-dimensional conformal radiotherapy based on intracranial tumor location. Cancers. 2018;10(11):401.

17. Kobayashi T. Long-term results of gamma knife radiosurgery for 100 consecutive cases of craniopharyngioma and a treatment strategy. Prog Neurol Surg. 2009;22:63–76.

18. Chiou S-H, Lunsford LD, Niranjan A, Kondziolka D, Flickinger J. Stereotactic radiosurgery of residual or recurrent craniopharyngioma, after surgery, with or without radiation therapy. Neuro-Oncology. 2001;3:159–66.

19. Niranjan A, Kano H, Mathieu D, Kondziolka D, Flickinger JC, Lunsford LD. Radiosurgery for craniopharyngioma. Int J Radiat Oncol. 2010;78(1):64–71.

20. Losa M, Pieri V, Bailo M, Gagliardi F, Barzaghi LR, Gioia L, et al. Single fraction and multisession Gamma Knife radiosurgery for craniopharyngioma. Pituitary. 2018;21(5):499–506.

21. Lee M, Larvie M, Cheshier S, Gibbs IC, Adler JR, Chang S. Radiation therapy and CyberKnife radiosurgery in the management of craniopharyngiomas. Neurosurg Focus. 2008;24(5):E4.

22. Iwata H, Tatewaki K, Inoue M, Yokota N, Baba Y, Nomura R, et al. Single and hypofractionated stereotactic radiotherapy with CyberKnife for craniopharyngioma. J Neurooncol. 2012;106(3):571–7.

23. Regine WF, Mohiuddin M, Kramer S. Long-term results of pediatric and adult craniopharyngiomas treated with combined surgery and radiation. Radiother Oncol. 1993;27(1):13–21.

24. Karavitaki N, Brufani C, Warner JT, Adams CBT, Richards P, Ansorge O, et al. Craniopharyngiomas in children and adults: systematic analysis of 121 cases with long-term follow-up. Clin Endocrinol (Oxf). 2005;62(4):397–409.

How to Manage Recurrent Craniopharyngiomas

8

Luigi M. Cavallo, Domenico Solari, Teresa Somma, Cinzia Baiano, Elena D'Avella, and Paolo Cappabianca

8.1 Introduction

Craniopharyngiomas are benign disembryogenetic tumors [1, 2] accounting for the 2–5% of all intracranial tumors in a bimodal fashion, most frequently involving the childhood (mean age 5–14 years) and the late adulthood (mean age 50–74 years) [3, 4]. The consistency could be cystic, solid, or a combination of both; intralesional calcifications represent a quite common finding (about 60 to 80% of cases). Histologically two major variants have been identified: the adamantinomatous type, which results the most frequent in childhood and the papillary, more common in adults. Thus far, according to such unpredictable features of aspects and biological behaviors, the surgical management of such disease is still a challenging matter [5].

Considering the above, the complete removal at primary surgery has been claimed as the most effective treatment [6–13], albeit this goal remains troublesome due the several tumor inner features, i.e., deep location and involvement of vital neurovascular structures—this is especially true in pediatric cases [14].

However, it should be underlined that craniopharyngiomas present high rates of recurrence even after radical resection and surgical treatment of these latter cases is more challenging with possibility of total removal decreases, ranging between 21 and 68% (mean 44.8%) [6–12, 15–17], being burdened by higher risk of incomplete resections and greater mortality and morbidity rates (0 to 41%; mean 18.8%) [6–8, 11, 12, 15, 16, 18].

The difficulties related with the surgical treatment of these tumors, particularly after recurrences, have lead surgeons to consider several alternative therapeutic modalities to achieve the long-term control of such pathology, namely radiation therapy [17, 19–32], stereotactic placement of a catheter [33, 34], intracystic radiotherapy [35–38], or chemotherapy [39].

L. M. Cavallo · D. Solari (✉) · T. Somma · C. Baiano · E. D'Avella · P. Cappabianca
Division of Neurosurgery, Università degli Studi di Napoli "Federico II", Naples, Italy
e-mail: domenico.solari@unina.it

© Springer Nature Switzerland AG 2020
E. Jouanneau, G. Raverot (eds.), *Adult Craniopharyngiomas*,
https://doi.org/10.1007/978-3-030-41176-3_8

131

Historically, several transcranial approaches have been described as possible surgical options for the treatment of craniopharyngiomas, with the use of transsphenoidal approach being reserved for those lesions, preferably with a cystic component, with a minimal supradiaphragmatic extension; besides, normal pituitary function was a contraindication for endonasal route. Recently, thanks to the evolution of surgical techniques and technology—above all to the widespread use of the endoscope—providing higher effectiveness and decreased morbidity [40–47], the endonasal corridor has been adopted to achieve the exposure of suprasellar area and though as a viable route for the removal of extrasellar craniopharyngiomas [48–62].

The endonasal technique offers a direct approach that permits access to the suprasellar, retrosellar, and retroclival space, obviating brain retraction and considering that the majority of craniopharyngiomas are midline tumors, the endonasal route provides the advantage of accessing the tumor immediately after suprasellar dural opening without optic nerve manipulation and/or retraction, through a straight surgical route [63]. This corridor is more valuable in cases of recurrent tumors after primary craniotomies, where it represents a naive route, providing the possibility to bypass the adherences and to avoid further brain manipulation [8, 64].

Based on our experience with this surgical technique, we herein details variations required to treat recurrent lesions, depending on the original surgical treatment: transcranial, transsphenoidal (standard microscopic or endoscopic) expanded endonasal approach [64], and the eventual alternative treatments.

8.2   Endoscopic Endonasal Surgical Management

The endonasal approach for the removal of craniopharyngiomas is performed using a rigid 0-degree endoscope, 18 cm in length 4 mm in diameter (Karl Storz), as the sole visualizing instrument of the surgical field; angled scope are used to further explore the suprasellar area and properly manage the lateral aspects of the lesion attached to the neurovascular structures. Dedicated surgical instruments with different angled tips are needed in order to permit movements in all the visible corners of the surgical field.

The endoscopic endonasal approach is a 2-surgeon, 3- or 4-handed technique procedure that requires a surgical team, experienced in endoscopic surgery [40, 62, 65, 66].

As any skull base procedure, the EEA for removal of craniopharyngiomas is formed of three portions: exposure, tumor resection, and reconstruction.

The patient, under general anesthesia, is placed supine (or in slight Trendelenburg position), turned 5–10° toward the surgeons (the patient's right). Before entering the endoscope, the nose is decongested with cotton pledgets soaked in a solution of 2 ml of adrenaline, 5 ml of 20% diluted lidocaine, and 4 ml of saline solution. The mid-face and the periumbilical area are prepped and draped and a third or fourth-generation cephalosporin antibiotic is administered for perioperative prophylaxis.

The procedure starts in the right nostril, where the middle turbinate is displaced laterally while in the left naris it is removed, whether the first surgeon is right handed; whether he/she is left handed the wider lateral corridor will be in the left nostril. Thereafter, a wide anterior sphenoidotomy and the posterior ethmoid air cells (bilaterally posterior ethmoidectomy) are performed to create a large single work cavity.

The harvesting of Hadad-Bassagasteguy naso-septal flap (HBF) (HBF) [67] should be performed at this point. However, we changed our attitudes and the flap is only drawn at this time: two parallel incisions are performed following the sagittal plane of the septum and joined anteriorly by a vertical cut. Elevation of the flap is realized at the end of the procedure, in order to reduce the nasal bleeding during surgery and avoid the twisting of the pedicle causing an ischemia [67].

Once the sphenoid sinus has been opened, the "3-4 hands technique" is mandatory to perform a bimanual dissection under dynamic visual control between close-up and panoramic views, provided by the in-and-out endoscope movements.

The bone removal starts with the drilling of the upper half of the sella and a complete removal of the tuberculum sellae—we named it suprasellar notch [68] according to its aspect as seen from endonasal perspective, including bilateral mOCRs is mandatory to expose the subarachnoid opticocarotid cistern in order to allow adequate suprasellar exposure for tumor resection and the identification of the subchiasmatic perforating vessels that eventually have been displaced, thus preventing devascularization of the optic nerves, chiasm, and infundibulum.

Finally, before the dura can be opened, the SIS should be coagulated with the bipolar and transected [50, 69].

The dissection and removal maneuvers in the endoscopic transsphenoidal approach for craniopharyngiomas are tailored to each lesion following the same principles and goals of transcranial microsurgery: internal debulking of the solid part and/or cystic evacuation followed by dissection from the main surrounding neurovascular structure. Nevertheless as compared to transcranial route, approaching the tumor from its ventral aspect, offers the great advantage to face the critical neurovascular structures on its dorsum and perimeter, providing direct visualization of the inferior aspect of the chiasm, the infundibulum, the third ventricle, and/or the retro and parasellar spaces.

Since craniopharyngiomas often adhere or invade the chiasm and/or hypothalamus, particularly in cases of recurrence [64], it is essential "not to force" the resection in order to preserve vital tissue integrity and function.

In case of infradiaphragmatic recurrent cystic lesion, this latter component is drained, while the solid component is to be sharply dissected from the sellar walls and/or from the suprasellar cistern trying to not damage it. Whether cyst wall dissection was not easy to obtain, due to thigh adherences and/or the eventual close relationships with the surrounding neurovascular structures, we adopted the so-called cystosphenoidostomy technique: after realizing maximum-allowed tumor removal, an "X" or "T" shaped silastic catheter was placed inside the tumor cavity, in order to create a direct communication between such cavity and the sphenoid sinus [34].

If a previous transcranial approach had been performed, the endonasal approach represents a naïve corridor. The suprasellar prechiasmatic portion of the lesion could result more troublesome to manage, due to the arachnoidal adherences, whereas the primary transcranial route did not allow reaching the most inferior and posterior portion of the tumor. This corridor provides a direct access to these portions of the lesions through the subchiasmatic and intraventricular corridors, which are along the same axis of the approach [70].

In cases in which a previous standard transsphenoidal approach has been performed, the nasal and sphenoidal steps need further refinement, and the bone opening starts at the level of the previous defect being enlarged as described previously. Concerning the tumor management, it should be considered that it is easier in case of intra-suprasellar prechiasmatic lesions because the cisternal spaces and the arachnoidal plane are intact, whereas in case of retrosellar or intraventricular craniopharyngioma it might be not, due to the presence of scar tissue. Finally, in recurrent craniopharyngiomas already operated on by the extended endonasal approach, the procedure is faster since a binostril corridor has been already created; the removal of the reconstruction material from the osteo-dural defect is the first step. Tumor removal is affected by the presence of a high concentration of arachnoidal scars but the endonasal corridor still allows the most direct route as it proceeds along to the same axis of the tumor.

After removal of the lesion, the osteo-dural defect must be accurately repaired. Reconstruction is properly achieved addressing the following principles: protection of the suprasellar cistern, filling of the "dead space," and closure of the osteo-dural defect.

In case of infradiaphragmatic lesions,, namely when the suprasellar cistern is intact collagen sponge or dural substitute foils along with fibrin glue are adopted to fill the dead space and protect it [71]. On the other hand craniopharyngiomas involving the subarachnoid space and/or third ventricle [72] require a meticulous repair of the defect after tumor removal: it starts with arachnoid sealing, continues with the closure of the osteo-dural defect, and thereafter covering of the breach and filling of the sphenoid cavity are accomplished. Different materials can be used either alone or in combination, as defined per proper techniques [73–75] and once a watertight barrier has been achieved, the pedicled naso-septal flap is placed over to enforce the reconstruction [67, 76, 77]; a further support is provided by filling the sphenoid sinus with oxidized cellulose and hemostatic sponges.

Differently from the transcranial route, the EEA provides a direct visualization of the neurovascular structures of the suprasellar region from below, avoiding any brain manipulation; this route seems to minimize the risk of postoperative visual loss, which is related to the integrity of the vascularization of the optic chiasm, especially when running a naive surgical route [64]. This different point of view gave a new understanding of tumor's position as related to the stalk and other main vital surrounding structures, nonetheless, it is not always possible to determine preoperatively these relationships, especially when dealing with large eccentric tumors.

Most of the benefits are gained when dealing with lesions whose original surgery was a transcranial approach [64], namely the surgeon will manage a "primary" tumor with a preserved arachnoidal plane and gliotic reaction and it will be possible to reach some areas like the subchiasmatic, the retrosellar, or the intraventricular in a direct way [70].

Beside these advantages, we nevertheless observed some factors, which, somehow, could affect the lesion dissection and removal, either related to the lesion and to the anatomy [40, 78, 79]. A more limited access to the suprachiasmatic areas is provided if the chiasm is anteriorly displaced, while concerning lesion-related conditions, it has to be said that encasement and adherence of neurovascular structures as one or both ICAs and/or the AcomA complex and/or optic apparatus and/or hypothalamus, could represent major concerns.

8.3 Alternative Treatment Strategies

Several other surgical techniques and/or combination of surgery with other therapeutic approaches can be taken into account for the management of recurrent craniopharyngiomas in order to achieve long-term control of the disease [24, 28, 29, 32, 34–38, 80–82]. Furthermore, the possibility of achieving a less risky subtotal resection (STR), followed by adjuvant radiation treatments has been advocated as a valid strategy [81, 83–90] backing upon the concept of safe "maximum-allowed" resection,, in accordance to patient's age, endocrine status, and preoperative goals.

Indeed, cyst drainage can be realized via a transcranial burr-hole approach with catheterization of the cyst connected to an Ommaya reservoir or with transsphenoidal insertion of the catheter into the cyst for the cyst content drainage [34] as well as wide marsupialization of the cysts into CSF spaces [91] with neuroendoscopic technique (Figs. 8.1, 8.2, and 8.3).

These techniques could be implemented with other therapeutic modalities, such as radiotherapy or, more recently, radiosurgery: the fractionated technique revealed to be the most suitable treatment [85, 86, 92–98], while stereotactic radiosurgery seems to provide favorable control rates at 5 years post-treatment [96, 99–103].

In these regards, it should be bear in mind that radiation therapy carries the risk—mostly dose-related—of secondary tumor development as well as eventual late impairment of neurological, vascular and endocrinological functions.

Therefore, a watchful waiting strategy can be adopted whether small residual tumors, adherent to neurovascular vital structures, eventually with calcified fragments, not growing, are observed at close neuroradiological follow-up;

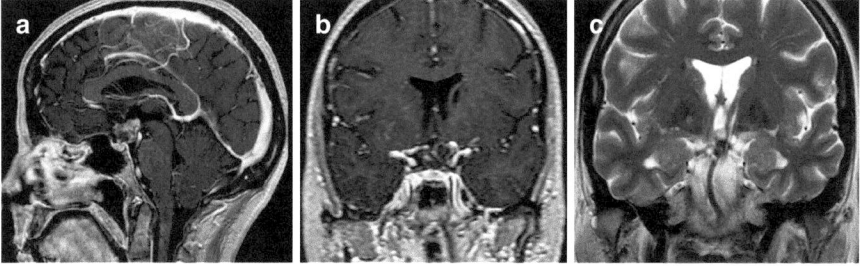

Fig. 8.1 Image showing the preoperative sagittal (**a**) and coronal (**b**) MRI scans of a recurrent retrosellar craniopharyngioma. Primary tumor was predominantly cystic, so that patient already underwent surgery via a transcranial burr-hole approach: cyst drainage was achieved and a catheter piercing the cyst and the third ventricle floor—the tip reaches the interpeduncular cistern (arrow)-connected to a Rickham reservoir was placed (**c**)

Fig. 8.2 Intraoperative endoscopic pictures showing the surgical cavity exploration after tumor removal. A close-up view of the retrosellar space discloses the tip of the catheter—placed at primary surgery—next to the basilar artery trunk and covered by the same arachnoidal bundles inside the interpeduncular cistern. A small residual tumor is observed within the floor of the third ventricle (asterisk)

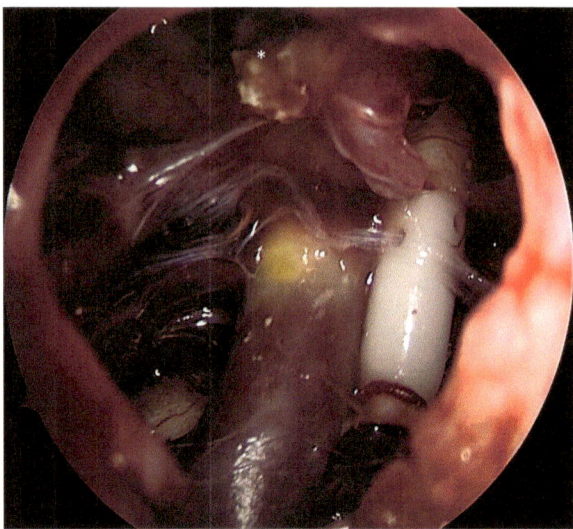

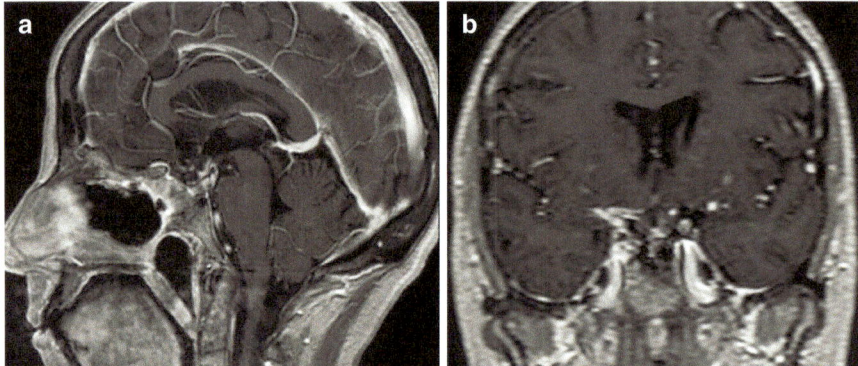

Fig. 8.3 Image showing the postoperative sagittal (**a**) and coronal (**b**) MRI scans of the recurrent retrosellar craniopharyngioma treated via endoscopic endonasal transplanum approach. A small remnant of the lesion can be identified infiltrating the third ventricle floor

contrariwise, in case of rapidly growing residual tumors an early second surgical procedure can be preferred prior than radiotherapy to achieve relief from mass effect symptoms [88, 90, 104, 105].

Several groups adopted the use of intralesional therapies, especially in pediatric patients, administered in the attempt of postponing or sparing the adverse effects of surgery—above all for the hypophyseal and hypothalamic functions—and/or avoid radiotherapy. The management of recurrent craniopharyngiomas via stereotactic aspiration of the cystic component with the instillation of antibiotics, radionucleo-tides, and/or cell-cycle inhibitors resulted in successful and effective minimally invasive strategies of treatment [106–112] (Fig. 8.4).

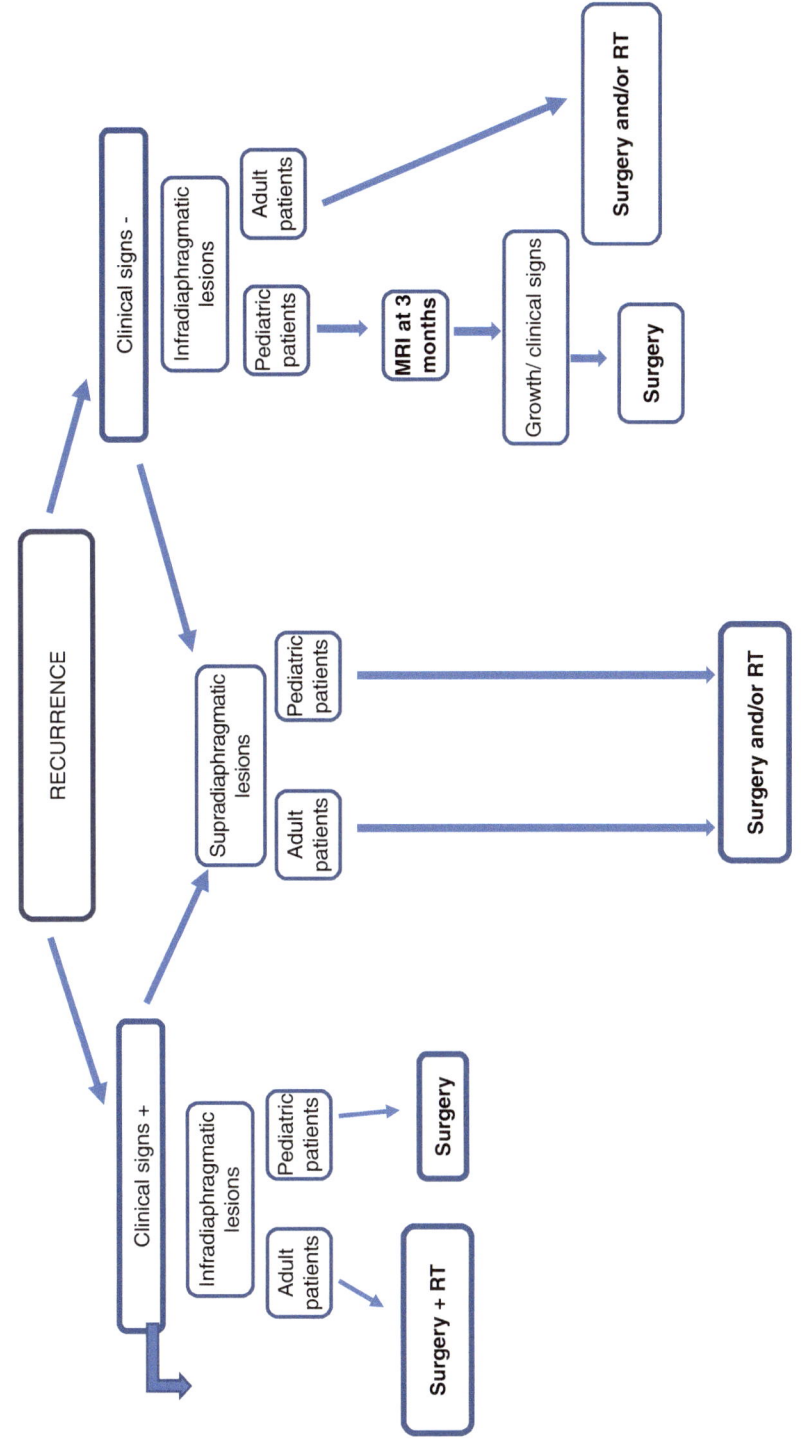

Fig. 8.4 Diagram illustrates alternative treatment strategies for recurrent craniopharyngiomas

Nowadays, upon the identification of exclusive clonal driver mutations in CTNNB1 [113–115] and BRAF genes [116] in the vast majority of ACPs and PCPs, targeted therapy—combined BRAF and MEK-targeted—have found effective in case of recurrent papillary craniopharyngioma with genetically confirmed BRAFV600E mutation [117].

It stands clear that treatment of recurrent craniopharyngiomas should back upon a multidisciplinary management; many adjuvant therapies have been found viable and effective: single treatment should not be considered definitive, and each of them has to be intended as a proper asset of a tailored management strategy.

References

1. Jane JA Jr, Laws ER. Craniopharyngioma. Pituitary. 2006;9(4):323–6.
2. Lewin R, Ruffolo E, Saraceno C. Craniopharyngioma arising in the pharyngeal hypophysis. South Med J. 1984;77(12):1519–23.
3. Bunin GR, Surawicz TS, Witman PA, Preston-Martin S, Davis F, Bruner JM. The descriptive epidemiology of craniopharyngioma. J Neurosurg. 1998;89(4):547–51.
4. Haupt R, Magnani C, Pavanello M, Caruso S, Dama E, Garre ML. Epidemiological aspects of craniopharyngioma. J Pediatr Endocrinol Metab. 2006;19(Suppl 1):289–93.
5. Cappabianca P, Cavallo LM, Esposito F, De Divitiis E. Craniopharyngiomas. J Neurosurg. 2008;109(1):1–3.
6. Fahlbusch R, Honegger J, Paulus W, Huk W, Buchfelder M. Surgical treatment of craniopharyngiomas: experience with 168 patients. J Neurosurg. 1999;90(2):237–50.
7. Hoffman HJ. Surgical management of craniopharyngioma. Pediatr Neurosurg. 1994;21(Suppl 1):44–9.
8. Minamida Y, Mikami T, Hashi K, Houkin K. Surgical management of the recurrence and regrowth of craniopharyngiomas. J Neurosurg. 2005;103(2):224–32.
9. Samii M, Bini W. Surgical treatment of craniopharyngiomas. Zentralbl Neurochir. 1991;52(1):17–23.
10. Symon L, Sprich W. Radical excision of craniopharyngioma. Results in 20 patients. J Neurosurg. 1985;62(2):174–81.
11. Van Effenterre R, Boch AL. Craniopharyngioma in adults and children: a study of 122 surgical cases. J Neurosurg. 2002;97(1):3–11.
12. Yasargil MG, Curcic M, Kis M, Siegenthaler G, Teddy PJ, Roth P. Total removal of craniopharyngiomas. Approaches and long-term results in 144 patients. J Neurosurg. 1990;73(1):3–11.
13. Zuccaro G. Radical resection of craniopharyngioma. Childs Nerv Syst. 2005;21(8–9):679–90.
14. Puget S, Garnett M, Wray A, Grill J, Habrand JL, Bodaert N, et al. Pediatric craniopharyngiomas: classification and treatment according to the degree of hypothalamic involvement. J Neurosurg. 2007;106(1 Suppl):3–12.
15. Wisoff JH. Surgical management of recurrent craniopharyngiomas. Pediatr Neurosurg. 1994;21(Suppl 1):108–13.
16. Caldarelli M, di Rocco C, Papacci F, Colosimo C Jr. Management of recurrent craniopharyngioma. Acta Neurochir. 1998;140(5):447–54.
17. Sung DI. Treatment results of craniopharyngiomas. Cancer. 1981;47:847–52.
18. Weiner HL, Wisoff JH, Rosenberg ME, Kupersmith MJ, Cohen H, Zagzag D, et al. Craniopharyngiomas: a clinicopathological analysis of factors predictive of recurrence and functional outcome. Neurosurgery. 1994;35(6):1001–10; discussion 10–11.
19. Baskin DS, Wilson CB. Surgical management of craniopharyngiomas. A review of 74 cases. J Neurosurg. 1986;65(1):22–7.

20. Cabezudo JM, Vaquero J, Areitio E, Martinez R, de Sola RG, Bravo G. Craniopharyngiomas: a critical approach to treatment. J Neurosurg. 1981;55(3):371–5.
21. Carmel PW, Antunes JL, Chang CH. Craniopharyngiomas in children. Neurosurgery. 1982;11(3):382–9.
22. Choux M, Lena G, Genitori L. Le craniopharyngiome de l'enfant. Neurochirurgie. 1991;37:132–43.
23. Duffner PK, Cohen ME, Parker MS. Prospective intellectual testing in children with brain tumors. Ann Neurol. 1988;23(6):575–9.
24. Fischer EG, Welch K, Shillito J Jr, Winston KR, Tarbell NJ. Craniopharyngiomas in children. Long-term effects of conservative surgical procedures combined with radiation therapy. J Neurosurg. 1990;73(4):534–40.
25. Hoogenhout J, Otten BJ, Kazem I, Stoelinga GB, Walder AH. Surgery and radiation therapy in the management of craniopharyngiomas. Int J Radiat Oncol Biol Phys. 1984;10(12):2293–7.
26. Kalapurakal JA, Goldman S, Hsieh YC, Tomita T, Marymont MH. Clinical outcome in children with recurrent craniopharyngioma after primary surgery. Cancer J. 2000;6(6):388–93.
27. Pierre-Kahn A, Brauner R, Renier D, Sainte-Rose C, Gangemi MA, Rappaport R, et al. Treatment of craniopharyngiomas in children. Retrospective analysis of 50 cases. Arch Fr Pediatr. 1988;45(3):163–7.
28. Regine WF, Mohiuddin M, Kramer S. Long-term results of pediatric and adult craniopharyngiomas treated with combined surgery and radiation. Radiother Oncol. 1993;27(1):13–21.
29. Scott RM, Hetelekidis S, Barnes PD, Goumnerova L, Tarbell NJ. Surgery, radiation, and combination therapy in the treatment of childhood craniopharyngioma--a 20-year experience. Pediatr Neurosurg. 1994;21(Suppl 1):75–81.
30. Thomsett MJ, Conte FA, Kaplan SL, Grumbach MM. Endocrine and neurologic outcome in childhood craniopharyngioma: review of effect of treatment in 42 patients. J Pediatr. 1980;97(5):728–35.
31. Tomita T, Bowman RM. Craniopharyngiomas in children: surgical experience at children's memorial hospital. Childs Nerv Syst. 2005;21(8–9):729–46.
32. Weiss M, Sutton L, Marcial V, Fowble B, Packer R, Zimmerman R, et al. The role of radiation therapy in the management of childhood craniopharyngioma. Int J Radiat Oncol Biol Phys. 1989;17(6):1313–21.
33. Spaziante R, de Divitiis E. Drainage techniques for cystic craniopharyngiomas. Neurosurg Quart. 1997;7:183–208.
34. Spaziante R, de Divitiis E, Irace C, Cappabianca P, Caputi F. Management of primary or recurring grossly cystic craniopharyngiomas by means of draining systems. Topic review and 6 case reports. Acta Neurochir. 1989;97(3–4):95–106.
35. Julow J, Lanyi F, Hajda M, Szeifert G, Simkovics M, Toth S, et al. Further experiences in the treatment of cystic craniopharyngeomas with yttrium 90 silicate colloid. Acta Neurochir Suppl. 1988;42:113–9.
36. Backlund EO. Treatment of craniopharyngiomas: the multimodality approach. Pediatr Neurosurg. 1994;21(Suppl 1):82–9.
37. Munari C, Landre E, Musolino A, Turak B, Habert MO, Chodkiewicz JP. Long term results of stereotactic endocavitary beta irradiation of craniopharyngioma cysts. J Neurosurg Sci. 1989;33(1):99–105.
38. Pollock BE, Lunsford LD, Kondziolka D, Levine G, Flickinger JC. Phosphorus-32 intracavitary irradiation of cystic craniopharyngiomas: current technique and long-term results. Int J Radiat Oncol Biol Phys. 1995;33(2):437–46.
39. Hargrave DR. Does chemotherapy have a role in the management of craniopharyngioma? J Pediatr Endocrinol Metab. 2006;19(Suppl 1):407–12.
40. de Divitiis E, Cavallo LM, Cappabianca P, Esposito F. Extended endoscopic endonasal transsphenoidal approach for the removal of suprasellar tumors: part 2. Neurosurgery. 2007;60(1):46–58; discussion 9.
41. Delashaw JB Jr, Tedeschi H, Rhoton AL. Modified supraorbital craniotomy: technical note. Neurosurgery. 1992;30(6):954–6.

42. Fatemi N, Dusick JR, de Paiva Neto MA, Malkasian D, Kelly DF. Endonasal versus supraorbital keyhole removal of craniopharyngiomas and tuberculum sellae meningiomas. Neurosurgery 2009;64(5 Suppl 2):269–284; discussion 84–6.
43. Fahlbusch R, Schott W. Pterional surgery of meningiomas of the tuberculum sellae and planum sphenoidale: surgical results with special consideration of ophthalmological and endocrinological outcomes. J Neurosurg. 2002;96(2):235–43.
44. Goel A, Muzumdar D, Desai KI. Tuberculum sellae meningioma: a report on management on the basis of a surgical experience with 70 patients. Neurosurgery. 2002;51(6):1358–63; discussion 63–4.
45. Jallo GI, Benjamin V. Tuberculum sellae meningiomas: microsurgical anatomy and surgical technique. Neurosurgery. 2002;51(6):1432–9. discussion 9–40.
46. Jarrahy R, Cha ST, Berci G, Shahinian HK. Endoscopic transglabellar approach to the anterior fossa and paranasal sinuses. J Craniofac Surg. 2000;11(5):412–7.
47. Reisch R, Perneczky A. Ten-year experience with the supraorbital subfrontal approach through an eyebrow skin incision. Neurosurgery. 2005;57(4 Suppl):242–55.
48. Laws ER Jr. Transsphenoidal microsurgery in the management of craniopharyngioma. J Neurosurg. 1980;52(5):661–6.
49. Laws ER Jr. Transsphenoidal removal of craniopharyngioma. Pediatr Neurosurg. 1994;21(Suppl 1):57–63.
50. de Divitiis E, Cappabianca P, Cavallo LM, Esposito F, de Divitiis O, Messina A. Extended endoscopic transsphenoidal approach for extrasellar craniopharyngiomas. Neurosurgery. 2007;61(5 Suppl 2):219–27; discussion 28.
51. de Divitiis E, Cappabianca P, Cavallo LM. Endoscopic transsphenoidal approach: adaptability of the procedure to different sellar lesions. Neurosurgery. 2002;51(3):699–705; discussion 7.
52. Frank G, Pasquini E, Mazzatenta D. Extended transsphenoidal approach. J Neurosurg. 2001;95(5):917–8.
53. Honegger J, Buchfelder M, Fahlbusch R, Daubler B, Dorr HG. Transsphenoidal microsurgery for craniopharyngioma. Surg Neurol. 1992;37(3):189–96.
54. Jho HD, Ha HG. Endoscopic endonasal skull base surgery: part 1--the midline anterior fossa skull base. Minim Invasive Neurosurg. 2004;47(1):1–8.
55. Kaptain GJ, Vincent DA, Sheehan JP, Laws ER Jr. Transsphenoidal approaches for the extracapsular resection of midline suprasellar and anterior cranial base lesions. Neurosurgery. 2001;49(1):94–101.
56. Kato T, Sawamura Y, Abe H, Nagashima M. Transsphenoidal-transtuberculum sellae approach for supradiaphragmatic tumours: technical note. Acta Neurochir. 1998;140(7):715–9.
57. Kim J, Choe I, Bak K, Kim C, Kim N, Jang Y. Transsphenoidal supradiaphragmatic intradural approach: technical note. Minim Invasive Neurosurg. 2000;43(1):33–7.
58. Kitano M, Taneda M. Extended transsphenoidal approach with submucosal posterior ethmoidectomy for parasellar tumors. Technical note. J Neurosurg. 2001;94(6):999–1004.
59. Kouri JG, Chen MY, Watson JC, Oldfield EH. Resection of suprasellar tumors by using a modified transsphenoidal approach. Report of four cases. J Neurosurg. 2000;92(6):1028–35.
60. Romano A, Zuccarello M, van Loveren HR, Keller JT. Expanding the boundaries of the transsphenoidal approach: a microanatomic study. Clin Anat. 2001;14(1):1–9.
61. Weiss MH. The transnasal transsphenoidal approach. In: Apuzzo MLJ, editor. Surgery of the third ventricle. Baltimore: Williams & Wilkins; 1987. p. 476–94.
62. Cappabianca P, Cavallo LM, Esposito F, de Divitiis O, Messina A, de Divitiis E. Extended endoscopic endonasal approach to the midline skull base: the evolving role of transsphenoidal surgery. In: Pickard JD, Akalan N, Di Rocco C, Dolenc VV, Lobo Antunes J, Mooij JJA, et al., editors. Advances and technical standards in neurosurgery. Wien, New York: Springer; 2008. p. 152–99.
63. Kassam AB, Prevedello DM, Thomas A, Gardner P, Mintz A, Snyderman C, et al. Endoscopic endonasal pituitary transposition for a transdorsum sellae approach to the interpeduncular cistern. Neurosurgery. 2008;62(3 Suppl 1):57–72; discussion 4.

64. Cavallo LM, Prevedello DM, Solari D, Gardner PA, Esposito F, Snyderman CH, et al. Extended endoscopic endonasal transsphenoidal approach for residual or recurrent craniopharyngiomas. J Neurosurg. 2009;111(3):578–89.
65. Prevedello DM, Kassam AB, Snyderman C, Carrau RL, Mintz AH, Thomas A, et al. Endoscopic cranial base surgery: ready for prime time? Clin Neurosurg. 2007;54:48–57.
66. Kassam A. Fully endoscopic endonasal resection of parasellar craniopharyngiomas: an early experience and review of literature. Skull Base. 2004;(abstract);12 Suppl I(21).
67. Hadad G, Bassagasteguy L, Carrau RL, Mataza JC, Kassam A, Snyderman CH, et al. A novel reconstructive technique after endoscopic expanded endonasal approaches: vascular pedicle nasoseptal flap. Laryngoscope. 2006;116(10):1882–6.
68. de Notaris M, Solari D, Cavallo LM, D'Enza AI, Ensenat J, Berenguer J, et al. The "suprasellar notch," or the tuberculum sellae as seen from below: definition, features, and clinical implications from an endoscopic endonasal perspective. J Neurosurg. 2012;116(3):622–9.
69. Kassam AB, Gardner PA, Snyderman CH, Carrau RL, Mintz AH, Prevedello DM. Expanded endonasal approach, a fully endoscopic transnasal approach for the resection of midline suprasellar craniopharyngiomas: a new classification based on the infundibulum. J Neurosurg. 2008;108(4):715–28.
70. Cavallo LM, de Divitiis O, Aydin S, Messina A, Esposito F, Iaconetta G, et al. Extended endoscopic endonasal transsphenoidal approach to the suprasellar area: anatomic considerations - part 1. Neurosurgery. 2007;61:ONS-24-ONS-34.
71. Cappabianca P, Esposito F, Magro F, Cavallo LM, Solari D, Stella L, et al. Natura abhorret a vacuo--use of fibrin glue as a filler and sealant in neurosurgical "dead spaces". Technical note. Acta Neurochir. 2010;152(5):897–904.
72. Zanation AM, Carrau RL, Snyderman CH, McKinney KA, Wheless SA, Bhatki AM, et al. Nasoseptal flap takedown and reuse in revision endoscopic skull base reconstruction. Laryngoscope. 2011;121(1):42–6.
73. Cavallo LM, Messina A, Esposito F, de Divitiis O, Dal Fabbro M, de Divitiis E, et al. Skull base reconstruction in the extended endoscopic transsphenoidal approach for suprasellar lesions. J Neurosurg. 2007;107(4):713–20.
74. Esposito F, Dusick JR, Fatemi N, Kelly DF. Graded repair of cranial base defects and cerebrospinal fluid leaks in transsphenoidal surgery. Neurosurgery. 2007;60(4 Suppl 2):295–303; discussion 4.
75. Leng LZ, Brown S, Anand VK, Schwartz TH. "Gasket-seal" watertight closure in minimal-access endoscopic cranial base surgery. Neurosurgery. 2008;62(5 Suppl 2).:ONSE342–3; discussion ONSE3.
76. Kassam A, Carrau RL, Snyderman CH, Gardner P, Mintz A. Evolution of reconstructive techniques following endoscopic expanded endonasal approaches. Neurosurg Focus. 2005;19(1):E8.
77. Kassam AB, Thomas A, Carrau RL, Snyderman CH, Vescan A, Prevedello D, et al. Endoscopic reconstruction of the cranial base using a pedicled nasoseptal flap. Neurosurgery. 2008;63(1 Suppl 1):ONS44–52; discussion ONS-ONS3.
78. Gardner PA, Kassam AB, Snyderman CH, Carrau RL, Mintz AH, Grahovac S, et al. Outcomes following endoscopic, expanded endonasal resection of suprasellar craniopharyngiomas: a case series. J Neurosurg. 2008;109(1):6–16.
79. Cappabianca P, Frank G, Pasquini E, de Divitiis O, Calbucci F. Extended endoscopic endonasal transsphenoidal approaches to the suprasellar region, planum sphenoidale and clivus. In: de Divitiis E, Cappabianca P, editors. Endoscopic endonasal transsphenoidal surgery. New York: Springer; 2003. p. 176–87.
80. Hussain I, Eloy JA, Carmel PW, Liu JK. Molecular oncogenesis of craniopharyngioma: current and future strategies for the development of targeted therapies. J Neurosurg. 2013;119(1):106–12.
81. Laws ER Jr, Vance ML. Radiosurgery for pituitary tumors and craniopharyngiomas. Neurosurg Clin N Am. 1999;10(2):327–36.

82. Lin LL, El Naqa I, Leonard JR, Park TS, Hollander AS, Michalski JM, et al. Long-term outcome in children treated for craniopharyngioma with and without radiotherapy. J Neurosurg Pediatr. 2008;1(2):126–30.
83. Chung WY, Pan DH, Shiau CY, Guo WY, Wang LW. Gamma knife radiosurgery for craniopharyngiomas. J Neurosurg. 2000;93(Suppl 3):47–56.
84. Kobayashi T, Kida Y, Hasegawa T. Long-term results of gamma knife surgery for craniopharyngioma. Neurosurg Focus. 2003;14(5):e13.
85. Minniti G, Saran F, Traish D, Soomal R, Sardell S, Gonsalves A, et al. Fractionated stereotactic conformal radiotherapy following conservative surgery in the control of craniopharyngiomas. Radiother Oncol. 2007;82(1):90–5.
86. Schulz-Ertner D, Frank C, Herfarth KK, Rhein B, Wannenmacher M, Debus J. Fractionated stereotactic radiotherapy for craniopharyngiomas. Int J Radiat Oncol Biol Phys. 2002;54(4):1114–20.
87. Ulfarsson E, Lindquist C, Roberts M, Rahn T, Lindquist M, Thoren M, et al. Gamma knife radiosurgery for craniopharyngiomas: long-term results in the first Swedish patients. J Neurosurg. 2002;97(5 Suppl):613–22.
88. Cavallo LM, Frank G, Cappabianca P, Solari D, Mazzatenta D, Villa A, et al. The endoscopic endonasal approach for the management of craniopharyngiomas: a series of 103 patients. J Neurosurg. 2014;121(1):100–13.
89. Koutourousiou M, Gardner PA, Fernandez-Miranda JC, Tyler-Kabara EC, Wang EW, Snyderman CH. Endoscopic endonasal surgery for craniopharyngiomas: surgical outcome in 64 patients. J Neurosurg. 2013;119(5):1194–207.
90. Leng LZ, Greenfield JP, Souweidane MM, Anand VK, Schwartz TH. Endoscopic, endonasal resection of craniopharyngiomas: analysis of outcome including extent of resection, cerebrospinal fluid leak, return to preoperative productivity, and body mass index. Neurosurgery. 2012;70(1):110–23; discussion 23–4.
91. Delitala A, Brunori A, Chiappetta F. Purely neuroendoscopic transventricular management of cystic craniopharyngiomas. Childs Nerv Syst. 2004;20(11–12):858–62.
92. Combs SE, Thilmann C, Huber PE, Hoess A, Debus J, Schulz-Ertner D. Achievement of long-term local control in patients with craniopharyngiomas using high precision stereotactic radiotherapy. Cancer. 2007;109(11):2308–14.
93. Varlotto JM, Flickinger JC, Kondziolka D, Lunsford LD, Deutsch M. External beam irradiation of craniopharyngiomas: long-term analysis of tumor control and morbidity. Int J Radiat Oncol Biol Phys. 2002;54(2):492–9.
94. Minniti G, Esposito V, Amichetti M, Enrici RM. The role of fractionated radiotherapy and radiosurgery in the management of patients with craniopharyngioma. Neurosurg Rev. 2009;32(2):125–32; discussion 32.
95. Cavallo LM, Solari D, Esposito F, Villa A, Minniti G, Cappabianca P. The role of the endoscopic endonasal route in the management of craniopharyngiomas. World Neurosurg. 2014;82(6 Suppl):S32–40.
96. Aggarwal A, Fersht N, Brada M. Radiotherapy for craniopharyngioma. Pituitary. 2013;16(1):26–33.
97. Moon SH, Kim IH, Park SW, Kim I, Hong S, Park CI, et al. Early adjuvant radiotherapy toward long-term survival and better quality of life for craniopharyngiomas--a study in single institute. Childs Nerv Syst. 2005;21(8–9):799–807.
98. Stripp DC, Maity A, Janss AJ, Belasco JB, Tochner ZA, Goldwein JW, et al. Surgery with or without radiation therapy in the management of craniopharyngiomas in children and young adults. Int J Radiat Oncol Biol Phys. 2004;58(3):714–20.
99. Chiou SM, Lunsford LD, Niranjan A, Kondziolka D, Flickinger JC. Stereotactic radiosurgery of residual or recurrent craniopharyngioma, after surgery, with or without radiation therapy. Neuro-Oncology. 2001;3(3):159–66.
100. Jackson AS, St George EJ, Hayward RJ, Plowman PN. Stereotactic radiosurgery. XVII: recurrent intrasellar craniopharyngioma. Br J Neurosurg. 2003;17(2):138–43.

101. Iannalfi A, Fragkandrea I, Brock J, Saran F. Radiotherapy in craniopharyngiomas. Clin Oncol. 2013;25(11):654–67.
102. Veeravagu A, Lee M, Jiang B, Chang SD. The role of radiosurgery in the treatment of cranio-pharyngiomas. Neurosurg Focus. 2010;28(4):E11.
103. Jeon C, Kim S, Shin HJ, Nam DH, Lee JI, Park K, et al. The therapeutic efficacy of fraction-ated radiotherapy and gamma-knife radiosurgery for craniopharyngiomas. J Clin Neurosci. 2011;18(12):1621–5.
104. Gardner PA, Prevedello DM, Kassam AB, Snyderman CH, Carrau RL, Mintz AH. The evolu-tion of the endonasal approach for craniopharyngiomas. J Neurosurg. 2008;108(5):1043–7.
105. Turel MK, Tsermoulas G, Gonen L, Klironomos G, Almeida JP, Zadeh G, et al. Management and outcome of recurrent adult craniopharyngiomas: an analysis of 42 cases with long-term follow-up. Neurosurg Focus. 2016;41(6):E11.
106. Derrey S, Blond S, Reyns N, Touzet G, Carpentier P, Gauthier H, et al. Management of cystic craniopharyngiomas with stereotactic endocavitary irradiation using colloidal 186Re: a ret-rospective study of 48 consecutive patients. Neurosurgery. 2008;63(6):1045–52; discussion 52–3.
107. Hasegawa T, Kondziolka D, Hadjipanayis CG, Lunsford LD. Management of cystic cranio-pharyngiomas with phosphorus-32 intracavitary irradiation. Neurosurgery. 2004;54(4):813–20; discussion 20–2.
108. Hukin J, Steinbok P, Lafay-Cousin L, Hendson G, Strother D, Mercier C, et al. Intracystic bleomycin therapy for craniopharyngioma in children: the Canadian experience. Cancer. 2007;109(10):2124–31.
109. Julow J, Backlund EO, Lanyi F, Hajda M, Balint K, Nyary I, et al. Long-term results and late complications after intracavitary yttrium-90 colloid irradiation of recurrent cystic craniopha-ryngiomas. Neurosurgery. 2007;61(2):288–95; discussion 95–6.
110. Cavalheiro S, Dastoli PA, Silva NS, Toledo S, Lederman H, da Silva MC. Use of inter-feron alpha in intratumoral chemotherapy for cystic craniopharyngioma. Childs Nerv Syst. 2005;21(8–9):719–24.
111. Mallucci C, Pizer B, Blair J, Didi M, Doss A, Upadrasta S, et al. Management of cranio-pharyngioma: the Liverpool experience following the introduction of the CCLG guidelines. Introducing a new risk assessment grading system. Childs Nerv Syst. 2012;28(8):1181–92.
112. Liu W, Fang Y, Cai B, Xu J, You C, Zhang H. Intracystic bleomycin for cystic craniopharyn-giomas in children (abridged republication of Cochrane systematic review). Neurosurgery. 2012;71(5):909–15.
113. Sekine S, Shibata T, Kokubu A, Morishita Y, Noguchi M, Nakanishi Y, et al. Craniopharyngiomas of adamantinomatous type harbor beta-catenin gene mutations. Am J Pathol. 2002;161(6):1997–2001.
114. Hofmann BM, Kreutzer J, Saeger W, Buchfelder M, Blumcke I, Fahlbusch R, et al. Nuclear beta-catenin accumulation as reliable marker for the differentiation between cystic cranio-pharyngiomas and Rathke cleft cysts: a clinico-pathologic approach. Am J Surg Pathol. 2006;30(12):1595–603.
115. Holsken A, Stache C, Schlaffer SM, Flitsch J, Fahlbusch R, Buchfelder M, et al. Adamantinomatous craniopharyngiomas express tumor stem cell markers in cells with acti-vated Wnt signaling: further evidence for the existence of a tumor stem cell niche? Pituitary. 2014;17(6):546–56.
116. Martinez-Gutierrez JC, D'Andrea MR, Cahill DP, Santagata S, Barker FG 2nd, Brastianos PK. Diagnosis and management of craniopharyngiomas in the era of genomics and targeted therapy. Neurosurg Focus. 2016;41(6):E2.
117. Brastianos PK, Taylor-Weiner A, Manley PE, Jones RT, Dias-Santagata D, Thorner AR, et al. Exome sequencing identifies BRAF mutations in papillary craniopharyngiomas. Nat Genet. 2014;46(2):161–5.

Craniopharyngioma: Endocrinological Aspects After Surgery

Mirela Diana Ilie and Gérald Raverot

Craniopharyngioma (CP), a midline epithelial tumor arising on the path of the craniopharyngeal duct (most commonly in the sellar and parasellar region), often has an infiltrative tendency and an aggressive behavior that is responsible for significant mortality and morbidity [1, 2]. Amongst the complications of CP, hypopituitarism, defined as complete or partial deficiency of at least one pituitary hormone, is in itself associated with significant morbidity and excess mortality. The risk factors for increased mortality in hypopituitary patients include: a diagnosis of CP, transcranial surgery, radiation therapy, hypogonadism, and diabetes insipidus (DI) [3].

Given the origin of CP and its localization and infiltrative nature, it would be expected that hypopituitarism would be frequently encountered preoperatively and be aggravated by the surgical treatment. Indeed, preoperatively more than 75% of these patients have at least one hormonal deficiency, with the most frequent deficiencies being growth hormone deficiency (GHD) and central hypogonadism [4]. Direct surgical insults during the surgical treatment, or rarer, postoperative hemorrhage or ischemia, may either exacerbate existing hypothalamic-pituitary dysfunction or create new endocrine deficiencies, with notably DI being a common complication of CP surgery [4, 5]. The recovery of preoperative pituitary deficiencies is relatively rare in CP [4], but generally speaking, in regard to pituitary surgery, the recovery rate of hypopituitarism is higher at 1 year compared with 3 months after surgery [5].

M. D. Ilie · G. Raverot (✉)
Fédération d'Endocrinologie, Groupement Hospitalier Est,
Centre de Référence Maladies Rares Hypophysaires (HYPO), Bron Cedex, France

Université Lyon 1, Lyon, France
e-mail: gerald.raverot@chu-lyon.fr

© Springer Nature Switzerland AG 2020
E. Jouanneau, G. Raverot (eds.), *Adult Craniopharyngiomas*,
https://doi.org/10.1007/978-3-030-41176-3_9

145

In this chapter, we will focus on the diagnosis and treatment of new-onset deficiencies appearing after the surgical treatment of adult CP and give key advice on how to improve the endocrinological management of these patients.

9.1   Central DI and SIADH

In major surgical series of CP, the reported incidence of postoperative DI varies from 4% to 100%, with authors reporting either higher or similar rates of postoperative DI when using the transcranial approach compared to the transsphenoidal approach [4]. In any case, DI remains the most frequent surgical complication, with a transient course in more than half of the patients [6].

DI usually occurs in the first 2 days postoperatively and it can sometimes evolve in a triphasic pattern: an initial polyuric phase, a second phase corresponding to the syndrome of inappropriate antidiuretic hormone secretion (SIADH) that usually develops between days 4–10 postoperatively and lasts for 2–5 days, and a final, and usually chronic, polyuric phase that returns in a matter of weeks [5, 7]. Conversely, the SIADH phase may not be present and DI may evolve in a single phase [7].

Diagnosis and monitoring include measurement of daily fluid intake and urinary output (polyuria being when >50 mL per kg of body weight per day), measurements of serum sodium and serum osmolarity (high or normal in DI) and of urine specific gravity (typically ≤1.005) or urine osmolality (<300 mOsm/kg) [4, 5, 7, 8].

For the treatment of the initial phase of DI, replacement therapy should be on an as-needed basis in order to avoid iatrogenic hyponatremia, especially that DI may revert to SIADH [4, 5, 8]. Some authors advise administering short acting subcutaneous vasopressin rather than desmopressin for this initial phase [5, 8], while others advise against administering antidiuretic hormone substitutes too early, because treating overhydration may be more difficult than managing established DI [6]. Many patients may not require any therapy as long as they are able to drink to their thirst and are normonatremic [7].

SIADH, characterized by euvolemic hyponatremia due to excess ADH release, can either be part of the triphasic phase of the DI or it can appear isolated, in the absence of DI, and it may be heightened by concomitant hypocortisolism [5]. The serum sodium level should be checked around days 5–8 postoperatively [7]. Mild hyponatremia (134–125 mmol/L) can be treated, in an outpatient setting, by stopping the vasopressin/desmopressin and with fluid restriction and subsequently monitored by performing frequent sodium checks [5]. Severe or symptomatic hyponatremia (usually <125 mmol/L) requires hospitalization for more aggressive management, which includes fluid restriction, hypertonic saline, or even vasopressin receptor antagonist drugs [5, 7].

The chronic phase of DI is treated with desmopressin orally, sublingually, or intranasally [5], (the intranasal form not generally being used until after the nose has healed and nasal congestion has improved [7]). The adaptation of the treatment is done depending on clinical evolution and individualized to the patient's needs: some patients who have only partial DI may even choose not to take any treatment if polyuria does not bother them, while for the rest of the patients, one should use the lowest dose of desmopressin that allows a good night's sleep and minimal disruption of activities during the daytime [8]. Patients should be advised to only drink to their thirst [5] and be educated on the signs and symptoms suggestive of reduced effectiveness of the treatment, such as increased thirst and increased urinary output, as well as the signs and symptoms suggestive of overdose such as headache, fatigue, and low urinary output [9]. Biochemical monitoring consists of measurement of serum sodium and urea levels [9]. If DI does occur postoperatively, patients should also be advised that during the first months after surgery they should periodically (every couple of weeks), or at least once, interrupt desmopressin treatment in order to check whether it is still required [5, 8].

9.1.1 The Particular Case of Adipsic DI

Adipsic DI is a very rare condition, consisting of the coexistence of DI and of adipsia (loss of the thirst perception) and has been described to occur, both preoperatively and postoperatively in CP cases [10]. There have also been both pediatric and adult cases of adipsic DI reported following surgery for CP, where patients regained their thirst perception, despite persistence of DI, within months (in the pediatric cases) or years (in the adult cases) after surgery [11, 12].

Compared to isolated DI where the thirst perception is preserved preventing hypernatremic dehydration, in the case of adipsic DI, there is a risk of significant hypernatremia if the patient is undertreated or during acute medical illnesses such as infection or vomiting. Conversely, there is also a risk of hyponatremia if the patient drinks excessively and/or is overtreated [10, 13, 14]. Both hyponatremia and hypernatremia can result in lethargy, weakness, irritability, nausea, vomiting, seizures, coma, and even death [13]. Moreover, a high rate of venous thromboembolism occurs as a complication of hypernatremic dehydration [10, 14]. Therefore, the management of adipsic DI represents a major clinical challenge [10].

Being a very rare disease, no established guidelines are available. The recommendations made by several experienced teams [10, 13, 14] are congruent and consist of:

1. Advise patients to have about 1.5–2 liters of fluid intake daily and start desmopressin at least twice daily, titrating the fluid intake/desmopressin to achieve eunatremia on an inpatient basis.
2. Determine the weight of the patient while euvolemic and normonatremic.
3. Advise patients to carry out daily weight measurements and that the patient adjusts their daily fluid intake in order to maintain his/her normonatremic weight. For example, if he/she is 1 kg below the normonatremic weight, to replace the deficit with an equivalent volume of fluid, i.e., to drink an additional 1 liter of fluid. However, Cuesta et al. [10] warn that patients show poor compliance with the daily weighing regimen and we personally fear that, especially in obese patients, the daily weight measurements may not be accurate enough to correctly detect small variations.

4. Plasma sodium level be regularly measured.
5. Educate the patient and his/her family on principles of water balance and management, for example, increasing fluid intake in times of increased exercise or increased ambient temperature.

Prophylactic anticoagulation therapy during episodes of hypernatremic dehydration has also been recommended by various authors [10, 14].

9.2   Central Adrenal Insufficiency

Patients with adrenal insufficiency (AI) already diagnosed before surgery should receive stress-dose glucocorticoids (GCs) both peri- and postoperatively [7]. As the chances of AI recovery after surgery are very low, a single postoperative morning cortisol can be enough to confirm persistent AI [5]. Interpretation depends on the authors and on the cortisol assays employed, but a cortisol level >14.5 to 15 µg/dL makes AI improbable [8, 15]. Newer assays will most probably modify this cut-off value in the future. It is important to bear in mind that for patients already on GCs, biochemical testing should be performed after waiting at least 18–24 h following the last dose of hydrocortisone (HC) or after an even longer period of time depending on the synthetic GCs used for substitution [8].

For patients without central AI before surgery and whose surgery involved stalk transection or hypophysectomy, stress-dose GCs should begin intraoperatively and then be tapered to reach maintenance replacement [4]. For the rest of the patients, protocols vary, ranging from administering empirical GC coverage to steroid sparing management [7]. In case of preventive GC coverage, GCs are administered until normal adrenal function is found postoperatively [5]. If a steroid sparing management is applied, treatment is started only if postoperative AI develops and this is tested usually with measurement of morning serum cortisol level on day 1–3 postoperatively [5, 15], and then interpretation is as above. The suspected AI is usually assessed further by dynamic testing, using either an insulin tolerance test (ITT) (preferred) or a corticotropin stimulation test, with peak cortisol levels <18.1 to 20 µg/dL depending on the assay, considered to be indicative of AI [8, 16]. However, Raverot et al. showed that when the new Elecsys Cortisol II assay (Roche Diagnostics, Meylan, France) is used, the cut-off for stimulation tests should be 374 nmol/L (13.55 µg/dL) [17]. If the ITT is used, adequate hypoglycemia (blood glucose <2.2 mmol/L or 40 mg/dL) must be obtained in order to validate the test [8, 15, 16]. If the corticotropin stimulation test is used, one should bear in mind that it can give false negative results for 4–6 weeks after surgery and in cases of partial AI [15, 16]. Other tests including a CRH stimulation test, a glucagon stimulation test, or a metyrapone stimulation test may also be used [15, 16, 18].

Where available, oral HC is the recommended treatment, administered either in a multidose (two-dose or three-dose) regimen or as a single dose [8]. Currently, the estimated dose of HC needed is 5.7–7.4 mg/m²/day, so a theoretical daily dose is usually between 10 and 25 mg [19]. If HC is not available or in selected cases, equivalent doses of other GCs may also be used [8]. If AI is only partial or the results of the dynamic testing are borderline normal/abnormal, only stress-dose GCs during intercurrent illness may be administered [15]. Alternatively, lower than conventional doses for replacement (5–10 mg HC daily) can be used in case of partial AI [9], but all cases should be treated since even mild AI may manifest as clinically important adrenal crisis (AC) in patients undergoing stress [8]. Patients should also be educated on stress-dose GCs administration, including the self-administration of injectable high-dose GCs and to always carry with them an emergency steroid card [9, 20]. Concerning the route for self-administering the high-dose GCs, it has been demonstrated that subcutaneous HC is absorbed with only a short delay (11 min) compared to intramuscular HC, and patients also prefer subcutaneous over intramuscular injection [20].

Adjusting the dose and its eventual repartition is done depending on clinical signs and symptoms and considering the clinical status, comorbidities, and patient preferences [5, 8]. The main risk of undertreatment is AC, while overtreatment increases the risks of metabolic, cardiovascular, and bone disease [8].

9.2.1 Impact of Other Hormones on AI Testing and Treatment

– Because conversion of cortisone to cortisol is suppressed by GH, commencing GH treatment may unmask an incipient AI, thus the presence of AI should be assessed before and then after starting GH treatment [8, 21]; additionally, depending on the replacement therapy, patients may need higher doses of GCs once GH treatment is initiated [8].
– Thyroid hormones accelerate cortisol clearance, so starting thyroid replacement therapy could unmask AI and precipitate an adrenal crisis (AC). Therefore, if exclusion of an AI cannot be made before starting thyroid replacement therapy, empirical GCs should also be administered until definitive testing is possible [8, 22].
– Oral (but not transdermal) estrogen therapy increases circulating cortisol binding globulin levels, leading to elevated total serum cortisol levels [8, 23]. Free cortisol levels do not appear to be affected by oral estrogen therapy, but given the difficulties in measuring free cortisol, it is standard practice to discontinue oral estrogens, for up to 6 weeks, in order to assess for AI [23].

9.2.2 The Particular Case of DHEA Deficiency in Women

DHEA supplementation is not part of standard care, however, a hormone supplementation therapy may be proposed to selected patients and maintained if clinical improvement is achieved [18]. Using a dose of 20–30 mg of DHEA in women with hypopituitarism who had severe androgen deficiency, Johannsson et al. noted effects mainly on the skin and on pubic and axillary hair, and improved stamina, initiative, and alertness, as reported by the partners of the patients. The authors suggested initiating treatment at a lower dose than that used in women with peripheral AI and to titrate this dose so that morning levels of DHEAS normalize and additionally by clinically monitoring the effects on skin and hair [24].

9.3   Central Hypothyroidism

If preoperative central hypothyroidism (CH) is present, replacement therapy should continue throughout the perioperative period; if CH is not present preoperatively, new-onset CH should be assessed at least 6 weeks postoperatively [7, 8].

A low free T4 (fT4) in combination with a low, normal, or only mildly elevated TSH confirms a CH diagnosis in the absence of non-thyroidal illness [8, 9]. A low-normal fT4 in combination with an inappropriately low serum TSH may also indicate CH, with suggested approaches including commencing trial replacement therapy if the patient is symptomatic (i.e., shows fatigue, cold intolerance, hair loss, constipation, etc.), or monitoring the evolution of fT4 and starting substitution if fT4 decreases by 20% [8, 25].

Replacement therapy should be with levothyroxine, at an average dose in CH of around 1.6 μg/kg/day. In order to avoid the cardiovascular risks of overtreatment or undertreatment and the fracture risk in the case of overtreatment, it is important to further adapt the levothyroxine dose so that the fT4 is in the mid to the upper half of the normal range [8].

9.3.1   Impact of Other Hormones on CH Testing and Treatment

– CH can be masked by GHD, so if a GHD patient is started on GH therapy, he/she can either develop CH if they were considered euthyroid before, or require an increase in their levothyroxine dose if already on levothyroxine. Therefore, thyroid function should be checked about 6 weeks after the patient has started or adjusted the GH therapy [5, 8].
– The required levothyroxine dose is increased by increased estrogen levels as the production of the thyroid-binding globulin is estrogen-dependent; therefore, in CH patients that have a change in their estrogen therapy, the levothyroxine dose should be also rechecked and adjusted [8].

9.4   Central Hypogonadism in Males

In males, central hypogonadism manifests with a low testosterone level with low or normal gonadotropins and with symptoms and signs of testosterone deficiency and/or with impaired spermatogenesis [8, 16].

Given the long duration of treatment that may be required to achieve an adequate sperm count for fertility, for men interested in future fertility, it would be prudent to perform a spermogram at the time the CP is diagnosed and to collect and freeze the sperm if there is an adequate sperm count [26]. After surgery, assessment for hypogonadism should start at least 6 weeks postoperatively [7]. Testing implies measuring FSH, LH and fasting morning serum testosterone [8]. Measurement of not only total testosterone, but also of free testosterone concentration (i.e., non-SHBG–non-albumin-bound testosterone) is recommended, using equilibrium dialysis or an estimation of it by using an accurate formula when testosterone values are borderline low or when free testosterone level is not expected to correlate with the total testosterone level [27]. Conditions or medications that interfere with the levels of testosterone by affecting SHBG and albumin levels include, amongst others, hypothyroidism/hyperthyroidism, obesity, GCs, and anticonvulsants [8]. Results should be confirmed by repeating fasting morning total and free testosterone [27].

Since hyperprolactinemia, in itself, can be responsible for functional central hypogonadism, before deciding there is a need for replacement therapy, hyperprolactinemia must be corrected using dopamine agonists that may restore gonadotropic function [8, 16]. There are also other possible causes of functional central hypogonadism and in patients with CP one of the most notable of these is severe obesity. However, these causes are less readily correctable than hyperprolactinemia thus waiting to treat them prior to starting the replacement therapy is not really an option.

In the absence of short-term paternity project, the replacement therapy is carried out with testosterone. Various formulations are available, including intramuscular injections, transdermal gels or patches, pellets, buccal and oral formulations; adaptation of the dose differs from one form to another, but the general rule is that therapy should raise testosterone to the middle of the normal range [27]. When fertility is desired, and, in the absence of available frozen sperm, spermatogenesis can be induced using equivalents of LH—human chorionic gonadotropin (hCG) or recombinant human LH (rhLH), alone when there is residual FSH secretion, or in combination with FSH-containing preparations such as human menopausal gonadotropin (hMG) or recombinant human FSH (rhFSH) [28]. However, this will take months and in some cases 2–3 years [9].

9.4.1 Impact of Other Hormones on Central Hypogonadism Testing and Treatment in Males

In men with hypopituitarism, concomitant testosterone and GH therapy is needed to achieve optimal effects on body composition, muscle function, and protein anabolism, but side effects such as edema, myalgia, and arthralgia are also more frequent when co-administered. For this reason, testosterone and GH treatment should be introduced stepwise and gradually adjusted [29].

9.5 Central Hypogonadism in Females

In premenopausal women, diagnosis should be suspected in the presence of menstrual cycle abnormalities (oligomenorrhea or amenorrhea); additionally signs of estrogen deprivation such as vaginal dryness and dyspareunia might also be present. Plasma estradiol concentrations are usually low-normal, similar to the beginning of the follicular phase, or sometimes undetectable, and those of gonadotropins, in particular of FSH, are not high [16]. In postmenopausal women not on hormonal replacement therapy, the absence of high FSH and LH concentrations is diagnostic for central hypogonadism [8].

As in the case of central hypogonadism in males, hyperprolactinemia can be responsible for functional central hypogonadism and correction of hyperprolactinemia by using dopamine agonists may restore gonadotropic function [8, 16]. Alternatively, if a woman with hypopituitarism does give birth to a child and she also has a prolactin deficiency, this could prevent lactation [28]. To date, there is no hormonal replacement therapy for the prolactin deficiency.

In premenopausal women, in the absence of short-term maternity project, the replacement therapy is with estrogens, with added progestins if the patient has an intact uterus [5]. Various formulations of estrogens with different potency are available, including oral, transdermal patches, topical lotions and gels, vaginal rings and intravaginal creams and tablets [8, 28]. There are no studies comparing the effects of the combined estrogen-progestin contraceptive pill and that of hormone replacement therapy (HRT) in premenopausal patients with central hypogonadism [8]. Oral estrogens (either natural or synthetic, with the natural estrogens carrying a lesser risk of thromboembolism and arterial hypertension) with cyclic addition of progestin remains the most common replacement regimen [9, 28]. However, especially in cases of combined pituitary deficiencies, as is usually the case in CP, transdermal estrogen formulations should be privileged [5]. If transdermal patches are used, approximately 100 μg estradiol daily for 3 weeks then 1 week off (which is similar to 2 mg oral 17ß-estradiol and with 1.25 mg oral conjugated estrogens) was suggested to be preferable in hypogonadal women [30]. Follow-up is done by evaluating symptoms and monitoring for side effects [8], with younger women usually needing higher doses than women approaching the normal age of menopause and then, after the age of 50, estrogens are usually withdrawn [9].

When fertility is desired, this may be achieved, similar to the case of males, via the administration of hCG and hMG or rhLH and rhFSH [31]. There is insufficient data to know the outcome in general, but rare cases have been reported of pregnancy and successful births in women with hypopituitarism secondary to CP. In addition, although there is limited available data on the outcome of pregnancy, there is no evidence to suggest that correctly substituted hypopituitarism would be associated with decreased frequency of livebirths, variation in birthweight or in the gestational week of delivery, nor with an increased risk of malformation [9].

9.6   GH Deficiency

Assessment of GH axis is performed at variable points starting at least 6 weeks after surgery [7] and is of real interest only in the perspective of getting GH replacement therapy started [16].

Strategies for GH replacement therapy in adults differ between countries with, in the UK, the treatment being offered to adults with severe GHD based solely on impairment of quality of life (QoL), while in the USA and in other European countries, GH replacement is proposed to severely GHD adults on holistic grounds [32]. Benefits attributed to the GH replacement therapy in adults include an improvement in body composition, lipid profile, bone mineral density, muscle mass and strength, exercise capacity, QoL, and a reduction in the increased standardized mortality ratio and fracture rate reported in hypopituitary adults [8, 32, 33]. Moreover, GHD impacts ovarian function and fertility and several studies have shown the potential benefit of GH therapy in women with GHD who are trying to fall pregnant [34].

Regarding the possible increased risk of neoplasia, a large study including 956 GH-treated and 102 GH-untreated patients with a history of CP found neither an increased risk of recurrence in the GH-treated group nor an increased risk for breast, prostate, or colorectal primary cancers in 8418 GH-treated versus 1268 GH-untreated hypopituitary patients [35]. However, speculation remains that GH treatment may confer an increased risk of neoplasia [35] and some authors have raised concerns about the potential role GH may have in CP recurrence, reporting that high expression of GH receptor in CP was associated with a shorter duration of stable disease postoperatively [36] or that GH and insulin-like growth factor (IGF)-1 could significantly promote CP cell growth in vitro [37].

The GH axis may be initially tested by measuring only serum IGF-1 levels, but unless IGF-1 is low in a patient with three other documented pituitary hormone deficiencies, the diagnosis of GHD requires failure of one or more GH stimulation tests [5, 8]. Dynamic tests generally recommended in adults are the insulin tolerance, glucagon, and GHRH-arginine tests [8, 16]. The ITT has the best sensitivity (100%), specificity (97%), positive (99%) and negative (100%) predictive values and provided that blood glucose falls below 2.2 mmol/L (0.40 g/L), a severe GHD is defined as a GH peak <3.3 µg/L (10UI/L) during the ITT [16]. However, obesity may blunt the GH response to stimulation, thus the cut-off values for the GH peak should be correlated to BMI [8].

Recombinant human GH (rhGH) is used for replacement therapy. The recommended starting dose is 0.2–0.4 mg/day in patients under 60 years and 0.1–0.2 mg/day in patients over 60 years, followed by dose titration: increasing the daily dose by 0.1–0.2 mg at 6-week intervals so that IGF-1 levels remain below the upper limit of normal or reducing the dose if side effects manifest. Women usually require higher doses than men, even in the absence of oral estrogens, and patients with morbid obesity may also require higher doses [8].

9.6.1   Impact of Other Hormones on GHD Testing and Treatment

- Untreated hypothyroidism may result in reduced IGF-1 levels and in a blunted response of GH to dynamic testing, leading to an over-diagnosis of GHD, thus CH should be treated before testing for GHD [5, 8].
- Oral estrogen treatment leads to decreased circulating IGF-1 levels in GHD women, so for untreated women with GHD, oral estrogen will worsen the

GH-deficient state, while for those being treated, the effectiveness of the treatment will be reduced, requiring a significant increase in the rhGH dose. This effect may be avoided by administration of estrogens via a non-oral route [8, 29].

9.7 Conclusions

Hypopituitarism is a common finding in adult patients with CP, occurring both pre- and postoperatively. Testing and treatment may not always be straightforward given the multiple pituitary deficiencies that may be present and the complex clinical situation. It is important not to underdiagnose and undertreat, but at the same time it is important to not overtreat. A schematized suggested approach for endocrinological management is presented in Table 9.1. It should be kept in mind that the clinical situation of the patient may change over time, as may the scientific evidence, available tests, and treatments, thus management of the patient needs to be adapted accordingly.

Table 9.1 Suggested approach for the endocrinological management of adult craniopharyngioma patients

Before surgery
Assess for hypopituitarism[a]
Start treatment for central AI, CH, and DI if necessary or even consider preventive GCs
In males, consider sperm count and freezing
In the immediate postoperative period
Monitor for central AI, DI, and SIADH
Start treatment if necessary or even consider preventive GCs
≥6 weeks after surgery
Reassess for hypopituitarism[a]
Stop preventive GCs if administered and are no longer needed
Start treatment for central AI, CH, DI, and hyperprolactinemia if necessary
3–6 months after surgery
Reassess for hypopituitarism[a]
Start treatment for central hypogonadism if necessary
1 year after surgery
Reassess for hypopituitarism[a] ± dynamic testing for the GHD
Start treatment for GHD if necessary
When all treatments are adapted
Monitor once or twice annually

[a]Testing for hypopituitarism: Cortisol 8 am ± dynamic testing; TSH, free T4; FSH, LH, estrogen in premenopausal females in presence of amenorrhea, +/− Prolactin; FSH, LH, morning total testosterone (± free testosterone/SHBG) in males +/− Prolactin; IGF1; Symptoms of DI ± biochemical testing
AI adrenal insufficiency, *DI* diabetes insipidus, *SIADH* syndrome of inappropriate antidiuretic hormone secretion, *GCs* glucocorticoids, *CH* central hypothyroidism, *GHD* growth hormone deficiency

References

1. Karavitaki N, Brufani C, Warner J, Adams C, Richards P, Ansorge O, et al. Craniopharyngiomas in children and adults: systematic analysis of 121 cases with long-term follow-up. Clin Endocrinol. 2005;62(4):397–409.
2. Zoicas F, Schöfl C. Craniopharyngioma in adults. Front Endocrinol (Lausanne). 2012;3:46.
3. Jasim S, Alahdab F, Ahmed A, Tamhane S, Prokop L, Nippoldt T, et al. Mortality in adults with hypopituitarism: a systematic review and meta-analysis. Endocrine. 2017;56(1):33–42.
4. Louis RG, Barkhoudarian G, Kelly DF. Chapter 18 - Surgical approaches: complications of surgical management. In: Kenning TJ, Evans JJ, editors. Craniopharyngiomas. 1st ed. San Diego: Academic Press; 2015. p. 281–301.
5. Prete A, Corsello S, Salvatori R. Current best practice in the management of patients after pituitary surgery. Ther Adv Endocrinol Metab. 2017;8(3):33–48.
6. Guinto G, Estrada E, Gallardo D, González JC, Orellana F. Craniopharyngiomas in adults: part II—treatment. Contemp Neuros. 2018;40(7):1–7.
7. Woodmansee W, Carmichael J, Kelly D, Katznelson L. American association of clinical endocrinologists and American college of endocrinology disease state clinical review: postoperative management following pituitary surgery. Endocr Pract. 2015;21(7):832–8.
8. Fleseriu M, Hashim I, Karavitaki N, Melmed S, Murad M, Salvatori R, et al. Hormonal replacement in hypopituitarism in adults: an endocrine society clinical practice guideline. J Clin Endocrinol Metab. 2016;101(11):3888–921.
9. Higham CE, Johannsson G, Shalet SM. Hypopituitarism. Lancet. 2016;388(10058): 2403–15.
10. Cuesta M, Hannon MJ, Thompson CJ. Adipsic diabetes insipidus in adult patients. Pituitary. 2017;20(3):372–80.
11. Sinha A, Ball S, Jenkins A, Hale J, Cheetham T. Objective assessment of thirst recovery in patients with adipsic diabetes insipidus. Pituitary. 2011;14(4):307–11.
12. Cuesta M, Gupta S, Salehmohamed R, Dineen R, Hannon M, Tormey W, et al. Heterogenous patterns of recovery of thirst in adult patients with adipsic diabetes insipidus. QJM. 2016;109(5):303–8.
13. Ball SG, Vaidja B, Baylis PH. Hypothalamic adipsic syndrome: diagnosis and management. Clin Endocrinol. 1997;47(4):405–9.
14. Crowley RK, Sherlock M, Agha A, Smith D, Thompson CJ. Clinical insights into adipsic diabetes insipidus: a large case series. Clin Endocrinol. 2007;66(4):475–82.
15. Garrahy A, Agha A. How should we interrogate the hypothalamic-pituitary-adrenal axis in patients with suspected hypopituitarism? BMC Endocr Disord. 2016;16(1):36.
16. Chanson P. Pathologies hypophysaires: quels tests utiliser? MCED. 2016;80:56–62.
17. Raverot V, Richet C, Morel Y, Raverot G, Borson-Chazot F. Establishment of revised diagnostic cut-offs for adrenal laboratory investigation using the new Roche Diagnostics Elecsys® Cortisol II assay. Ann Endocrinol (Paris). 2016;77(5):620–2.
18. Crowley RK, Argese N, Tomlinson JW, Stewart PM. Central hypoadrenalism. J Clin Endocrinol Metab. 2014;99(11):4027–36.
19. Castinetti F, Guignat L, Bouvattier C, Samara-Boustani D, Reznik Y. Group 4: Replacement therapy for adrenal insufficiency. Ann Endocrinol (Paris). 2017;78(6):525–34.
20. Allolio B. Extensive expertise in endocrinology. Adrenal crisis. Eur J Endocrinol. 2015;172(3):R115–24.
21. Filipsson H, Johannsson G. GH replacement in adults: interactions with other pituitary hormone deficiencies and replacement therapies. Eur J Endocrinol. 2009;161(Suppl 1):S85–95.
22. Persani L. Clinical review: central hypothyroidism: pathogenic, diagnostic, and therapeutic challenges. J Clin Endocrinol Metab. 2012;97(9):3068–78.
23. Qureshi AC, Bahri A, Breen LA, Barnes SC, Powrie JK, Thomas SM, et al. The influence of the route of oestrogen administration on serum levels of cortisol-binding globulin and total cortisol. Clin Endocrinol. 2007;66(5):632–5.

24. Johannsson G, Burman P, Wirén L, Engström BE, Nilsson AG, Ottosson M, et al. Low dose dehydroepiandrosterone affects behavior in hypopituitary androgen-deficient women: a placebo-controlled trial. J Clin Endocrinol Metab. 2002;87(5):2046–52.
25. Feldt-Rasmussen U, Klose M. Central hypothyroidism and its role for cardiovascular risk factors in hypopituitary patients. Endocrine. 2016;54(1):15–23.
26. Stewart PM, Vance ML. Hypopituitarism (Internet). The pituitary society. 2018. [cited 29 September 2018]. https://www.pituitarysociety.org/sites/all/pdfs/Pituitary_Society_Hypopituitarism_brochure.pdf.
27. Bhasin S, Brito JP, Cunningham GR, Hayes FJ, Hodis HN, Matsumoto AM, et al. Testosterone therapy in men with hypogonadism: an Endocrine Society∗ clinical practice guideline. J Clin Endocrinol Metab. 2018;103(5):1715–44.
28. Ascoli P, Cavagnini F. Hypopituitarism. Pituitary. 2006;9(4):335–42.
29. Birzniece V, Ho KKY. Sex steroids and the GH axis: implications for the management of hypopituitarism. Best Pract Res Clin Endocrinol Metab. 2017;31(1):59–69.
30. Pozo J, Argente J. Ascertainment and treatment of delayed puberty. Horm Res. 2003;60(Suppl 3):35–48.
31. Kim SY. Diagnosis and treatment of hypopituitarism. Endocrinol Metab (Seoul). 2015;30(4):443–55.
32. Shalet SM. Extensive expertise in endocrinology: UK stance on adult GH replacement: the economist vs the endocrinologist. Eur J Endocrinol. 2013;169(4):R81–7.
33. Díez JJ, Sangiao-Alvarellos S, Cordido F. Treatment with growth hormone for adults with growth hormone deficiency syndrome: benefits and risks. Int J Mol Sci. 2018;19(3):893.
34. Vila G, Luger A. Growth hormone deficiency and pregnancy: any role for substitution? Minerva Endocrinol. 2018;43:451. https://doi.org/10.23736/S0391-1977.18.02834-1. [Epub ahead of print].
35. Child CJ, Conroy D, Zimmermann AG, Woodmansee WW, Erfurth EM, Robison LL. Incidence of primary cancers and intracranial tumour recurrences in GH-treated and untreated adult hypopituitary patients: analyses from the Hypopituitary Control and Complications Study. Eur J Endocrinol. 2015;172(6):779–90.
36. Ogawa Y, Watanabe M, Tominaga T. Prognostic factors of craniopharyngioma with special reference to autocrine/paracrine signaling: underestimated implication of growth hormone receptor. Acta Neurochir. 2015;157(10):1731–40.
37. Li Q, You C, Liu L, Rao Z, Sima X, Zhou L, et al. Craniopharyngioma cell growth is promoted by growth hormone (GH) and is inhibited by tamoxifen: involvement of growth hormone receptor (GHR) and IGF-1 receptor (IGF-1R). J Clin Neurosci. 2013;20(1):153–7.

Disease and Treatment-Related
Hypothalamic Alterations
in Craniopharyngioma: Clinical
Presentation, Prognostic Impact,
and Implications for Treatment
Strategies

10

Hermann L. Müller

10.1 Introduction

Disease and/or treatment-related alterations of hypothalamic structures have major impact on prognosis after childhood-onset craniopharyngioma (CP) [1–4] (Fig. 10.1).

10.2 Neuroendocrine Deficiencies

Neuroendocrine pituitary and hypothalamic hormonal deficiencies are frequently observed in CP. At diagnosis, 40–87% of pediatric patients [5–8] are presenting with at least a single endocrine deficit and 17–27% [6, 7, 9, 10] are initially diagnosed with insipidus neurohormonalis. Due to tumor involvement of hypothalamic–pituitary axes, the rate of postsurgical endocrine deficiencies is significantly higher [5, 7, 9, 11–15]. Transient diabetes insipidus neurohormonalis is observed in 80–100% of all CP cases after surgery [5, 16], whereas the incidence of permanent diabetes insipidus neurohormonalis ranges between 40 and 93% after surgery [5, 7, 9, 13, 14, 16–19].

Deficiencies of the anterior pituitary lobe and diabetes insipidus neurohormonalis are most frequently observed as initial presentations in adult-onset CP patients and the majority of CP patients are primarily diagnosed with hypopituitarism [8, 20–22]. Mortini et al. [23] observed that 82%, 76%, 73%, and 67% of adult-onset

H. L. Müller (✉)
Department of Pediatrics and Pediatric Hematology/Oncology,
University Children's Hospital, Klinikum Oldenburg AöR, Oldenburg, Germany
e-mail: mueller.hermann@klinikum-oldenburg.de

© Springer Nature Switzerland AG 2020
E. Jouanneau, G. Raverot (eds.), *Adult Craniopharyngiomas*,
https://doi.org/10.1007/978-3-030-41176-3_10

157

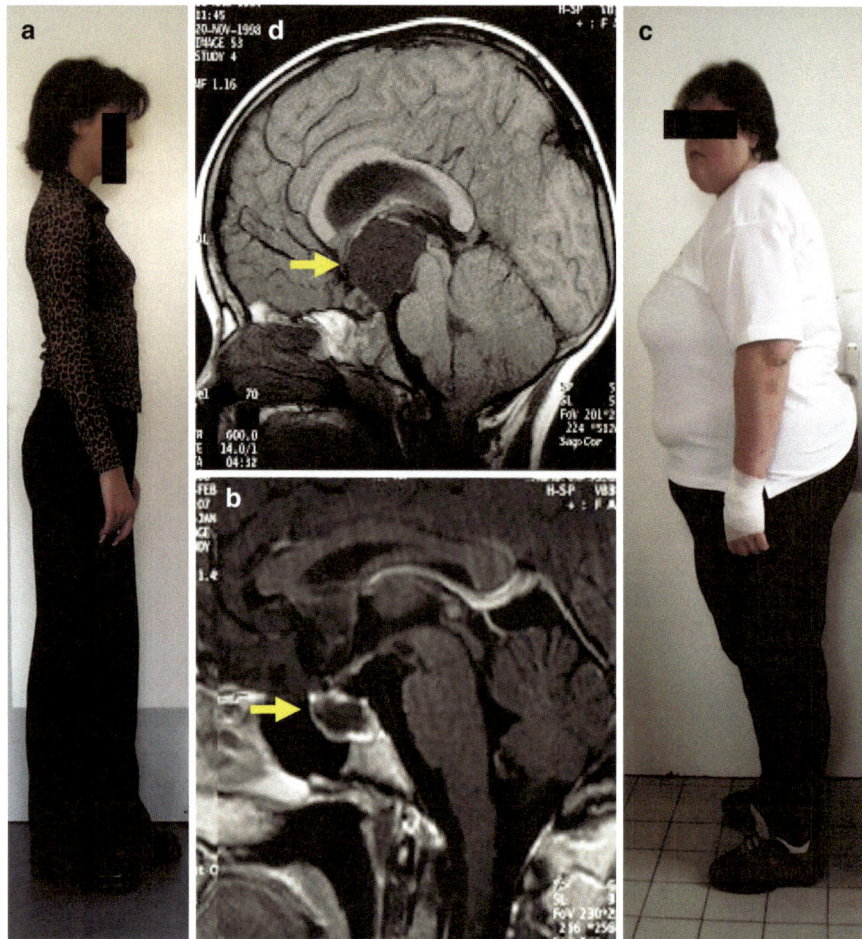

Fig. 10.1 Degree of obesity with regard to location of childhood-onset craniopharyngioma (CP). In both patients, CP (as indicated by arrow on MRI before surgery) could be completely resected. Both patients had complete hypopituitarism after surgery, requiring endocrine substitution of all hypothalamic–pituitary axes. The patient depicted in (**c**) developed severe obesity due to hypotha-lamic lesions of suprasellar parts of CP (**d**). The patient depicted in (**a**) presented with a small tumor confined to the sellar region (**b**). After complete resection she kept normal weight without any eating disorders. (Modified and reproduced from Müller et al., Monatsschr Kinderhlkd, 2003;151:1056–1063 with the kind permission of Springer)

CP patients with normal baseline findings for growth hormone (GH), adrenocorti-cotropin hormone (ACTH), thyroid-stimulating hormone (TSH), and gonadotropins developed new neuroendocrine deficiencies of the hypothalamic–pituitary axes postsurgically. In 70% of their patients, the authors diagnosed diabetes insipidus neurohormonalis after surgery. The rate of new endocrine deficiencies seems to be lower in CP patients operated via transsphenoidal surgical approach [8, 23]. Postsurgical recovery of preexisting endocrine deficiencies is rare. Most adult-onset

CP patients develop partial or complete hypopituitarism as well as diabetes insipidus neurohormonalis. Substitution of more than two pituitary hormones is required in approximately 80% of these CP patients [21, 24].

GH deficiency is observed in 26–75% of childhood-onset CP at the time of diagnosis [6, 18]. Impaired growth velocity—a primary manifestation of CP—often occurs during early infancy several years before CP diagnosis [15]. GH deficiency after treatment for childhood-onset CP is observed in 70–92% of CP patients [15, 19, 25, 26]. Positive responses to GH treatment with regard to growth velocity and QoL are found in most cases [27–29]. Normal growth rates in childhood-onset CP patients with proven GH deficiency are reported [30]. CP patients with hypothalamic syndrome were shown to reach normal adult height more often than those without hypothalamus involvement of CP [15]. This phenomenon of "growth without GH" was first reported in childhood-onset CP five decades ago [31]. However, the pathophysiology of growth in these CP cases is still not fully understood, although leptin and/or insulin are hypothesized to play a compensating major role in this phenomenon. Both hormones are supposed to support growth in obese children [32–34]. Leptin has been reported to function as a bone growth factor acting directly and independently of GH [32]. It is well known that insulin is stimulating growth by its anabolic effects. At high serum levels, insulin is hypothesized to bind to the type 1 insulin-like growth factor (IGF) receptor thereby inducing growth, mediated by a decrease of IGF-binding protein 1 levels and an increase of free IGF-1 concentrations [32]. In support of this concept, obese childhood-onset CP patients were observed to present with increased height SDS at the time of CP diagnosis and at last follow-up visit with no difference in terms of hormonal substitution, including GH substitution therapy [35]. In contrast, Srinivasan et al. reported that childhood-onset CP patients with normal growth despite GH deficiency had similar body composition, auxiological measures, and metabolic parameters as those under GH substitution therapy [30].

10.3 Hypothalamic Dysfunction

Approximately 35% of childhood-onset CP patients initially present with symptoms related to hypothalamic dysfunction, such as daytime sleepiness, disturbed circadian rhythm, obesity, behavioral changes, and imbalances with regard to temperature regulation, thirst, blood pressure, and/or heart rate [9]. The incidence of hypothalamic syndrome dramatically increases after radical surgical treatment—in some series up to 65–80% [9, 11, 16]. Obstructive hydrocephalus and CP involvement of the third ventricle are suggestive findings for hypothalamic syndrome [5]. Several clinical and neuroradiological grading systems for hypothalamic dysfunction have been reported [11, 14, 19, 36–46] (Table 10.1). These grading systems frequently represent algorithms for decision on treatment strategies based on hypothalamic involvement and the degree of obesity.

Surgical removal of suprasellar CP parts involving mammillary bodies (i.e., the posterior hypothalamic areas) frequently results in lesions of posterior hypothalamus structures and severe hypothalamic obesity [19, 47]. Incidence and degree of

Table 10.1 Novel grading systems and treatment algorithms for childhood-onset craniopharyngioma patients based on MRI

Author	n	FU (year)	Grade 0 (0°)	Grade 1 (I°)	Grade 2 (II°)	Treatment recommendation	Outcome parameters
Puget [44]	66 ped	7	No HI	Contact with HI (distortion/elevation) the hypothalamus is still visible	Tumor spread to the hypothalamus, which was no longer identifiable	0°: GTR I°: GTR; if not achieved: Second OP ± XRT II°: STR w/o HD + XRT	Grading correlated with BMI, HUI, neuropsychological disorders
Elowe-Gruau [37]	65 ped	3	No HI	Contact with HI (distortion/elevation) the hypothalamus is still visible	Tumor spread to the hypothalamus, which was no longer identifiable	0°: GTR I°: GTR; if not achieved: Second OP ± XRT II°: STR w/o HD + XRT	Lower BMI in cohort treated per algorithm
Müller [19, 38]	120 ped	3	No HI	HI/HD of the anterior hypothalamus not involving MB	HI/HD of the anterior + posterior hypothalamic area, i.e., involving MB	0°: GTR I°: STR w/o HD + XRT II°: STR w/o HD + XRT	Higher BMI and lower QoL in II° cohort treated by GTR with posterior HD
Fjalldal [39]	42 ped	20	No HI	Suprasellar growth, not towards or into the third ventricle (non-TGTV)	Suprasellar growth towards or into the third ventricle (TGTV)	Non-TGTV: GTR TGTV: STR w/o HD + XRT	Lower cognitive performance in TGTV patients treated by GTR
Van Gom-pel [40]	28 adults	1	No HI	Degree of hypothalamic T2 signal change and irregular hypothalamic contrast enhancement in MRI		Risk-adapted surgical strategies according to MRI findings on HI	Post-OP weight gain correlated with degree of HI

Reference	n	FU	Grading of HI			Surgical strategy	Findings
Elliott [41]	80 ped	9	Preoperative clinical status assessed with standardized scale (CCSS) including vision, pituitary function, hypothalamic dysfunction, educational/occupational status			Risk-adapted surgical strategies according to preoperative CCSS findings	Pre-OP CCSS predicted outcome better than MRI-assessed HI/HD
Steno [11]	41 ped	10	No HI	Outside the third ventricle	Inside the third ventricle	GTR only in case of location outside the third ventricle recommended	Better outcome after GTR in extraventricular cases
Mallucci [42]	20 ped	3	No HI	Tumor size (<2 to 4 cm), no hydrocephalus, no breech third ventricle	Retrochiasmatic tumor, (>4 cm), hydrocephalus, breech third ventricle	0°: GTR I°: Consider GTR II°: STR w/o HD + XRT	Reassessment of HI after endoscopic cyst shrinkage, improved surgical strategy
Roth [36]	41 ped	5	No HI	HD score including assessment of pituitary gland and stalk, ventriculomegaly, and residual tumor		Risk-adapted surgical strategies according to HD score	HD score correlated ($p = 0.02$) with BMI post OP
Mortini [23]	47 20% ped	3.2	Grade of HI according to hypothalamic hyperintensity in T2-weighted MRI, MB involvement, unidentifiable pituitary stalk, dislocated chiasm, unrecognizable supraoptic recess, retrochiasmatic extension			Risk-adapted surgical strategies according to grade of HI	Outcome related ($p < 0.01$) to published grading systems [19, 38, 44]

n size of cohort, *FU* follow-up, *HI* hypothalamic involvement, *HD* hypothalamic damage, *n.a.* not analyzed, *HUI* Health Utility Index, *GTR* gross total resection, *STR* subtotal resection, *MB* mammillary bodies, *XRT* irradiation, *BMI* body mass index, *TGTV* growth towards third ventricle, *MRI* magnetic resonance imaging, *w/o* without, *ped* pediatric patients. Reproduced from Müller et al. [1] with kind permission of Nature Publishing

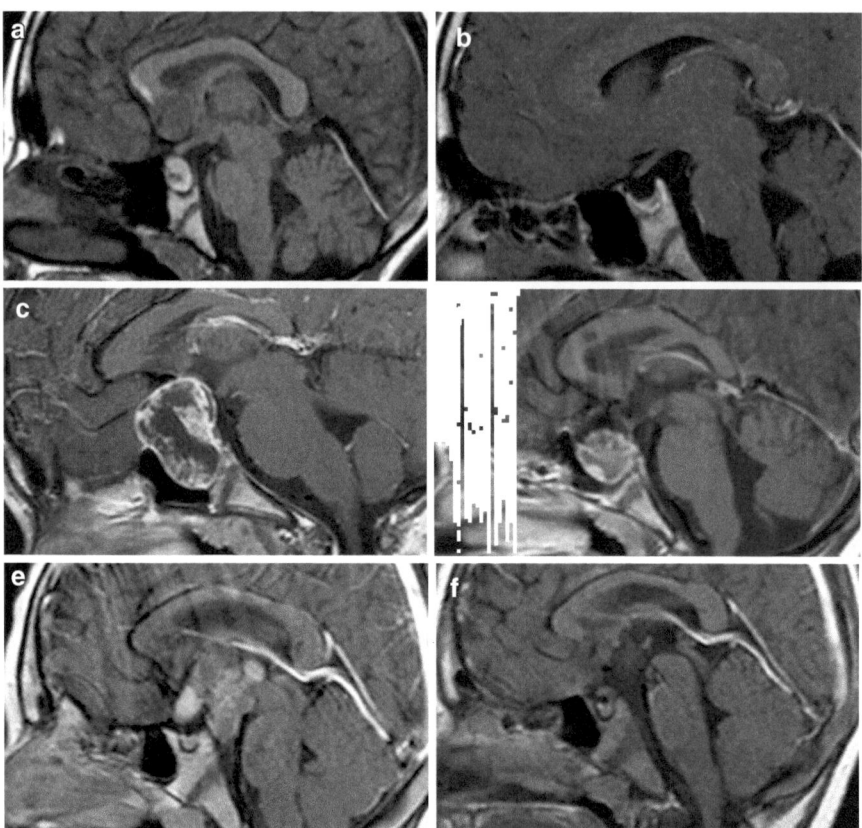

Fig. 10.2 BMI SDS [51] and MRI imaging at diagnosis and 36 months after surgery in three cases of childhood craniopharyngiomas (CP) with different grade of hypothalamic involvement/lesion. (**a, b**) Patient with CP confined to the intrasellar space (0° no hypothalamic involvement (**a**)/surgical lesion (**b**)). BMI at diagnosis: −1.96 S.D.; BMI 36 months after complete resection: −1.62 S.D. (**c, d**) Patient with CP involving the anterior hypothalamus (I° hypothalamic involvement (**c**)/surgical lesion of the anterior hypothalamic area (**d**)). BMI at diagnosis: +1.01 S.D.; BMI 36 months after complete resection: +0.59 S.D. (**e, f**) Patient with CP involving the anterior and posterior hypothalamus (II° hypothalamic involvement (**e**)/surgical lesion of the anterior and posterior hypothalamic area (**f**)). BMI at diagnosis: +6.08 S.D.; BMI 36 months after complete resection: +6.79 S.D. Mammillary bodies are defining the border between anterior and posterior involvement/lesion. Modified and reproduced from Müller et al. [19] with kind permission of Bioscientifica

long-term hypothalamic obesity after CP are positively correlated with the extent of hypothalamic lesions [19, 48–50] (Fig. 10.2). Fjalldal et al. [39] analyzed cognitive performance and psychosocial health in 42 childhood-onset CP patients at a median follow-up of 20 years (1–40 years) after CP diagnosis. The authors found impaired processing speed and disturbed attention. The observed deficits were most pronounced in CP patients presenting with hypothalamic tumor involvement [39, 52]. Based on these findings, a novel MRI-based grading of presurgical hypothalamic involvement and postsurgical hypothalamic damage has been published [46].

This classification of Flitsch et al. is intended to help establish risk-appropriate neurosurgical strategies based on a grading of pre- and postsurgical hypothalamic alterations.

10.4 Obesity and Eating Disorders

Rapid and severe weight gain, starting during the first year after surgery, and severe long-term obesity are frequently observed sequelae caused by involvement of hypothalamic structures and/or treatment-related hypothalamic lesions in CP patients. Frequently, clinical significant weight occurs years before CP diagnosis [15]. Twelve to nineteen percentage of CP patients are reported to present with obesity at the time of diagnosis [6, 7, 16, 18]. Weight gain occurs despite adequate hormonal replacement therapy. The development of morbid obesity is exacerbated by comorbidities limiting physical activity such as disturbances of circadian rhythms, marked daytime sleepiness, and neurological deficits [18, 35, 49, 53]. Following treatment, a 55% prevalence rate of severe obesity is reported [7, 16, 17, 30, 35, 54–56]. Eating disorders and severe obesity result in increased risks of metabolic syndrome [30] and cardiovascular morbidities [50], including increased multisystem morbidity [22] and mortality [16, 57–65].

The pathogenic mechanisms responsible for cardiometabolic complications in CP patients are still not fully understood [49, 50, 66, 67]. Adipose tissue shows a rich innervation by sympathetic nerve fibers controlling lipolysis. Furthermore, lipogenesis is regulated via parasympathetic innervation of adipose tissue originating from distinct neurons in the suprachiasmatic and periventricular nucleus [68]. Accordingly, the suprachiasmatic nucleus plays a major role in balancing circadian activity of both branches of the autonomous nervous system. It is most likely that in CPs with disease and/or treatment-related hypothalamus alterations the functionality of the suprachiasmatic hypothalamic nucleus is frequently impaired. This might affect central clock mechanisms, which predisposes to metabolic alterations. Accordingly, surgical treatment strategies aiming at hypothalamic integrity are recommended for prevention of sequelae such as severe hypothalamic obesity.

In CP with a suprasellar tumor extension, increased serum leptin concentrations relative to body mass index (BMI) were observed [69]. Roth et al. postulated that normal satiety sensation failed to occur in these patients due to dysfunction of hypothalamic receptors that regulate the negative feedback loop in which leptin of adipocyte origin binds to hypothalamic leptin receptors. However, Harz et al. analyzed self-assessment of caloric intake by nutritional diaries and found that hypothalamic obesity was observed after CP even when caloric intake was comparable to BMI-matched controls [70].

10.5 Physical Activity and Energy Expenditure

Studies on physical activity using accelerometric assessments found that physical activity was significantly lower in childhood-onset CP patients when compared with healthy controls matched for BMI [70]. Concomitant visual and/or neurological compromise should also be taken into account for the observed reduction of physical activity in CP patients. Additionally, disturbances of circadian rhythms and increased daytime sleepiness have been observed in childhood-onset CP patients suffering from hypothalamic obesity [53]. These findings were significantly associated with decreased nocturnal and early morning melatonin concentrations in saliva. The suspected pathogenic mechanism of impaired hypothalamic regulation of circadian melatonin secretion was supported by experiences with oral melatonin substitution in CP patients: daytime sleepiness improved and melatonin levels normalized [71]. However, reports on a long-term effect of melatonin medication on daytime sleepiness and weight development have not been published.

Typical polysomnographic patterns for secondary narcolepsy, i.e., high frequency of sleep-onset REM phases (SOREM) have been found in childhood-onset CP patients suffering from severe daytime sleepiness [54, 72, 73]. Daytime sleepiness was significantly improved under medication with central stimulating agents (modafinil, methylphenidate) [72]. Mason et al. [74] treated five CP patients with severe hypothalamic obesity with dextroamphetamine and reached a stabilization of BMI and improvement in physical activity.

A reduced metabolic rate, in terms of total and resting energy expenditure, has been suggested to contribute to the development of severe obesity in CP patients. When compared to controls, lower resting–energy expenditure (REE) was observed in adult and childhood-onset CP [49, 75, 76] and these differences were not associated with body composition. The energy intake/REE ratio was lower in patients with CPs involving the third ventricle [49]. Impaired physical activity is also likely to contribute to lowering of total energy expenditure [49, 50, 70, 75].

10.6 Autonomous Nervous System

Lustig et al. [77, 78] suggested that hypothalamic disinhibition of vagal output is a major cause of β-cell stimulation in childhood-onset CP patients leading to hyperinsulinism and severe obesity. The authors studied treatment with the somatostatin analogue octreotide, which suppresses β-cell activity [77]. Several reports [79, 80] hypothesized that impaired central sympathetic output exerts significant pathogenic impact on physical activity and the development of obesity in patients with childhood-onset CP. Roth et al. reported on reduced catecholamine metabolite urine concentrations, correlating with the level of physical activity and the degree of obesity [81].

10.7 Appetite Regulation

Roth et al. analyzed peptide YY, ghrelin, and brain-derived neurotrophic factor and their effects on satiety regulation in CP patients with hypothalamic obesity [82, 83]. The authors observed that reduced ghrelin secretion and impaired postprandial suppression of ghrelin in severely obese CP patients result in dysregulation of satiety and appetite. Differences with regard to peptide YY serum concentrations between normal weight, obese, and severely obese CP patients were not found. A pathogenic role of peripheral α-melanocyte-stimulating hormone in childhood-onset CP obesity has also been reported [84].

Hoffmann et al. [85] studied eating behavior and eating disorders in childhood-onset CP patients and BMI-matched healthy controls. Severely obese CP patients showed pathological eating behavior and more eating disorders when compared with obese and normal or overweight CP patients. However, CP patients with different degree of obesity showed similar or even less pathological findings for eating behavior when compared with BMI-matched healthy controls. Associations between eating behavior and oxytocin concentrations have been recently reported in CP patients [86].

Pre-and post-meal responses to visual food cues **were** analyzed by Roth et al. [87] in CP patients using functional magnetic resonance imaging (fMRI). In BMI-matched healthy controls, suppression of activation due to high calorie food cues was demonstrated, whereas CP patients presented with higher activation. The authors conclude that perception of food cues after food intake is disturbed in CP patients with hypothalamic obesity.

Although hypothalamic obesity is the most common sequelae after childhood-onset CP [82], also diencephalic syndrome leading to severe weight loss and cachexia has been reported as a rare hypothalamic disturbance of body composition [88, 89]. Hoffmann et al. [89] studied the incidence, clinical manifestations of diencephalic syndrome, and outcome in 485 CP patients. 4.3% of CP patients presented with clinical signs of diencephalic syndrome at the time of CP diagnosis. Significant differences between CP patients with diencephalic syndrome at diagnosis and normal weight CP patients at diagnosis were initially observed at 5 years of age. Within the first 2 years after CP diagnosis, the BMI of diencephalic syndrome patients and normal weight patients converged to a similar level. Hoffmann et al. concluded that diencephalic syndrome clinically present at the time of CP diagnosis does not preclude subsequent weight gain caused by hypothalamic involvement.

10.8 Pharmacological Treatment of Hypothalamic Obesity

Due to impairments in satiety regulation, central sympathetic output, and energy expenditure CP patients suffering from hypothalamic syndrome typically develop morbid obesity, which is unresponsive to conventional treatment such as lifestyle modifications. Based on the observed impairment of sympathetic activation leading to reduced hormonal response to hypoglycemia, treating this disorder with amphetamine derivatives has been supposed [90, 91]. Dextroamphetamine medication was shown to diminish continuous weight gain, to stabilize BMI [74], and to increase physical activity. Even short-term dextroamphetamine treatment resulted in subjective improvement of daytime sleepiness [92]. Elfers et al. observed beneficial effects of a medication with central stimulating agents (particularly methylphenidate) on weight development in CP patients [93].

CP patients suffering from hypothalamic obesity present with a so-called parasympathetic predominance due to vagal activation and manifesting with lowering of heart rate, reduced body temperature, and increased daytime sleepiness [94]. Parasympathetic stimulation results in insulin hypersecretion by direct activation of β cells. The somatostatin analogue octreotide is a somatostatin analogue reducing insulin secretion. In a double-blind randomized controlled study in children with hypothalamic obesity, Lustig et al. demonstrated that octreotide medication resulted in moderate reductions in weight gain [77]. Insulin levels during a proof-of-concept oral glucose tolerance test decreased without leading to major changes in glucose tolerance. A larger trial performed using octreotide LAR in 60 patients with hypothalamic obesity (http://clinicaltrials.gov/ct2/show/NCT00076362) showed no changes in BMI. Due to increased risk of gallstone formation, the open label segment of the trial was terminated.

Dual therapy with diazoxide and metformin was hypothesized to lower insulin secretion and the risk for hyperglycemia [95]. Diazoxide decreases insulin secretion via binding to the KATP channel of the ß-cell. Metformin decreases hepatic gluconeogenesis and improves insulin sensitivity. A combination therapy of diazoxide and metformin was studied in 9 pediatric patients with hypothalamic obesity following CP. The synergy of enhanced insulin action and lower insulin levels resulted in improved weight gain of +1.2 ± 5.9 kg compared to +9.5 ± 2.7 kg in the 6 months prior to therapy. Of the seven CP patients who completed the study, the two with the highest pretreatment insulin levels responded best with the most robust weight loss [95]. The study was limited by its small size and adverse events with one patient withdrawing due to development of peripheral edema, and another due to emesis and elevated liver enzymes.

Zoicas et al. [96] treated 8 adult patients (6 CP) with hypothalamic obesity with GLP-1 analogues and observed a sustained weight loss associated with improvements in metabolic and cardiovascular risk profiles.

Triiodothyronine (T3) increases energy expenditure through induction of thermogenesis. In a case series, three patients (one adult, two children) exhibited weight loss and improved daytime lethargy with T3 supplementation for up to 2 years [97]. These patients had suprasellar tumors but not CPs. It is unclear if they had significant hypothalamic damage. Van Santen et al. measured metabolic brown adipose tissue activity in a patient with hypothalamic obesity following CP treated with T3 [98]. Perhaps because the hypothalamic pathways were damaged, no changes in energy expenditure or brown adipose tissue activity were seen, suggesting that this adjunct therapy is not beneficial.

Methionine aminopeptidase 2 (MetAP2) inhibitors were initially developed as oncological agents for anti-angiogenesis therapy. MetAP2 inhibitors were subsequently found to cause weight loss with decreased leptin and increased adiponectin concentrations, resulting in increased lipolysis, decreased lipogenesis, and increased fat oxidation. Changes in extracellular signal regulated kinase hypophosphorylation are suggested as pathogenic mechanisms. A study analyzing 14 adult patients with hypothalamic obesity, treated for 8 weeks with the MetAP2 inhibitor beloranib observed an average decrease in body weight of 3.2 kg in the first 4 weeks, and 6.2 kg at 8 weeks of treatment [99]. Additionally, patients were observed to have significantly decreased leptin levels after 4 weeks of therapy. Unfortunately, although consistent weight loss was seen in all patients treated, further development of the pharmaceutical agent was stopped due to venous thromboembolic events seen in clinical studies on patients with hypothalamic obesity different from CP origin treated with the MetAP2 inhibitor beloranib [100].

The serotonin and noradrenaline uptake inhibitor sibutramine is known to decrease appetite and prevent reduced energy expenditure after weight loss [101, 102]. However, sibutramine induced weight loss in children with hypothalamic obesity was less efficient when compared with non-hypothalamic obesity [90]. Further studies with sibutramine as a pharmaceutical agent are not expected as sibutramine was withdrawn from major markets in 2010 due to concerns over increased cardiovascular risk [103].

Dexamphetamine has been used to decrease appetite and improve concentration in patients with hypothalamic obesity. In a series of 12 patients treated for an average of 13 months, dexamphetamine improved daytime wakefulness and resulted in weight loss or weight stabilization [92]. Similarly, dextroamphetamine resulted in weight stabilization in five patients treated for 24 months [74].

A combination therapy with fenofibrate and metformin was studied in 22 CP children [104]. Fenofibrate is a peroxisome proliferator activated receptor alpha (PPARa) agonist. PPARa is expressed throughout the body and has been hypothesized to improve insulin sensitivity [105] and decrease triglycerides concentrations. Treated patients did not present with significant weight or BMI improvement; however, improved lipid profiles and insulin resistance were observed.

Daubenbüchel et al. [106] recently reported that CP patients with specific hypothalamic damage limited to anterior hypothalamic areas presented with lower fasting oxytocin levels. Changes in oxytocin saliva concentrations before and after standardized breakfast correlated with BMI, indicating that CP patients with hypothalamic obesity show impaired variation in oxytocin secretion due to nutrition. The authors speculated that oxytocin medication might have beneficial effects on hypothalamic obesity and/or neurobehavioral deficits due to specific anterior hypothalamus damage. In a small pilot study on 11 CP patients, Hoffmann et al. tested this hypothesis by single nasal oxytocin application [107]. All patients presented with detectable oxytocin levels before nasal oxytocin administration. Nasal oxytocin administration was well tolerated and led to increased oxytocin saliva and urine concentrations. After oxytocin administration, CP patients with surgical hypothalamic lesions limited to anterior hypothalamic areas presented improvements with regard to emotional identification compared to CP patients with anterior and posterior hypothalamic lesions. Focusing on correct assignments to positive and negative emotion categories, CP patients improved assignment to negative emotions.

Reports on long-term effects of oxytocin treatment in CP are rare. Parental observed neurobehavioral and pro-social behavior improved after 22 months of oxytocin treatment in a case [108]. In a second case, weight loss and improvement of hyperphagia was observed under oxytocin therapy (10 weeks) followed by a combined 38 weeks therapy with oxytocin and naltrexone [109].

A controlled randomized trial (ClinicalTrials.gov Identifier: NCT 02849743) is currently testing if nasal administration of oxytocin promotes weight loss in children, adolescents, and adults with hypothalamic obesity.

10.9 Bariatric Treatment of Hypothalamic Obesity

Early studies on bariatric surgery in childhood-onset CP patients with hypothalamic obesity demonstrated sufficient tolerability and short-term BMI reduction [110–112]. An instant improvement of binge-eating behavior immediately after laparoscopic adjustable gastric banding (LAGB) was observed in CP patients. However, long-term weight reduction was not achieved [113].

Bretault et al. [114] reported on the 12-month outcome after bariatric surgery for hypothalamic obesity due to CP based on a meta-analysis of the literature. At 1 year, 6 of 18 cases presented with a 20% loss of initial body weight; all had undergone either Roux Y gastric bypass (n = 3), biliopancreatic diversion (n = 1), or sleeve gastrectomy (n = 2). All CP patients presenting with a loss of less than 5% of their initial body weight were treated by LAGB, except one Roux Y gastric bypass case. The authors could show that Roux Y gastric bypass, sleeve gastrectomy, and biliopancreatic diversion are the most efficient bariatric treatment options for weight reduction in hypothalamic obesity due to childhood-onset CP. However, treatment with non-reversible bariatric methods is controversial in the pediatric age cohort because of legal, medical, and ethical considerations [113, 115, 116].

It should be emphasized that currently no bariatric or pharmacological therapy for hypothalamic obesity in CP has been proven to be effective in randomized controlled studies [117].

10.10 Quality of Life, Neurocognitive Outcome, and Psychosocial Functioning

Studies assessing physical and psychosocial function after CP report on variable results, ranging from excellent in a majority of subjects to impaired function in almost half of CP patients [7, 16, 118–121]. The most frequently observed impairments include emotional and social functioning, with patients rating their psychosocial status to be lower than their physical health [16]. Other reported complaints include somatic symptoms such as pain, reduced mobility, and self-care [13, 16]. Behavioral studies found a high rate of psychopathological symptoms, including withdrawal, depression, and anxiety. Difficulties in learning, emotional control, unsatisfactory peer relationships, and concerns regarding body image and physical appearance are frequent problems in children's everyday functioning [26, 122].

Younger age at time of diagnosis and preoperative functional impairments are known factors associated with impaired QoL as well as psychosocial and neurocognitive functioning. Larger tumor volume, hypothalamic and third ventricle involvement are known risk factors for survival and QoL after CP [14, 38, 47, 123].

Endocrine, neurological, and ophthalmological sequelae adversely affect QoL [7, 9, 11, 13, 16, 118, 119]. Hypothalamic dysfunction has been found to have the most important negative impact on social functioning, physical ability, and body image [16, 35, 119].

Long-term neurocognitive complications after CP include cognitive problems, particularly those affecting executive function, attention, episodic memory, and working memory [16, 26, 122, 124–129]. Özyurt et al. [130] reported on reduced performance scores for memory and executive functioning in childhood CP patients when compared with normal controls. The degree of hypothalamic involvement and damage had negative impact on executive functions and functional capabilities.

Psychological and educational deficits were also observed in long-term CP survivors after primary subtotal surgical resection followed by radiation therapy [26]. Reported neurocognitive impairments include memory disturbances, slower cognitive speed, attention problems, and behavioral instability [26, 122, 124, 126, 127, 131]. Intact intellectual functioning has been reported in up to 82% of patients [26, 122].

Studies analyzing intervention efforts with regard to neurocognitive deficits are rare. Efficacy of cognitive rehabilitation for dysexecutive problems and behavioral lability have been analyzed in recent case studies [132, 133]. These case studies demonstrate that goal management therapy and functional behavioral analysis seem to be useful diagnostic and therapeutic options for cognitive rehabilitation, compensating for psychosocial and cognitive impairments [134].

10.11   Survival and Late Morbidity

Overall mortality rates in CP are reported to be three to five times higher than those observed in general population [22, 135]. The overall survival rates described in pediatric series range from 83 to 96% at 5 years [6, 35, 59, 60, 136–138] and 65–100% at 10 years [6, 7, 14, 16, 58, 59, 62–65, 136, 137, 139, 140] and average 62% at 20 years [141]. In cohorts with mixed-age range (adults and children), the overall survival rates range from 54 to 96% at 5 years [20, 22, 118, 137, 142–147], from 40 to 93% at 10 years [9, 20, 22, 118, 135, 137, 143–147], and from 66 to 85% at 20 years [22, 146, 147]. It is still a matter of debate, whether age at CP diagnosis is a prognostic factor for survival. Several studies found that the youngest patients have better survival rates [135, 137, 142, 145]; others report on better outcome in older CP patients [123, 147], or similar survival rates in pediatric and adult cohorts [20, 143, 146, 148, 149]. Some authors found higher mortality rates among females [22, 135], whereas others did not observe any gender differences in terms of survival [20, 59, 143, 149].

Causes of late mortality include those directly related to the tumor or its treatment such as progressive disease with multiple recurrences, chronic neuroendocrine deficiencies, cerebrovascular disease [9, 11, 14, 16, 58], and non-alcoholic steatohepatitis leading to liver cirrhosis [5, 16, 55, 58, 150–154]. The standardized overall mortality rate varied from 2.88 to 9.28 in cohort studies performed by Erfurth et al. The authors report that, CP patients have a 3 to 19-fold increased cardiovascular mortality rate when compared with general population, and female CP patients have an even higher risk [21].

The histological tumor type as a prognostic factor is also a matter of debate. Better 5-year overall survival has been observed in the papillary type vs. the adamantinomatous and combined histological types [155]. Higher perioperative mortality has been reported in adult adamantinomatous tumors [156], but other authors have not found prognostic differences between both histological subtypes [157, 158]. In adult-onset CP patients, a more favorable prognosis has been described in CPs lacking calcification [148, 156], although no specific pathological feature predicted survival in childhood-onset CP patients [60]. The prognostic impact of an initial hydrocephalus is also still a matter of debate. Increased mortality due to primary hydrocephalus has been reported [123] as well as a lack of association between hydrocephalus and mortality [20, 59, 60, 143, 159].

Sterkenburg et al. [3] observed that 20-year overall survival was significantly reduced in CP with hypothalamic involvement. On the other hand, the authors found that 20-year progression-free survival rate was not associated with the degree of surgical resection, supporting their conclusion that radical resection had no advantage in terms of tumor recurrence (Fig. 10.3).

10.12 Neuropsychological Deficiencies

Animal studies have demonstrated that electrical stimulation of the amygdala, septal nuclei, and posterior hypothalamus causes aggression attacks and intermittent, explosive behavior. Cat models showed that electrical stimulation of the posterior lateral hypothalamus can lead to hyperphagia in addition to the abovementioned aggressive behavior attacks. It turned out that several cases where the ventromedial nucleus was affected resulted in both hyperphagia and disinhibited aggressive behavior [160, 161].

In humans, hypothalamic lesions can bring about emotional lability, fury attacks, abnormal sexual behavior, and deficits in memory and intellectual capacities [162]. Flynn et al. [160] report a *neurobehavioral syndrome* with the four main symptoms. (1) episodic tantrums, (2) emotional instability, (3) hyperphagia with attendant obesity, and (4) intellectual impairment. According to Flynn, this syndrome is especially germane to lesions of the ventromedial nucleus. Flynn also states that thus far, attempted treatments of this *neurobehavioral syndrome* such as high doses of an antipsychotic neuroleptic and/or psychotherapeutic behavior interventions are ineffective.

Related to this work, Cohen has documented observed problems in the area of attention spans and deficits in impulse control and motivation [163]. Children with tumors of the third ventricle display symptoms of amnesia, confusion, and consciousness impairment [164]. Lesions of the ventromedial prefrontal cortex whose victims display symptoms of poor impulse control and attention deficits have also been documented [165].

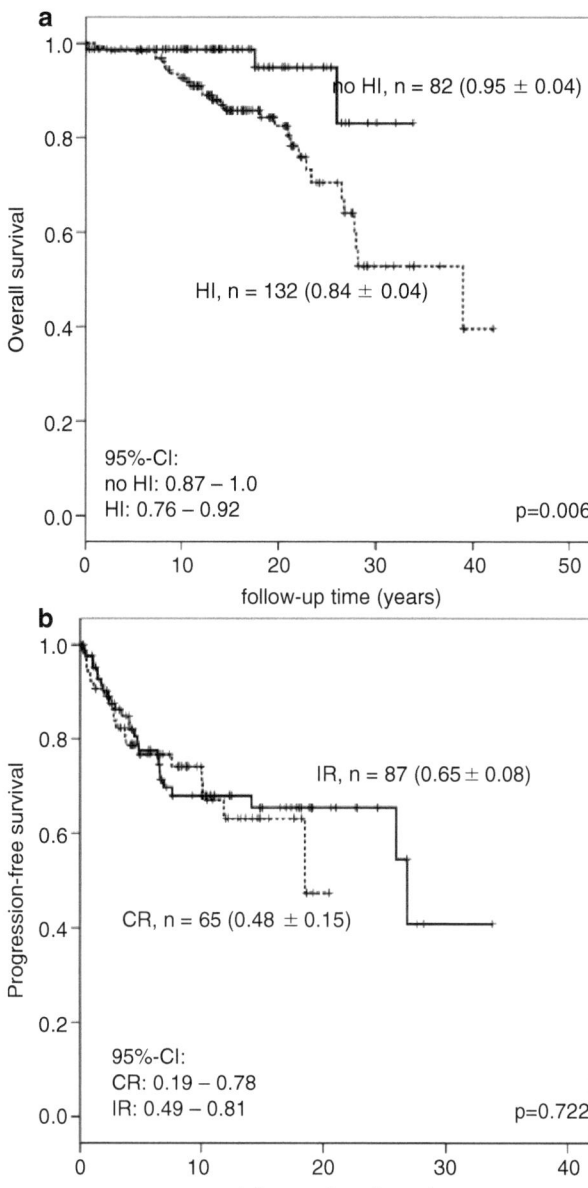

Fig. 10.3 Twenty-years overall survival in regard to hypothalamic involvement (**a**) and 20-years progression-free survival (PFS) in regard to the degree of surgical resection (**b**) of patients with childhood-onset craniopharyngioma recruited in the German Craniopharyngioma Registry (HIT Endo). *CR* complete resection, *IR* incomplete resection; as confirmed by neuroradiological reference assessment. Reproduced from Sterkenburg et al. [3] with kind permission of Oxford University Press

Tonkonogy et al. [166] attribute the posterior hypothalamus and its relationship to components of the limbic system as having significant importance as it is from there that socialized inhibition of aggressive behavior occurs. In the opinion of these authors, aggressive behavior attacks are due to tumor size and/or scar tissue-disrupted connections between the posterior hypothalamus and limbic system from surgical intervention.

The literature on neuropsychological conditions of CP patients appears to be controversial based on a small investigative collective and a variety of study methodologies [167]. Data on preoperative neuropsychological conditions are rare and studies on postoperative, neuropsychological outcomes are frequently extremely difficult to interpret in the absence of preoperative baseline investigations. Comparative evaluations of pre- and postoperative neuropsychological deficits are key to planning surgical strategies (gross total resection vs. partial resection plus immediate irradiation) with regard to long-term QoL effects.

The predominant indicator found in the literature is postoperative normal intelligence quotients for adult-onset CP patients [7, 168], yet only anecdotal reports have been published on diminished postoperative intelligence results [169, 170]. Honegger and colleagues prospectively studied a small collective ($n = 13$) of adult-onset CP patients following mostly transsphenoidal resections and found no impairments regarding their neuropsychological status [171]. However, several studies of children with CP yielded disturbances of memory, attention, impulse control, motivation, and socialization [124, 131, 172–175]. The correlation between cognitive interferences and radical resection remains controversial [174, 176]. It is generally agreed that neuropsychological consequences following irradiation are dependent upon the child's age, irradiation volume, individual dosages, fractionated method, and the total dosage, as well as illness-contingent and other therapy-associated variables. Neuropsychological deficits appear more serious in patients following relapses and/or relapse surgery [177]. As of yet there are no published prospective investigations regarding neuropsychological prognoses of children and adolescents with CP.

In a first review on cognitive performance in patients with childhood-onset CP, Özyurt et al. [129] recently summarized and systemized findings obtained with formalized neuropsychological testing. Notably, detailed neuroradiological assessment of the tumor or lesion site with respect to the hypothalamus was only performed in few of the studies [39, 130, 178]. A systematic assignment of test results to subcomponents of cognition contributed to a comprehensive picture of spared and impaired cognitive functions associated with CPs or their removal. With few exceptions [179, 180], IQ scores were shown to be in the normal range [7, 122, 130, 167, 168, 178, 181–183], albeit [182] found significantly lower IQ scores when compared to a healthy control group. Despite well-preserved overall cognitive abilities, several studies obtained significant deficits in tests assessing memory, attention, processing speed, and executive functioning.

In accordance with frequent complaints of children and their caregivers [184], memory is the most investigated cognitive domain in childhood-onset CP. Typically, deficits were shown for episodic memory, which is a consciously accessible memory system that allows to re-experience past events or episodes in life including their spatial and temporal context [185]. Tests used to assess episodic memory most frequently include list-learning tasks, story memory tasks, or complex geometric designs [186]. In several studies, encoding in long-term memory and/or episodic long-term retention were shown to be impaired, including verbal as well as visual/visuo-spatial information [39, 122, 130, 178], (but see [182, 187]). Waber et al. [181] reported on severe impairments in a narrative task (story memory) but not in a word list or visual memory task. In one of the studies [39], additional analyses indicated that patients with hypothalamic involvement were mainly responsible for the deficits reported for the whole patient group. Noteworthy, in the two studies that tested delayed recognition memory, performance was found to be preserved, despite findings of deficient episodic memory recall [130, 178]. Where tested, verbal and visuo-spatial short-term memory were also found to be in the normal range [167, 178, 181] or not different from controls [130].

Only few studies tested executive functions with formalized questionnaires or tests. In a study that used a standardized questionnaire to assess everyday problems with executive functions, Laffond et al. [188] reported a high proportion of children to suffer from deficits. In studies using neuropsychological testing, cognitive flexibility, which is of vital importance for the ability to adapt to changing situations and goals, was often shown to be impaired [124, 130, 167]. However, Bawden et al. [182] did not find any deficits in tasks assessing executive performance (cognitive flexibility, verbal and figural fluency, and concept formation). Results on sustained attention are inconsistent, with findings of both, impaired [39, 130] and unimpaired performance [181, 182]. Studies that tested cognitive processing speed found abnormal slow performance in the patient groups [39, 181]. The inconsistent results, for attentional control in particular, may be partly due to the small and heterogeneous patient samples in the currently available studies on cognitive performance in childhood-onset CP.

10.13 Social-Emotional Performance

Aside from cognitive deficits, CP patients often suffer from emotional dysregulation and social impairments, severely affecting health-related quality of life. Those impairments significantly challenge families, friends, and the patients' ability to perform in school and working environments [16, 122, 189]. Frequently reported abnormalities include depression, anxiety, mood swings, emotional outburst and irritability in the emotional domain, and hostility and aggressiveness in the social domain [190]. In a systematic literature review, emotional dysfunctions were reported for 40% of the childhood-onset CP patients. Social withdrawal was reported for 35% of the patients [191]. The relevance of acquiring both, self- and other-reports, is nicely illustrated in a study by Poretti et al. [16]. By using the Child Behavior Checklist (CBCL) and the Youth Self Report [192], they found that 33% of the pediatric patients reported social problems in their everyday interactions. Interestingly, parents' ratings of children's social problems were much higher

(58%), a discrepancy which they also reported for other dimensions, such as externalizing behavior. It should be noted, however, that studies on social-emotional functioning are all based on questionnaires. Hence, objective data based on experimental tasks or neuropsychological testing are not available yet.

Disease-related changes such as severe obesity and loss of functional abilities may trigger significant social-emotional reactions, including anxiety, depression, and social withdrawal. At the same time, neuropathological changes in the hypothalamus and associated limbic networks clearly increase the likelihood of adverse outcomes in mood and behavior [193]. However, most of the studies investigating social-emotional abnormalities in CP patients did not report tumor or lesion location with respect to the hypothalamus and some of them not even considered the relevance of these factors (e.g., [122, 181]). This is remarkable, as some of the patients' deficits are similar to or at least reminiscent of abnormalities reported for hypothalamic lesions in single-case studies of humans, and in animals [194, 195]. In studies, which explicitly considered the role of the hypothalamus for neurobehavioral performance, deficits in emotion and interpersonal relationships were shown to be worse in patients with hypothalamic involvement, compared to those without hypothalamic involvement [16, 188, 189]. A further shortcoming of the current literature is the virtual lack of a detailed assessment of specific social and emotional domains. Almost all studies in the field used quality of life questionnaires and the Child Behavior Checklist, which both provide a first valuable assessment, but are not suitable for providing detailed information on specific subdomains of social-emotional functions. Moreover, several functional domains, which may be impaired due to the location of the tumor and potential damage in associated limbic networks, have not been considered yet (e.g., emotion regulation strategies and social cognition).

10.14 Quality of Life (QoL)

CP and treatment of affected children and adolescents means long-term somatic and psychosocial consequences continually affecting their QoL. Additional factors are social reintegration and rehabilitation back into school and occupation, as they impact patients' long-term life planning. Systematic detection of health-related QoL and long-term consequences has not yet been established. Existing reports are on single-center, cross-sectional investigations of small collectives that provide rough estimates regarding somatic and neuropsychiatric long-term consequences based on the QoL conclusions drawn from the respective studies [196]. Systematic analysis of long-term health-related QoL has not yet been established. Eveslage et al. [197] recently reported on short-term QoL during the first 3 years after CP diagnosis in patients recruited in the multinational trial KRANIOPHARYNGEOM 2007 [198]. CP patients treated with radical surgical strategies such as GTR resulting in surgical lesions of posterior hypothalamic areas presented with significant lower self- and parental-assessed QoL during short-term follow-up of 3 years after CP diagnosis.

10.15 Brain Abnormalities in Childhood-Onset CP

CPs bear a significant risk for the integrity of fronto-limbic networks, even beyond the damage directly resulting from tumor growth. First, as in other brain tumors, a number of treatment-related factors such as surgical approaches, radiation therapy, and complications may worsen tumor-related damage and may also result in damage to other areas [199]. Second, hypothalamic lesions may trigger proximal and distal changes in connected brain areas (through diaschisis or transneuronal degeneration), which then add to impairments in cognitive, social, and emotional performance often observable in patients [200]. Such secondary processes are likely to be spread along hypothalamic connections with fronto-limbic subsystems: a posterior subsystem that constitutes a neural system supporting episodic memory and an anterior subsystem supporting emotional, motivational, and social functioning [201, 202]. Notably, neurobehavioral deficiencies frequently observed in CP patients strikingly correspond with the functional range of these two subsystems.

Brain abnormalities associated with CP surgery have only been investigated recently. In a PET-study with childhood-onset CP patients, several tumor- and treatment-related metabolic abnormalities were found after surgery and before proton therapy. A hypometabolism was observed in parts of the frontal lobe, medial/inferior temporal lobe, limbic areas, caudate nucleus, and cingulate gyrus, together with a hypermetabolism in parts of the contralateral temporal and parietal lobes [199]. Main predictors for the hypometabolism were hydrocephalus, sex, and the number of surgical interventions. Interestingly, the authors also reported results of a patient with transsphenoidal surgery only, i.e., without operative trauma to limbic or frontal areas. For this patient, hypometabolism was observed in fronto-limbic areas, indicating the potential consequences of hypothalamic lesions for the integrity of connected brain areas. This result is well in line with findings of an fMRI study, which focused on childhood-onset CP patients with hypothalamic involvement and was the first to provide evidence for distal effects of hypothalamic injury in humans [130]. As patients in this study were highly selected due to our exclusion criteria, they had a very low rate of complications and additional surgeries compared to those in the PET study. Nevertheless, when compared to age- and intelligence-matched healthy controls, patients with hypothalamic involvement had a failure of task-related deactivation in orbital and adjacent medial frontal cortex during memory recognition. This failure of deactivation was assumed to be functionally related to the altered functional coupling, which was observed between CP patients' rostral medial prefrontal cortex and the thalamus [203]. Findings of these two imaging studies motivated a retrospective analysis with voxel-based morphometry (VBM) to investigate whether hypothalamic lesions also impact brain structure in areas strongly connected to the hypothalamus. Patients compared to healthy controls revealed significantly reduced gray and white matter volumes in anterior and posterior limbic networks. Within the CP patient group, worse long-term memory retrieval was correlated with smaller gray matter volumes in the posterior cingulate cortex. The volumetric differences between patients and controls were also observed when lesions caused by surgical pathways and complications were accounted for as far as possible. Thus, these results provided the first evidence for gray and white matter volume reductions outside the area of tumor growth in patients with childhood-onset CP and hypothalamic involvement.

10.16 Conclusions

Hypothalamic involvement and/or treatment-related hypothalamic lesions have major negative impact on long-term prognosis after childhood-onset CP. As long as proven therapeutic options for hypothalamic syndrome are not available, hypothalamus-sparing treatment approaches with special regard to avoid lesions of posterior hypothalamic structures are currently the treatment of choice to prevent further hypothalamic damage and adverse sequelae [204].

References

1. Muller HL, Merchant TE, Puget S, Martinez-Barbera JP. New outlook on the diagnosis, treatment and follow-up of childhood-onset craniopharyngioma. Nat Rev Endocrinol. 2017;13(5):299–312.
2. van Iersel L, Brokke KE, Adan RAH, Bulthuis LCM, van den Akker ELT, van Santen HM. Pathophysiology and individualized treatment for hypothalamic obesity following craniopharyngioma and other suprasellar tumors: a systematic review. Endocr Rev. 2019;40:193.
3. Sterkenburg AS, Hoffmann A, Gebhardt U, Warmuth-Metz M, Daubenbuchel AM, Muller HL. Survival, hypothalamic obesity, and neuropsychological/psychosocial status after childhood-onset craniopharyngioma: newly reported long-term outcomes. Neuro-Oncology. 2015;17(7):1029–38.
4. Bogusz A, Muller HL. Childhood-onset craniopharyngioma: latest insights into pathology, diagnostics, treatment and follow-up. Expert Rev Neurother. 2018;18:793.
5. Caldarelli M, Massimi L, Tamburrini G, Cappa M, Di Rocco C. Long-term results of the surgical treatment of craniopharyngioma: the experience at the Policlinico Gemelli, Catholic University, Rome. Childs Nerv Syst. 2005;21(8–9):747–57.
6. Muller HL. Childhood craniopharyngioma. Recent advances in diagnosis, treatment and follow-up. Horm Res. 2008;69(4):193–202.
7. Hoffman HJ, De Silva M, Humphreys RP, Drake JM, Smith ML, Blaser SI. Aggressive surgical management of craniopharyngiomas in children. J Neurosurg. 1992;76(1):47–52.
8. Honegger J, Buchfelder M, Fahlbusch R. Surgical treatment of craniopharyngiomas: endocrinological results. J Neurosurg. 1999;90(2):251–7.
9. Elliott RE, Wisoff JH. Surgical management of giant pediatric craniopharyngiomas. J Neurosurg Pediatr. 2010;6(5):403–16.
10. Boekhoff S, Bison B, Eveslage M, Sowithayasakul P, Muller HL. Craniopharyngiomas presenting as incidentalomas: results of KRANIOPHARYNGEOM 2007. Pituitary. 2019;22:532.
11. Steno J, Bizik I, Steno A, Matejcik V. Craniopharyngiomas in children: how radical should the surgeon be? Childs Nerv Syst. 2011;27(1):41–54.
12. Jung TY, Jung S, Moon KS, Kim IY, Kang SS, Kim JH. Endocrinological outcomes of pediatric craniopharyngiomas with anatomical pituitary stalk preservation: preliminary study. Pediatr Neurosurg. 2010;46(3):205–12.
13. Merchant TE, Kiehna EN, Sanford RA, Mulhern RK, Thompson SJ, Wilson MW, et al. Craniopharyngioma: the St. Jude Children's Research Hospital experience 1984-2001. Int J Radiat Oncol Biol Phys. 2002;53(3):533–42.

14. De Vile CJ, Grant DB, Kendall BE, Neville BG, Stanhope R, Watkins KE, et al. Management of childhood craniopharyngioma: can the morbidity of radical surgery be predicted? J Neurosurg. 1996;85(1):73–81.
15. Muller HL, Emser A, Faldum A, Bruhnken G, Etavard-Gorris N, Gebhardt U, et al. Longitudinal study on growth and body mass index before and after diagnosis of childhood craniopharyngioma. J Clin Endocrinol Metab. 2004;89(7):3298–305.
16. Poretti A, Grotzer MA, Ribi K, Schonle E, Boltshauser E. Outcome of craniopharyngioma in children: long-term complications and quality of life. Dev Med Child Neurol. 2004;46(4):220–9.
17. Elliott RE, Jane JA Jr, Wisoff JH. Surgical management of craniopharyngiomas in children: meta-analysis and comparison of transcranial and transsphenoidal approaches. Neurosurgery. 2011;69:630.
18. Ahmet A, Blaser S, Stephens D, Guger S, Rutkas JT, Hamilton J. Weight gain in craniopharyngioma—a model for hypothalamic obesity. J Pediatr Endocrinol Metab. 2006;19(2):121–7.
19. Muller HL, Gebhardt U, Teske C, Faldum A, Zwiener I, Warmuth-Metz M, et al. Postoperative hypothalamic lesions and obesity in childhood craniopharyngioma: results of the multinational prospective trial KRANIOPHARYNGEOM 2000 after 3-year follow-up. Eur J Endocrinol. 2011;165(1):17–24.
20. Karavitaki N, Brufani C, Warner JT, Adams CB, Richards P, Ansorge O, et al. Craniopharyngiomas in children and adults: systematic analysis of 121 cases with long-term follow-up. Clin Endocrinol. 2005;62(4):397–409.
21. Erfurth EM, Holmer H, Fjalldal SB. Mortality and morbidity in adult craniopharyngioma. Pituitary. 2013;16(1):46–55.
22. Pereira AM, Schmid EM, Schutte PJ, Voormolen JH, Biermasz NR, van Thiel SW, et al. High prevalence of long-term cardiovascular, neurological and psychosocial morbidity after treatment for craniopharyngioma. Clin Endocrinol. 2005;62(2):197–204.
23. Mortini P, Losa M, Pozzobon G, Barzaghi R, Riva M, Acerno S, et al. Neurosurgical treatment of craniopharyngioma in adults and children: early and long-term results in a large case series. J Neurosurg. 2011;114(5):1350–9.
24. Kendall-Taylor P, Jonsson PJ, Abs R, Erfurth EM, Koltowska-Haggstrom M, Price DA, et al. The clinical, metabolic and endocrine features and the quality of life in adults with childhood-onset craniopharyngioma compared with adult-onset craniopharyngioma. Eur J Endocrinol. 2005;152(4):557–67.
25. Halac I, Zimmerman D. Endocrine manifestations of craniopharyngioma. Childs Nerv Syst. 2005;21(8–9):640–8.
26. Crom D, Smith D, Xiong Z, Onar A, Hudson M, Merchant T, et al. Health status in long-term survivors of pediatric craniopharyngiomas. J Neurosurg Nurs. 2010;42(6):323–8.
27. Geffner M, Lundberg M, Koltowska-Haggstrom M, Abs R, Verhelst J, Erfurth EM, et al. Changes in height, weight, and body mass index in children with craniopharyngioma after three years of growth hormone therapy: analysis of KIGS (Pfizer International Growth Database). J Clin Endocrinol Metab. 2004;89(11):5435–40.
28. Boekhoff S, Bogusz A, Sterkenburg AS, Eveslage M, Muller HL. Long-term effects of growth hormone replacement therapy in childhood-onset craniopharyngioma: results of the German Craniopharyngioma Registry (HIT-Endo). Eur J Endocrinol. 2018;179:331.
29. Heinks K, Boekhoff S, Hoffmann A, Warmuth-Metz M, Eveslage M, Peng J, et al. Quality of life and growth after childhood craniopharyngioma: results of the multinational trial KRANIOPHARYNGEOM 2007. Endocrine. 2018;59(2):364–72.
30. Srinivasan S, Ogle GD, Garnett SP, Briody JN, Lee JW, Cowell CT. Features of the metabolic syndrome after childhood craniopharyngioma. J Clin Endocrinol Metab. 2004;89(1):81–6.
31. Matson DD. Craniopharyngioma. Clin Neurosurg. 1964;10:14.
32. Phillip M, Moran O, Lazar L. Growth without growth hormone. J Pediatr Endocrinol Metab. 2002;15(Suppl 5):1267–72.
33. Geffner ME. The growth without growth hormone syndrome. Endocrinol Metab Clin N Am. 1996;25(3):649–63.

34. Costin G, Kogut MD, Phillips LS, Daughaday WH. Craniopharyngioma: the role of insulin in promoting postoperative growth. J Clin Endocrinol Metab. 1976;42(2):370–9.
35. Muller HL, Bueb K, Bartels U, Roth C, Harz K, Graf N, et al. Obesity after childhood craniopharyngioma—German multicenter study on pre-operative risk factors and quality of life. Klin Padiatr. 2001;213(4):244–9.
36. Roth CL, Eslamy H, Werny D, Elfers C, Shaffer ML, Pihoker C, et al. Semiquantitative analysis of hypothalamic damage on MRI predicts risk for hypothalamic obesity. Obesity (Silver Spring). 2015;23(6):1226–33.
37. Elowe-Gruau E, Beltrand J, Brauner R, Pinto G, Samara-Boustani D, Thalassinos C, et al. Childhood craniopharyngioma: hypothalamus-sparing surgery decreases the risk of obesity. J Clin Endocrinol Metab. 2013;98(6):2376–82.
38. Muller HL, Gebhardt U, Faldum A, Warmuth-Metz M, Pietsch T, Pohl F, et al. Xanthogranuloma, Rathke's cyst, and childhood craniopharyngioma: results of prospective multinational studies of children and adolescents with rare sellar malformations. J Clin Endocrinol Metab. 2012;97(11):3935–43.
39. Fjalldal S, Holmer H, Rylander L, Elfving M, Ekman B, Osterberg K, et al. Hypothalamic involvement predicts cognitive performance and psychosocial health in long-term survivors of childhood craniopharyngioma. J Clin Endocrinol Metab. 2013;98(8):3253–62.
40. Van Gompel JJ, Nippoldt TB, Higgins DM, Meyer FB. Magnetic resonance imaging-graded hypothalamic compression in surgically treated adult craniopharyngiomas determining postoperative obesity. Neurosurg Focus. 2010;28(4):E3.
41. Elliott RE, Sands SA, Strom RG, Wisoff JH. Craniopharyngioma clinical status scale: a standardized metric of preoperative function and posttreatment outcome. Neurosurg Focus. 2010;28(4):E2.
42. Mallucci C, Pizer B, Blair J, Didi M, Doss A, Upadrasta S, et al. Management of craniopharyngioma: the Liverpool experience following the introduction of the CCLG guidelines. Introducing a new risk assessment grading system. Childs Nerv Syst. 2012;28(8):1181–92.
43. Mortini P, Gagliardi F, Bailo M, Spina A, Parlangeli A, Falini A, et al. Magnetic resonance imaging as predictor of functional outcome in craniopharyngiomas. Endocrine. 2016;51(1):148–62.
44. Puget S, Garnett M, Wray A, Grill J, Habrand JL, Bodaert N, et al. Pediatric craniopharyngiomas: classification and treatment according to the degree of hypothalamic involvement. J Neurosurg. 2007;106(1 Suppl):3–12.
45. Garre ML, Cama A. Craniopharyngioma: modern concepts in pathogenesis and treatment. Curr Opin Pediatr. 2007;19(4):471–9.
46. Flitsch J, Muller HL, Burkhardt T. Surgical strategies in childhood craniopharyngioma. Front Endocrinol. 2011;2:96.
47. Muller HL. Consequences of craniopharyngioma surgery in children. J Clin Endocrinol Metab. 2011;96(7):1981–91.
48. de Vile CJ, Grant DB, Hayward RD, Kendall BE, Neville BG, Stanhope R. Obesity in childhood craniopharyngioma: relation to post-operative hypothalamic damage shown by magnetic resonance imaging. J Clin Endocrinol Metab. 1996;81(7):2734–7.
49. Holmer H, Pozarek G, Wirfalt E, Popovic V, Ekman B, Bjork J, et al. Reduced energy expenditure and impaired feeding-related signals but not high energy intake reinforces hypothalamic obesity in adults with childhood onset craniopharyngioma. J Clin Endocrinol Metab. 2010;95(12):5395–402.
50. Holmer H, Ekman B, Bjork J, Nordstom CH, Popovic V, Siversson A, et al. Hypothalamic involvement predicts cardiovascular risk in adults with childhood onset craniopharyngioma on long-term GH therapy. Eur J Endocrinol. 2009;161(5):671–9.
51. Rolland-Cachera MF, Cole TJ, Sempe M, Tichet J, Rossignol C, Charraud A. Body Mass Index variations: centiles from birth to 87 years. Eur J Clin Nutr. 1991;45(1):13–21.
52. Bogusz A, Boekhoff S, Warmuth-Metz M, Calaminus G, Eveslage M, Muller HL. Posterior hypothalamus-sparing surgery improves outcome after childhood craniopharyngioma. Endocr Connect. 2019;8:481.

53. Muller HL, Handwerker G, Wollny B, Faldum A, Sorensen N. Melatonin secretion and increased daytime sleepiness in childhood craniopharyngioma patients. J Clin Endocrinol Metab. 2002;87(8):3993–6.
54. O'Gorman CS, Simoneau-Roy J, Pencharz P, MacFarlane J, MacLusky I, Narang I, et al. Sleep-disordered breathing is increased in obese adolescents with craniopharyngioma compared with obese controls. J Clin Endocrinol Metab. 2010;95(5):2211–8.
55. Muller HL, Heinrich M, Bueb K, Etavard-Gorris N, Gebhardt U, Kolb R, et al. Perioperative dexamethasone treatment in childhood craniopharyngioma—influence on short-term and long-term weight gain. Exp Clin Endocrinol Diabetes. 2003;111(6):330–4.
56. Lek N, Prentice P, Williams RM, Ong KK, Burke GA, Acerini CL. Risk factors for obesity in childhood survivors of suprasellar brain tumours: a retrospective study. Acta Paediatr. 2010;99(10):1522–6.
57. Mong S, Pomeroy SL, Cecchin F, Juraszek A, Alexander ME. Cardiac risk after craniopharyngioma therapy. Pediatr Neurol. 2008;38(4):256–60.
58. Visser J, Hukin J, Sargent M, Steinbok P, Goddard K, Fryer C. Late mortality in pediatric patients with craniopharyngioma. J Neuro-Oncol. 2010;100(1):105–11.
59. Tomita T, Bowman RM. Craniopharyngiomas in children: surgical experience at Children's Memorial Hospital. Childs Nerv Syst. 2005;21(8–9):729–46.
60. Fisher PG, Jenab J, Gopldthwaite PT, Tihan T, Wharam MD, Foer DR, et al. Outcomes and failure patterns in childhood craniopharyngiomas. Childs Nerv Syst. 1998;14(10):558–63.
61. Habrand JL, Saran F, Alapetite C, Noel G, El Boustany R, Grill J. Radiation therapy in the management of craniopharyngioma: current concepts and future developments. J Pediatr Endocrinol Metab. 2006;19(Suppl 1):389–94.
62. Lin LL, El Naqa I, Leonard JR, Park TS, Hollander AS, Michalski JM, et al. Long-term outcome in children treated for craniopharyngioma with and without radiotherapy. J Neurosurg Pediatr. 2008;1(2):126–30.
63. Kalapurakal JA, Goldman S, Hsieh YC, Tomita T, Marymont MH. Clinical outcome in children with craniopharyngioma treated with primary surgery and radiotherapy deferred until relapse. Med Pediatr Oncol. 2003;40(4):214–8.
64. Scott RM, Hetelekidis S, Barnes PD, Goumnerova L, Tarbell NJ. Surgery, radiation, and combination therapy in the treatment of childhood craniopharyngioma—a 20-year experience. Pediatr Neurosurg. 1994;21(Suppl 1):75–81.
65. Khafaga Y, Jenkin D, Kanaan I, Hassounah M, Al Shabanah M, Gray A. Craniopharyngioma in children. Int J Radiat Oncol Biol Phys. 1998;42(3):601–6.
66. Lustig RH, Post SR, Srivannaboon K, Rose SR, Danish RK, Burghen GA, et al. Risk factors for the development of obesity in children surviving brain tumors. J Clin Endocrinol Metab. 2003;88(2):611–6.
67. Swaab DF, Gooren LJ, Hofman MA. The human hypothalamus in relation to gender and sexual orientation. Prog Brain Res. 1992;93:205–17; discussion 17–9
68. Kreier F, Fliers E, Voshol PJ, Van Eden CG, Havekes LM, Kalsbeek A, et al. Selective parasympathetic innervation of subcutaneous and intra-abdominal fat—functional implications. J Clin Invest. 2002;110(9):1243–50.
69. Roth C, Wilken B, Hanefeld F, Schroter W, Leonhardt U. Hyperphagia in children with craniopharyngioma is associated with hyperleptinaemia and a failure in the downregulation of appetite. Eur J Endocrinol. 1998;138(1):89–91.
70. Harz KJ, Muller HL, Waldeck E, Pudel V, Roth C. Obesity in patients with craniopharyngioma: assessment of food intake and movement counts indicating physical activity. J Clin Endocrinol Metab. 2003;88(11):5227–31.
71. Muller HL, Handwerker G, Gebhardt U, Faldum A, Emser A, Kolb R, et al. Melatonin treatment in obese patients with childhood craniopharyngioma and increased daytime sleepiness. Cancer Causes Control. 2006;17(4):583–9.
72. Muller HL, Muller-Stover S, Gebhardt U, Kolb R, Sorensen N, Handwerker G. Secondary narcolepsy may be a causative factor of increased daytime sleepiness in obese childhood craniopharyngioma patients. J Pediatr Endocrinol Metab. 2006;19(Suppl 1):423–9.

73. Muller HL. Increased daytime sleepiness in patients with childhood craniopharyngioma and hypothalamic tumor involvement: review of the literature and perspectives. Int J Endocrinol. 2010;2010:519607.

74. Mason PW, Krawiecki N, Meacham LR. The use of dextroamphetamine to treat obesity and hyperphagia in children treated for craniopharyngioma. Arch Pediatr Adolesc Med. 2002;156(9):887–92.

75. Shaikh MG, Grundy RG, Kirk JM. Reductions in basal metabolic rate and physical activity contribute to hypothalamic obesity. J Clin Endocrinol Metab. 2008;93(7):2588–93.

76. Kim RJ, Shah R, Tershakovec AM, Zemel BS, Sutton LN, Grimberg A, et al. Energy expenditure in obesity associated with craniopharyngioma. Childs Nerv Syst. 2010;26(7):913–7.

77. Lustig RH, Hinds PS, Ringwald-Smith K, Christensen RK, Kaste SC, Schreiber RE, et al. Octreotide therapy of pediatric hypothalamic obesity: a double-blind, placebo-controlled trial. J Clin Endocrinol Metab. 2003;88(6):2586–92.

78. Lustig RH. Hypothalamic obesity after craniopharyngioma: mechanisms, diagnosis, and treatment. Front Endocrinol. 2011;2:60.

79. Roth CL, Hunneman DH, Gebhardt U, Stoffel-Wagner B, Reinehr T, Muller HL. Reduced sympathetic metabolites in urine of obese patients with craniopharyngioma. Pediatr Res. 2007;61(4):496–501.

80. Cohen M, Syme C, McCrindle BW, Hamilton J. Autonomic nervous system balance in children and adolescents with craniopharyngioma and hypothalamic obesity. Eur J Endocrinol. 2013;168(6):845–52.

81. Roth CL. Hypothalamic obesity in patients with craniopharyngioma: profound changes of several weight regulatory circuits. Front Endocrinol. 2011;2:49.

82. Roth CL, Gebhardt U, Muller HL. Appetite-regulating hormone changes in patients with craniopharyngioma. Obesity (Silver Spring). 2011;19(1):36–42.

83. Roth CL, Elfers C, Gebhardt U, Muller HL, Reinehr T. Brain-derived neurotrophic factor and its relation to leptin in obese children before and after weight loss. Metab Clin Exp. 2013;62(2):226–34.

84. Roth CL, Enriori PJ, Gebhardt U, Hinney A, Muller HL, Hebebrand J, et al. Changes of peripheral alpha-melanocyte-stimulating hormone in childhood obesity. Metab Clin Exp. 2010;59(2):186–94.

85. Hoffmann A, Postma FP, Sterkenburg AS, Gebhardt U, Muller HL. Eating behavior, weight problems and eating disorders in 101 long-term survivors of childhood-onset craniopharyngioma. J Pediatr Endocrinol Metab. 2015;28(1–2):35–43.

86. Daubenbuchel AM, Ozyurt J, Boekhoff S, Warmuth-Metz M, Eveslage M, Muller HL. Eating behaviour and oxytocin in patients with childhood-onset craniopharyngioma and different grades of hypothalamic involvement. Pediatr Obes. 2019;14:e12527.

87. Roth CL, Aylward E, Liang O, Kleinhans NM, Pauley G, Schur EA. Functional neuroimaging in craniopharyngioma: a useful tool to better understand hypothalamic obesity? Obes Facts. 2012;5(2):243–53.

88. Kilday JP, Bartels U, Huang A, Barron M, Shago M, Mistry M, et al. Favorable survival and metabolic outcome for children with diencephalic syndrome using a radiation-sparing approach. J Neuro-Oncol. 2014;116(1):195–204.

89. Hoffmann A, Gebhardt U, Sterkenburg AS, Warmuth-Metz M, Muller HL. Diencephalic syndrome in childhood craniopharyngioma-results of German multicenter studies on 485 long-term survivors of childhood craniopharyngioma. J Clin Endocrinol Metab. 2014;99(11):3972–7.

90. Schofl C, Schleth A, Berger D, Terkamp C, von zur Muhlen A, Brabant G. Sympathoadrenal counterregulation in patients with hypothalamic craniopharyngioma. J Clin Endocrinol Metab. 2002;87(2):624–9.

91. Coutant R, Maurey H, Rouleau S, Mathieu E, Mercier P, Limal JM, et al. Defect in epinephrine production in children with craniopharyngioma: functional or organic origin? J Clin Endocrinol Metab. 2003;88(12):5969–75.

92. Ismail D, O'Connell MA, Zacharin MR. Dexamphetamine use for management of obesity and hypersomnolence following hypothalamic injury. J Pediatr Endocrinol Metab. 2006;19(2):129–34.
93. Elfers CT, Roth CL. Effects of methylphenidate on weight gain and food intake in hypothalamic obesity. Front Endocrinol. 2011;2:78.
94. Lustig RH. Hypothalamic obesity: causes, consequences, treatment. Pediatr Endocrinol Rev. 2008;6(2):220–7.
95. Hamilton JK, Conwell LS, Syme C, Ahmet A, Jeffery A, Daneman D. Hypothalamic obesity following Craniopharyngioma surgery: results of a pilot trial of combined diazoxide and metformin therapy. Int J Pediatr Endocrinol. 2011;2011:417949.
96. Zoicas F, Droste M, Mayr B, Buchfelder M, Schofl C. GLP-1 analogues as a new treatment option for hypothalamic obesity in adults: report of nine cases. Eur J Endocrinol. 2013;168(5):699–706.
97. Fernandes JK, Klein MJ, Ater JL, Kuttesch JF, Vassilopoulou-Sellin R. Triiodothyronine supplementation for hypothalamic obesity. Metab Clin Exp. 2002;51(11):1381–3.
98. van Santen HM, Schouten-Meeteren AY, Serlie M, Meijneke RW, van Trotsenburg AS, Verberne H, et al. Effects of T3 treatment on brown adipose tissue and energy expenditure in a patient with craniopharyngioma and hypothalamic obesity. J Pediatr Endocrinol Metab. 2015;28(1–2):53–7.
99. Simmons JH, Shoemaker AH, Roth CL. Treatment with glucagon-like Peptide-1 agonist exendin-4 in a patient with hypothalamic obesity secondary to intracranial tumor. Horm Res Paediatr. 2012;78(1):54–8.
100. McCandless SE, Yanovski JA, Miller J, Fu C, Bird LM, Salehi P, et al. Effects of MetAP2 inhibition on hyperphagia and body weight in Prader-Willi syndrome: a randomized, double-blind, placebo-controlled trial. Diabetes Obes Metab. 2017;19(12):1751–61.
101. Walsh KM, Leen E, Lean ME. The effect of sibutramine on resting energy expenditure and adrenaline-induced thermogenesis in obese females. Int J Obes Relat Metab Disord. 1999;23(10):1009–15.
102. Rolls BJ, Shide DJ, Thorwart ML, Ulbrecht JS. Sibutramine reduces food intake in non-dieting women with obesity. Obes Res. 1998;6(1):1–11.
103. James WP, Caterson ID, Coutinho W, Finer N, Van Gaal LF, Maggioni AP, et al. Effect of sibutramine on cardiovascular outcomes in overweight and obese subjects. N Engl J Med. 2010;363(10):905–17.
104. Kalina MA, Wilczek M, Kalina-Faska B, Skala-Zamorowska E, Mandera M, Malecka TE. Carbohydrate-lipid profile and use of metformin with micronized fenofibrate in reducing metabolic consequences of craniopharyngioma treatment in children: single institution experience. J Pediatr Endocrinol Metab. 2015;28(1–2):45–51.
105. Wysocki J, Belowski D, Kalina M, Kochanski L, Okopien B, Kalina Z. Effects of micronized fenofibrate on insulin resistance in patients with metabolic syndrome. Int J Clin Pharmacol Ther. 2004;42(4):212–7.
106. Daubenbuchel AM, Hoffmann A, Eveslage M, Ozyurt J, Lohle K, Reichel J, et al. Oxytocin in survivors of childhood-onset craniopharyngioma. Endocrine. 2016;54:524.
107. Hoffmann A, Ozyurt J, Lohle K, Reichel J, Thiel CM, Muller HL. First experiences with neuropsychological effects of oxytocin administration in childhood-onset craniopharyngioma. Endocrine. 2017;56(1):175–85.
108. Cook N, Miller J, Hart J. Parent observed neuro-behavioral and pro-social improvements with oxytocin following surgical resection of craniopharyngioma. J Pediatr Endocrinol. 2016;29(8):995–1000.
109. Hsu EA, Miller JL, Perez FA, Roth CL. Oxytocin and naltrexone successfully treat hypothalamic obesity in a boy post-craniopharyngioma resection. J Clin Endocrinol Metab. 2018;103(2):370–5.
110. Muller HL, Gebhardt U, Wessel V, Schroder S, Kolb R, Sorensen N, et al. First experiences with laparoscopic adjustable gastric banding (LAGB) in the treatment of patients with childhood craniopharyngioma and morbid obesity. Klin Padiatr. 2007;219(6):323–5.

111. Inge TH, Pfluger P, Zeller M, Rose SR, Burget L, Sundararajan S, et al. Gastric bypass surgery for treatment of hypothalamic obesity after craniopharyngioma therapy. Nat Clin Pract Endocrinol Metab. 2007;3(8):606–9.
112. Bingham NC, Rose SR, Inge TH. Bariatric surgery in hypothalamic obesity. Front Endocrinol. 2012;3:23.
113. Muller HL, Gebhardt U, Maroske J, Hanisch E. Long-term follow-up of morbidly obese patients with childhood craniopharyngioma after laparoscopic adjustable gastric banding (LAGB). Klin Padiatr. 2011;223(6):372–3.
114. Bretault M, Boillot A, Muzard L, Poitou C, Oppert JM, Barsamian C, et al. Bariatric surgery following treatment for craniopharyngioma: a systematic review and individual-level data meta-analysis. J Clin Endocrinol Metab. 2013;98(6):2239–46.
115. Schultes B, Ernst B, Schmid F, Thurnheer M. Distal gastric bypass surgery for the treatment of hypothalamic obesity after childhood craniopharyngioma. Eur J Endocrinol. 2009;161(1):201–6.
116. Rottembourg D, O'Gorman CS, Urbach S, Garneau PY, Langer JC, Van Vliet G, et al. Outcome after bariatric surgery in two adolescents with hypothalamic obesity following treatment of craniopharyngioma. J Pediatr Endocrinol Metab. 2009;22(9):867–72.
117. Bereket A, Kiess W, Lustig RH, Muller HL, Goldstone AP, Weiss R, et al. Hypothalamic obesity in children. Obes Rev. 2012;13(9):780–98.
118. Van Effenterre R, Boch AL. Craniopharyngioma in adults and children: a study of 122 surgical cases. J Neurosurg. 2002;97(1):3–11.
119. Muller HL, Faldum A, Etavard-Gorris N, Gebhardt U, Oeverink R, Kolb R, et al. Functional capacity, obesity and hypothalamic involvement: cross-sectional study on 212 patients with childhood craniopharyngioma. Klin Padiatr. 2003;215(6):310–4.
120. Muller HL, Bruhnken G, Emser A, Faldum A, Etavard-Gorris N, Gebhardt U, et al. Longitudinal study on quality of life in 102 survivors of childhood craniopharyngioma. Childs Nerv Syst. 2005;21(11):975–80.
121. Muller HL, Gebhardt U, Faldum A, Emser A, Etavard-Gorris N, Kolb R, et al. Functional capacity and body mass index in patients with sellar masses—cross-sectional study on 403 patients diagnosed during childhood and adolescence. Childs Nerv Syst. 2005;21(7):539–45.
122. Ondruch A, Maryniak A, Kropiwnicki T, Roszkowski M, Daszkiewicz P. Cognitive and social functioning in children and adolescents after the removal of craniopharyngioma. Childs Nerv Syst. 2011;27(3):391–7.
123. Yasargil MG, Curcic M, Kis M, Siegenthaler G, Teddy PJ, Roth P. Total removal of craniopharyngiomas. Approaches and long-term results in 144 patients. J Neurosurg. 1990;73(1):3–11. Epub 1990/07/01.
124. Cavazzuti V, Fischer E, Welch K, Belli J, Winston K. Neurological and psychophysiological sequelae following different treatments of craniopharyngioma in children. J Neurosurg. 1983;59(3):409–17.
125. Riva D, Pantaleoni C, Devoti M, Saletti V, Nichelli F, Giorgi C. Late neuropsychological and behavioral outcome of children surgically treated for craniopharyngioma. Childs Nerv Syst. 1998;14:179–84.
126. Kiehna E, Mulhern R, Li C, Xiong X, Merchant T. Changes in attentional performance of children and young adults with localized primary brain tumors after conformal radiation therapy. J Clin Oncol. 2006;24(33):5283–90.
127. Carpentieri S, Waber D, Scott R, Goumnerova L, Kieran M, Cohen L, et al. Memory deficits among children with craniopharyngioma. Neurosurgery. 2001;49(5):1053–8.
128. Sands S, Milner J, Goldberg J, Mukhi V, Moliterno J, Maxfield C, et al. Quality of life and behavioral follow-up study of pediatric survivors of craniopharyngioma. J Neurosurg Pediatr. 2005;103:302–11.
129. Ozyurt J, Muller HL, Thiel CM. A systematic review of cognitive performance in patients with childhood craniopharyngioma. J Neuro-Oncol. 2015;125(1):9–21.

130. Ozyurt J, Thiel CM, Lorenzen A, Gebhardt U, Calaminus G, Warmuth-Metz M, et al. Neuropsychological outcome in patients with childhood craniopharyngioma and hypothalamic involvement. J Pediatr. 2014;164(4):876–81.e4.
131. Colangelo M, Ambrosio A, Ambrosio C. Neurological and behavioral sequelae following different approaches to craniopharyngioma. Long-term follow-up review and therapeutic guidelines. Childs Nerv Syst. 1990;6(7):379–82.
132. Metzler-Baddeley C, Jones R. Brief communication: cognitive rehabilitation of executive functioning in a case of craniopharyngioma. Appl Neuropsychol. 2010;17:299–304.
133. Hammond J, Hall S. Functional analysis and treatment of aggressive behavior following resection of a craniopharyngioma. Developmental Medicine & Child Neurology. 2011;53:369–74.
134. Cohen M, Guger S, Hamilton J. Long term sequelae of pediatric craniopharyngioma - literature review and 20 years of experience. Front Endocrinol. 2011;2:81.
135. Bulow B, Attewell R, Hagmar L, Malmstrom P, Nordstrom CH, Erfurth EM. Postoperative prognosis in craniopharyngioma with respect to cardiovascular mortality, survival, and tumor recurrence. J Clin Endocrinol Metab. 1998;83(11):3897–904.
136. Habrand JL, Ganry O, Couanet D, Rouxel V, Levy-Piedbois C, Pierre-Kahn A, et al. The role of radiation therapy in the management of craniopharyngioma: a 25-year experience and review of the literature. Int J Radiat Oncol Biol Phys. 1999;44(2):255–63.
137. Regine WF, Mohiuddin M, Kramer S. Long-term results of pediatric and adult craniopharyngiomas treated with combined surgery and radiation. Radiother Oncol. 1993;27(1):13–21.
138. Muller HL, Gebhardt U, Pohl F, Flentje M, Emser A, Warmuth-Metz M, et al. Relapse pattern after complete resection and early progression after incomplete resection of childhood craniopharyngioma. Klin Padiatr. 2006;218(6):315–20. Epub 2006/11/03.
139. Hetelekidis S, Barnes PD, Tao ML, Fischer EG, Schneider L, Scott RM, et al. 20-year experience in childhood craniopharyngioma. Int J Radiat Oncol Biol Phys. 1993;27(2):189–95.
140. Cohen M, Bartels U, Branson H, Kulkarni AV, Hamilton J. Trends in treatment and outcomes of pediatric craniopharyngioma, 1975-2011. Neuro-Oncology. 2013;15(6):767–74.
141. Regine WF, Kramer S. Pediatric craniopharyngiomas: long term results of combined treatment with surgery and radiation. Int J Radiat Oncol Biol Phys. 1992;24(4):611–7.
142. Bunin GR, Surawicz TS, Witman PA, Preston-Martin S, Davis F, Bruner JM. The descriptive epidemiology of craniopharyngioma. Neurosurg Focus. 1997;3(6):e1.
143. Stripp DC, Maity A, Janss AJ, Belasco JB, Tochner ZA, Goldwein JW, et al. Surgery with or without radiation therapy in the management of craniopharyngiomas in children and young adults. Int J Radiat Oncol Biol Phys. 2004;58(3):714–20.
144. Bartlett JR. Craniopharyngiomas—a summary of 85 cases. J Neurol Neurosurg Psychiatry. 1971;34(1):37–41.
145. Fahlbusch R, Honegger J, Paulus W, Huk W, Buchfelder M. Surgical treatment of craniopharyngiomas: experience with 168 patients. J Neurosurg. 1999;90(2):237–50.
146. Pemberton LS, Dougal M, Magee B, Gattamaneni HR. Experience of external beam radiotherapy given adjuvantly or at relapse following surgery for craniopharyngioma. Radiother Oncol. 2005;77(1):99–104.
147. Rajan B, Ashley S, Gorman C, Jose CC, Horwich A, Bloom HJ, et al. Craniopharyngioma—a long-term results following limited surgery and radiotherapy. Radiother Oncol. 1993;26(1):1–10.
148. Petito CK, DeGirolami U, Earle KM. Craniopharyngiomas: a clinical and pathological review. Cancer. 1976;37(4):1944–52.
149. Wara WM, Sneed PK, Larson DA. The role of radiation therapy in the treatment of craniopharyngioma. Pediatr Neurosurg. 1994;21(Suppl 1):98–100.
150. Altuntas B, Ozcakar B, Bideci A, Cinaz P. Cirrhotic outcome in patients with craniopharyngioma. J Pediatr Endocrinol Metab. 2002;15(7):1057–8.
151. Basenau D, Stephani U, Fischer G. Entwicklung einer kompletten Lebercirrhose bei Hyperphagie-bedingter Fettleber. Klin Padiatr. 1994;206(1):62–4.

152. Holmer H, Popovic V, Ekman B, Follin C, Siversson AB, Erfurth EM. Hypothalamic involvement and insufficient sex steroid supplementation are associated with low bone mineral density in women with childhood onset craniopharyngioma. Eur J Endocrinol. 2011;165(1):25–31.
153. Muller HL, Schneider P, Bueb K, Etavard-Gorris N, Gebhardt U, Kolb R, et al. Volumetric bone mineral density in patients with childhood craniopharyngioma. Exp Clin Endocrinol Diabetes. 2003;111(3):168–73.
154. Hoffmann A, Bootsveld K, Gebhardt U, Daubenbuchel AM, Sterkenburg AS, Muller HL. Nonalcoholic fatty liver disease and fatigue in long-term survivors of childhood-onset craniopharyngioma. Eur J Endocrinol. 2015;173(3):389–97.
155. Szeifert GT, Sipos L, Horvath M, Sarker MH, Major O, Salomvary B, et al. Pathological characteristics of surgically removed craniopharyngiomas: analysis of 131 cases. Acta Neurochir. 1993;124(2–4):139–43.
156. Adamson TE, Wiestler OD, Kleihues P, Yasargil MG. Correlation of clinical and pathological features in surgically treated craniopharyngiomas. J Neurosurg. 1990;73(1):12–7.
157. Crotty TB, Scheithauer BW, Young WF Jr, Davis DH, Shaw EG, Miller GM, et al. Papillary craniopharyngioma: a clinicopathological study of 48 cases. J Neurosurg. 1995;83(2):206–14.
158. Weiner HL, Wisoff JH, Rosenberg ME, Kupersmith MJ, Cohen H, Zagzag D, et al. Craniopharyngiomas: a clinicopathological analysis of factors predictive of recurrence and functional outcome. Neurosurgery. 1994;35(6):1001–10; discussion 10–1.
159. Daubenbuchel AM, Hoffmann A, Gebhardt U, Warmuth-Metz M, Sterkenburg AS, Muller HL. Hydrocephalus and hypothalamic involvement in pediatric patients with craniopharyngioma or cysts of Rathke's pouch: impact on long-term prognosis. Eur J Endocrinol. 2015;172(5):561–9.
160. Flynn FG, Cummings JL, Tomiyasu U. Altered behavior associated with damage to the ventromedial hypothalamus: a distinctive syndrome. Behav Neurol. 1988;1(1):49–58.
161. Haugh RM, Markesbery WR. Hypothalamic astrocytoma. Syndrome of hyperphagia, obesity, and disturbances of behavior and endocrine and autonomic function. Arch Neurol. 1983;40(9):560–3.
162. Bray GA, Gallagher TF Jr. Manifestations of hypothalamic obesity in man: a comprehensive investigation of eight patients and a review of the literature. Medicine. 1975;54(4):301–30.
163. Cohen RA, Albers HE. Disruption of human circadian and cognitive regulation following a discrete hypothalamic lesion: a case study. Neurology. 1991;41(5):726–9.
164. Ellenberg L, McComb JG, Siegel SE, Stowe S. Factors affecting intellectual outcome in pediatric brain tumor patients. Neurosurgery. 1987;21(5):638–44.
165. Eslinger PJ, Damasio AR. Severe disturbance of higher cognition after bilateral frontal lobe ablation: patient EVR. Neurology. 1985;35(12):1731–41.
166. Tonkonogy JM, Geller JL. Hypothalamic lesions and intermittent explosive disorder. J Neuropsychiatry Clin Neurosci. 1992;4(1):45–50.
167. Riva D, Pantaleoni C, Devoti M, Saletti V, Nichelli F, Giorgi C. Late neuropsychological and behavioural outcome of children surgically treated for craniopharyngioma. Childs Nerv Syst. 1998;14(4–5):179–84.
168. Clopper RR, Meyer WJ 3rd, Udvarhelyi GB, Money J, Aarabi B, Mulvihill JJ, et al. Postsurgical IQ and behavioral data on twenty patients with a history of childhood craniopharyngioma. Psychoneuroendocrinology. 1977;2(4):365–72.
169. Katz EL. Late results of radical excision of craniopharyngiomas in children. J Neurosurg. 1975;42(1):86–93.
170. Weiss M, Sutton L, Marcial V, Fowble B, Packer R, Zimmerman R, et al. The role of radiation therapy in the management of childhood craniopharyngioma. Int J Radiat Oncol Biol Phys. 1989;17(6):1313–21.
171. Honegger J, Barocka A, Sadri B, Fahlbusch R. Neuropsychological results of craniopharyngioma surgery in adults: a prospective study. Surg Neurol. 1998;50(1):19–28; discussion 9.
172. Stelling MW, McKay SE, Carr WA, Walsh JW, Baumann RJ. Frontal lobe lesions and cognitive function in craniopharyngioma survivors. Am J Dis Child. 1986;140(7):710–4.

173. Fischer EG, Welch K, Belli JA, Wallman J, Shillito JJ Jr, Winston KR, et al. Treatment of craniopharyngiomas in children: 1972-1981. J Neurosurg. 1985;62(4):496–501.
174. Fischer EG, Welch K, Shillito J Jr, Winston KR, Tarbell NJ. Craniopharyngiomas in children. Long-term effects of conservative surgical procedures combined with radiation therapy. J Neurosurg. 1990;73(4):534–40.
175. Galatzer A, Nofar E, Beit-Halachmi N, Aran O, Shalit M, Roitman A, et al. Intellectual and psychosocial functions of children, adolescents and young adults before and after operation for craniopharyngioma. Child Care Health Dev. 1981;7(6):307–16.
176. Anderson CA, Wilkening GN, Filley CM, Reardon MS, Kleinschmidt-DeMasters BK. Neurobehavioral outcome in pediatric craniopharyngioma. Pediatr Neurosurg. 1997;26(5):255–60.
177. Scott RM. Craniopharyngioma: a personal (Boston) experience. Childs Nerv Syst. 2005;21(8–9):773–7.
178. Carpentieri SC, Waber DP, Scott RM, Goumnerova LC, Kieran MW, Cohen LE, et al. Memory deficits among children with craniopharyngiomas. Neurosurgery. 2001;49(5):1053–7; discussion 7–8.
179. Pedreira CC, Stargatt R, Maroulis H, Rosenfeld J, Maixner W, Warne GL, et al. Health related quality of life and psychological outcome in patients treated for craniopharyngioma in childhood. J Pediatr Endocrinol. 2006;19(1):15–24.
180. Dhellemmes P, Vinchon M. Radical resection for craniopharyngiomas in children: surgical technique and clinical results. J Pediatr Endocrinol Metab. 2006;19(Suppl 1):329–35.
181. Waber DP, Pomeroy SL, Chiverton AM, Kieran MW, Scott RM, Goumnerova LC, et al. Everyday cognitive function after craniopharyngioma in childhood. Pediatr Neurol. 2006;34(1):13–9.
182. Bawden HN, Salisbury S, Eskes G, Morehouse R. Neuropsychological functioning following craniopharyngioma removal. J Clin Exp Neuropsychol. 2009;31(1):140–4.
183. Flick T, Michel M. Rehabilitation jugendlicher Kraniopharyngeom-Patienten. Rehabilitation. 1986;25(2):45–52.
184. Bellhouse J, Holland A, Pickard J. Psychiatric, cognitive and behavioural outcomes following craniopharyngioma and pituitary adenoma surgery. Br J Neurosurg. 2003;17(4):319–26.
185. Tulving E. Episodic memory: from mind to brain. Annu Rev Psychol. 2002;53:1–25.
186. Lezak MD, Howieson DB, Bigler ED, Tranel D. Neuropsychological assessment. 5th ed. Oxford: Oxford University Press; 2012.
187. Di Pinto M, Conklin HM, Li C, Merchant TE. Learning and memory following conformal radiation therapy for pediatric craniopharyngioma and low-grade glioma. Int J Radiat Oncol Biol Phys. 2012;84(3):e363–9.
188. Laffond C, Dellatolas G, Alapetite C, Puget S, Grill J, Habrand JL, et al. Quality-of-life, mood and executive functioning after childhood craniopharyngioma treated with surgery and proton beam therapy. Brain Inj. 2012;26(3):270–81.
189. Pierre-Kahn A, Recassens C, Pinto G, Thalassinos C, Chokron S, Soubervielle JC, et al. Social and psycho-intellectual outcome following radical removal of craniopharyngiomas in childhood. A prospective series. Childs Nerv Syst. 2005;21(8–9):817–24.
190. Mehren A, Ozyurt J, Zu Klampen P, Boekhoff S, Thiel CM, Muller HL. Self- and informant-rated apathy in patients with childhood-onset craniopharyngioma. J Neuro-Oncol. 2018;140(1):27–35.
191. Zada G, Kintz N, Pulido M, Amezcua L. Prevalence of neurobehavioral, social, and emotional dysfunction in patients treated for childhood craniopharyngioma: a systematic literature review. PLoS One. 2013;8(11):e76562.
192. Achenbach T. Manual for the child behavior checklist 4–18 and 1991 profile. Burlington, VT: University of Vermont Department of Psychiatry; 1991.
193. Zasler ND, Martelli MF, Jacobs HE. Neurobehavioral disorders. Handb Clin Neurol. 2013;110:377–88.
194. Alpers BJ. Personality and emotional disorders associated with hypothalamic lesions. Psychosom Med. 1940;11(3):286–303.

195. Haller J. The neurobiology of abnormal manifestations of aggression--a review of hypothalamic mechanisms in cats, rodents, and humans. Brain Res Bull. 2013;93:97–109.
196. Villani RM, Tomei G, Bello L, Sganzerla E, Ambrosi B, Re T, et al. Long-term results of treatment for craniopharyngioma in children. Childs Nerv Syst. 1997;13(7):397–405.
197. Eveslage M, Calaminus G, Warmuth-Metz M, Kortmann RD, Pohl F, Timmermann B, et al. The postoperative quality of life in children and adolescents with craniopharyngioma. Dtsch Arztebl Int. 2019;116(18):321–8.
198. Hoffmann A, Warmth-Metz M, Gebhardt U, Pietsch T, Pohl F, Kortmann RD, et al. Childhood craniopharyngioma - changes of treatment strategies in the trials KRANIOPHARYNGEOM 2000/2007. Klin Padiatr. 2014;226(3):161–8.
199. Hua C, Shulkin BL, Indelicato DJ, Li Y, Li X, Boop FA, et al. Postoperative cerebral glucose metabolism in pediatric patients receiving proton therapy for craniopharyngioma. J Neurosurg Pediatr. 2015;16:567–73.
200. Fornito A, Zalesky A, Breakspear M. The connectomics of brain disorders. Nat Rev Neurosci. 2015;16(3):159–72.
201. Rolls ET. Limbic systems for emotion and for memory, but no single limbic system. Cortex. 2015;62:119–57.
202. Catani M, Dell'acqua F, Thiebaut de Schotten M. A revised limbic system model for memory, emotion and behaviour. Neurosci Biobehav Rev. 2013;37(8):1724–37.
203. Ozyurt J, Lorenzen A, Gebhardt U, Warmuth-Metz M, Muller HL, Thiel CM. Remote effects of hypothalamic lesions in the prefrontal cortex of craniopharyngioma patients. Neurobiol Learn Mem. 2014;111:71–80.
204. Muller HL. Management of endocrine disease: childhood-onset craniopharyngioma: state of the art of care in 2018. Eur J Endocrinol. 2019;180:R159.

Adult Versus Paediatric Craniopharyngiomas: Which Differences?

K. J. Sweeney, C. Mottolese, C. Villanueva, P. A. Beuriat, A. Szathmari, and F. Di Rocco

11.1 Introduction

Craniopharyngioma is a rare benign epithelial tumour. The WHO classification of CNS tumours has designated this tumour as grade I [1]. The incidence of craniopharyngioma displays a bimodal age distribution, paediatric and adult. They share a putative common embryology and are thought to occur anywhere along remnants of the primitive craniopharyngeal duct. There are two distinct histological subtypes, adamantinomatous (aCP) and papillary (pCP) form. The adamantinomatous form is distinct from the papillary form, in all respects, histologically, macroscopically, molecularly/genetics, age profile of the patient, natural history, location etc. (see Table 11.1).

Although the WHO classification of CNS tumours has designated these tumours as grade 1 and potentially curable with surgery, craniopharyngiomas by virtue of

K. J. Sweeney
Department of Paediatric Neurosurgery, Children's University Hospital,
Temple Street and the Royal College of Surgeons in Ireland, Dublin, Ireland

Service de Neurochirurgie Pédiatrique, Hôpital Mère Femme, Hospices Civils de Lyon,
Université de Lyon, Centre de Référence Maladies Rares, Lyon, France
e-mail: KieronJSweeney@rcsi.ie

C. Mottolese · P. A. Beuriat · A. Szathmari · F. Di Rocco (✉)
Service de Neurochirurgie Pédiatrique, Hôpital Mère Femme, Hospices Civils de Lyon,
Université de Lyon, Centre de Référence Maladies Rares, Lyon, France
e-mail: carmine.mottolese@chu-lyon.fr; pierre-aurelien.beuriat@chu-lyon.fr;
alexandru.szathmari@chu-lyon.fr; federico.dirocco@chu-lyon.fr

C. Villanueva
Service Endocrinologie Pédiatrique, Hôpital Mère Femme, Hospices Civils de Lyon,
Université de Lyon, Lyon, France
e-mail: carine.villanueva@chu-lyon.fr

© Springer Nature Switzerland AG 2020
E. Jouanneau, G. Raverot (eds.), *Adult Craniopharyngiomas*,
https://doi.org/10.1007/978-3-030-41176-3_11

187

Table 11.1 Synopsis of the differences between adult and paediatric craniopharyngiomas

	Paediatric	Adult	
Histology	Almost exclusively adamantinomatous	50–80% adamantinomatous	20–50% papillary
Origin	Infra-diaphragmatic	Intraventricular	Extraventricular
Macroscopic	Cystic with solid components		Predominately solid
Microscopic			
Genetic	Wnt/B-catenin, Ep-CAM, PTTG-1	Wnt/B-catenin, Ep-CAM, PTTG-1	BRAF V600E
Adhesions	Forms strong adhesions in the form of interdigitations		Unlikely to form adhesions
Plane of cleavage	Depends on origin and intervening lepto-meninges		Depends on origin and intervening lepto-meninges
Endoscopy possible	Yes in ages >3	Yes	
Recurrence rate	Higher	Lower	
Hypothalamic obesity	Higher	Lower	
Neurobehavioural	Emotional control	Memory disturbance	
Endocrinopathy	Higher	Lower	
Presenting symptom	Various systemic symptoms, typically headache, raised ICP or endocrinopathy	Usually visual	
Mortality	Higher	Lower	

their location behave in a "malignant" fashion and are plagued by recurrence. There are a little over 20 case reports of malignant transformation [2]. In this chapter we will focus on the relevant differences between adult and paediatric CPs.

11.2   Same Tumour (Location, Extension, Histology)

In this section we will discuss the differences between the two histological subtypes of craniopharyngioma based on epidemiology, location, radiological appearance, histology, genetics/pathogenesis (role of inflammation/calcifications), and adherence/infiltration and growth patterns.

Two recent epidemiological studies put standardised incidence rate for all age ranges from 1.7 to 1.86 per 100,000 [3, 4]. Although craniopharyngiomas can be diagnosed at any age, both studies describe a bimodal age distribution 0–19 and 40–79 years. There appears to be a slightly higher incidence among African and Asian populations [4–6]. The incidence rate for the sexes is almost identical with one study indicating the peak incidence rate in adults is marginally earlier, by 1 year, for females than in males [3]. CPs are the most common non-neuroepithelial tumour in children accounting for 5–11% of paediatric intracranial tumours and 2–5% of adult intracranial tumours. The total distribution of CPs is 76–90% aCPs and 9.7–24% pCPs.

Craniopharyngiomas can occur in the sellar, parasellar, or suprasellar regions. Several studies have identified significant associations between the location of the tumour, age group, and histological subtype [7, 8]. To understand this relationship we would need to understand the embryogenesis of the sellar region, pituitary gland, and oral cavity and the proposed cell of origin of craniopharyngiomas. Briefly, at approximately 4.5 weeks of development (Carnegie stage 11) when the neural tube has divided into five secondary vesicles there are several outpouchings from the diencephalic vesicle one of which gives rise to the neurohypophysis. The other outpouchings give rise to such structures as the optic stalks and the pineal gland. At the same time there is an outpouching from the oral ectoderm (also known as stomodeum). This outpouching, which is anterior to but in continuity with the buccopharyngeal membrane, is induced by BMP4 and FGF8, inhibited by SHH and is known as Rathke's pouch [9, 10]. The neurohypophysis and Rathke's pouch grow towards each other and come in contact by the fourth week and fuse by the eighth week forming a tubular structure called the hypophyseal–pharyngeal, craniopharyngeal or craniostomadeal duct. The anterior portion of Rathke's pouch forms the pars distalis and pars tuberalis of the anterior pituitary gland. The posterior portion of Rathke's pouch forms the pars intermedia. The oral ectoderm, from which Rathke's pouch is derived, also gives rise to cells that are involved in tooth formation such as ameloblasts and oral mucosa which is a stratified squamous epithelium.

11.2.1 Location/Origin

Several studies have demonstrated a strong relationship between site of origin, histology, and age group and in turn site of origin and attachment to surrounding neurovascular structures. As previously mentioned, CPs can develop along any remnants of Rathke's pouch. The main sites can be classified as (1) infra-diaphragmatic, (2) extra-arachnoid/supra-diaphragmatic/lower pituitary stalk, (3) intra-arachnoid/upper pituitary stalk, and (4) sub-arachnoid/tubero-infundibulum. The site of origin predicts the tumour growth pattern and which layers of the leptomeninges, if any, will interpose between the tumour and surrounding neurovascular structures. The histology of the tumour and the presence or absence of intervening lepto-meningeal membranes contribute to the tumours adherence to surrounding neurovascular structures and the degree of surgical difficultly in removal (see Fig. 11.1) [8, 11, 12]. Two notable studies describe CPs origin in relationship to the lepto-meninges [8, 13]. Qi et al. showed that location and growth pattern differed significantly between adults and children. They developed a growth pattern classification based on the tumours' likely origin and its relationship with the lepto-meninges. To understand this classification they refer to studies detailing the layers of arachnoid around the pituitary stalk. Essentially, the distal third of the

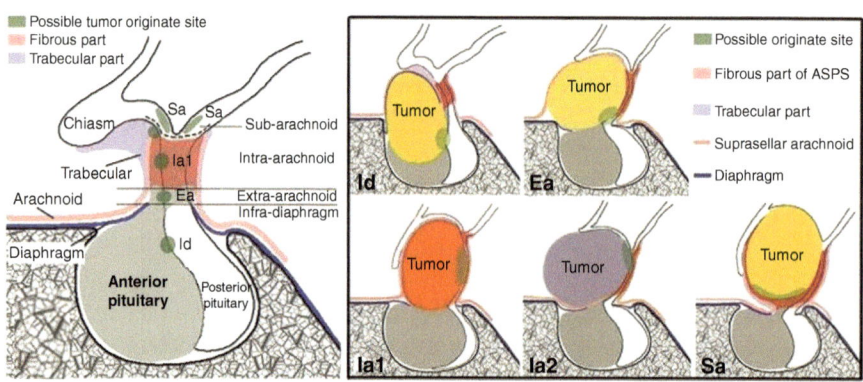

Fig. 11.1 Anatomic relations of the arachnoidea around the pituitary stalk: relevance for surgical removal of craniopharyngiomas: This is from a Springer publication

pituitary stalk is extra-arachnoidien. Both studies identify two layers to the arachnoid membrane: a basal or fibrous layer and a trabecular layer. Both studies describe the fibrous or basal layer forming a tight sleeve around the proximal 2/3 of the pituitary stalk and a circumferential trabecular layer that is attached to inner arachnoid membranes. Qi et al. found that the infra-diaphragmatic tumours predominated in the paediatric group and extra-ventricular tumours predominated in adults. Pascual et al. also confirmed the infra-diaphragmatic location was predominately in the paediatric group and the suprasellar-infundibular topography predominated in the adult group [12, 14]. However, there was no significant difference in the distribution of extra- and intraventricular tumours or trans-infundibular tumours. Tumours with an infra-diaphragmatic origin tend to have all layers of the lepto-meninges between the tumour and neurovascular structures such the optic nerves/chiasm and the floor of the third ventricle/tubero-infundibulum and therefore a plane of cleavage. Tumours originating in the extra-arachnoid zone of distal third of the pituitary stay will grow in an extra-arachnoid fashion and will have both layers of arachnoid between the tumour and neurovascular structures. Tumours originating from the proximal two-thirds or intra-arachnoid layer can be divided into tumours growing in the fibrous layer or the trabecular layer. Tumours originating in the fibrous sleeve of the pituitary stalk will have no significant plane of cleavage between the tumour and the PS but should have intact trabecular arachnoid at the interface with the carotid and chiasm. Tumours originating from within the trabecular arachnoid of the medial carotid membrane will have a plane of cleavage with the pituitary stalk but not the carotid. Conversely, tumours originating in the trabecular layer of Liliequist membrane will have a good plane of cleavage with all neurovascular structures. Tumours originating from the tubero-infundibular area or sub-arachnoid area will grow within the ventricle and form adhesions to the hypothalamus where no plane of dissection will be evident [8, 13]. It should be noted that induction of a significant inflammatory or fibrotic reaction can have an impact on delicate arachnoid planes.

11.2.2 Extension

Obstructive hydrocephalus is common in case of craniopharyngiomas filling the anterior part of the third ventricle. Children are more likely to present with hydrocephalus than adults. Hydrocephalus is present in approximately 50–63% of paediatric craniopharyngiomas compared to approximately 20% of adults [15, 16].

Giant craniopharyngiomas are defined as greater than 5 cm and can grow in any direction. They can grow anteriorly into the subfrontal area, superiorly into the third ventricle causing obstructive hydrocephalus, laterally into the middle cranial fossa, or posteriorly into the posterior cranial fossa [17]. These tend to be more common in the paediatric population. Despite an infra-diaphragmatic location, the larger size in the paediatric population which could extend superiorly to cause obstructive hydrocephalus can be explained by the fact that the ACP tend to form large cystic areas due to an active inflammatory process secreting a viscous oily substance into the cystic cavity.

11.2.3 Histology

It should be reminded that the adamantinomatous subtypes (aCPs) can occur in any age group but the papillary subtype (pCPs) occurs almost exclusively in the adult age range, with only case reports of pCPs in children [18, 19].

Macroscopically, aCPs are described as lobulated mixed solid and cystic mass. The cysts may contain dark greenish-brown turbid liquid resembling machinery oil which is a cholesterol-rich fluid. There may be macroscopic evidence of calcifications, ossification, fibrotic reaction with or invasion/adherence to neighbouring structures. On a microscopic level the histology of aCP has a complex tissue architecture with many different cell types such as epithelial, reactive glial, and inflammatory cells [20]. The squamous epithelium is disposed in cords, nodules, and irregular trabeculae bordered by palisaded columnar epithelium which forms whorls of small tissue islands. These whorls merge with loosely cohesive aggregates of squamous cells known as stellate reticulum. Nodules of "wet keratin" representing remnants of pale nuclei embedded within an eosinophilic keratinous mass are found in either the compact or looser areas. The cystic cavities are lined by flattened epithelium and can contain squamous debris. Non-caseating granulomatous inflammation associated with cholesterol clefts and giant cells may be found [1, 21]. aCP shares morphological and genetic features with ameloblastoma or calcifying cystic odontogenic tumour of the jaw suggesting a shared developmental origin with these tumours [21].

pCPs, on the other hand, resemble a Rathke's cleft cyst with squamous metaplasia [22, 23]. pCPs are solid, homogenous, well-circumscribed masses that rarely are cystic or contain calcifications. Microscopically, they are composed of well-differentiated squamous epithelium which covers a fibrovascular core. pCPs lack the three main characteristics that define the aCP, notably, wet keratin nodules, surface maturation, the picket-fence-like palisades. On small biopsies, some pCPs can be difficult to distinguish from other suprasellar and infundibulotuberal masses such as non-neoplastic Rathke's cleft cysts. These cysts are often lined by ciliated cuboidal or columnar epithelium, but prominent squamous metaplasia can also occur, resembling the epithelium of pCP and therefore it is recommended to analyse the sample for the BRAF V600E mutation [18, 23, 24].

There is increasing evidence that the two subtypes of craniopharyngiomas represent two separate biological entities. Not only do they differ macroscopically, microscopically, and with respect to their natural history, recent studies have demonstrated that each subtype has virtually mutually exclusive genetic alterations. Mutations in the gene CTNNB1 which codes for beta-catenin have been demonstrated via immunohistochemistry and gene sequencing techniques to occur in up to 96% aCPs, whereas mutations in BRAFV600E can occur in up to 100% of pCPs. Not only can these mutations support the accurate diagnosis, they can also be used in targeted treatment [22, 25–28].

The canonical or beta-catenin/Wnt signalling pathway is a regulator or modulator of gene transcription involved with progenitor cell proliferation and differentiation [29]. The pathway is activated when Wnt proteins bind to the extracellular domain of G-protein coupled transmembrane receptor. Wnt proteins are molecules involved in cell-to-cell signalling and play a major role in embryonic development and tissue homeostasis [30]. Normally, when the canonical Wnt pathway is not activated, cytosolic beta-catenin is phosphorylated by GSK 3B and destroyed by the ubiquitin-proteasome system. Once the Wnt protein bind to its receptor, several intracellular processes occur and via activation of the PI3K/MAPK pathway, GSK 3B is phosphorylated. This prevents the destruction of beta-catenin, which in turn leads to cytosolic accumulation and nuclear translocation where it regulates downstream gene expression by binding to Lef/Tcf factors [29, 30]. Beta-catenin is a cytoplasmic protein encoded by CTNNB1 gene located at 3p21. The gene is composed of 16 exons. Exon 3 encodes for the phosphorylation site of GSK3B. A missense mutation at this site leads to the constitutive activation of this pathway. A recent study has demonstrated pathway activation of inflammatory and odontogenic pathways which can explain the earlier ascertain that these tumours can macroscopically resemble ameloblastoma, and microscopically why we find evidence of inflammation, calcification, and reactive gliosis [31]. It must be noted that there was no significant difference in the methylation and genetic expression of paediatric and adult aCPs [26]. Another feature that is almost unique to aCPs is its ability to adhere to or invade surrounding structures. This has been reported by many studies. On a microscopic level, this adhesion is explained by interdigitations formed at the advancing edge of the brain–tumour interface. Within these interdigitations are specific cell niches that form clusters in a whorl like pattern that is not found in pCPS or other non-neuroepithelial tumours of the CNS [32–34].

Moreover, some studies have analysed the cystic content of the CPs by proteomics. Massami et al. identified proteins involved in inflammation, cytoskeletal organisation, and migration of tumour cells. This underlies the hypothesis that the generation of the cystic component of the aCPs is inflammatory driven. This hypothesis underpins the rationale for the use of intracystic interferon α, which has both anti-proliferative and anti-inflammatory properties [35–37].

BRAF protein is a serine/threonine-protein kinase and is encoded by the proto-oncogene BRAF which is located at 7q34. This protein is involved in the RAS-RAF-MEK-ERK pathway. This pathway acts as a signal transducer between the extracellular environment and the nucleus. Extracellular signals such as hormones, cytokines, and various growth factors interact with their membrane receptors to activate the small G-proteins of the RAS family. This leads to recruitment and activation of RAF proteins to the cell membrane. Active BRAF signals through a kinases cascade of MEK and ERK to activate downstream transcription which influences cell differentiation, proliferation, growth, and apoptosis. BRAF V600E is a point mutation where a valine is substituted by a glutamic acid at position 600. This causes constitutive activation of the RAS-RAF-MEK-ERK signalling pathway, independent of extracellular signals [38]. To date there have only been 2 case reports of targeted therapy using BRAF inhibitors in BRAF V600E mutated pCPS [39, 40].

In summary, the differences in biology between paediatric and adult craniopharyngiomas can be best explained by the histological mix that is found in these two age groups: in the paediatric group which contains virtually all aCPs and the adult group which can contain up to 50% aCPs and pCPs with no evidence of genetic or epigenetic difference between paediatric or adult-onset aCPs.

11.3   Tumour Resection vs Endocrine Development

Pre-operative endocrinopathy is present in to up 52–87% of paediatric patients and 26% of adult patients as either a presenting complaint or found on pre-operative investigations [41]. In children the symptoms may be polydipsia/polyuria, delayed or precocious puberty, and short stature. In adults the symptoms may be more subtle and only discovered on pre-operative investigations. The vast majority of long-term survivors will have pituitary dysfunction and polyendocrinopathy and this is the most common long-term morbidity. In children, this can have particular consequences for growth, development, and fertility. There are also secondary consequences such as obesity and a poor lipid profile and features of the metabolic syndrome are frequently seen after childhood craniopharyngioma. There is considerable overlap between the metabolic syndrome due to endocrinopathy and hypothalamic syndrome which causes obesity from hyperphagia and lethargy.

Of special interest to the paediatric neurosurgeon is the handling of the pituitary gland and stalk during surgery. The maintenance of the pituitary stalk could reduce the risk of anterior and posterior pituitary dysfunction after surgery; however, this would depend on whether pre-operative loss of function is permanent due to the invasion by craniopharyngioma or reversible due to compression by the craniopharyngioma. On the other hand, attempted preservation of the pituitary stalk for a possible unknown benefit may increase the risk of recurrence. Several studies have attempted to answer this question [41–44]. In order to begin to answer this question one must understand the relationship of the CP to the pituitary stalk, its origin, likely histology, and the potential intervening lepto-meningeal membranes between the CP and the PS. In essence, CPs arising from within the fibrous sleeve of arachnoid surrounding the pituitary stalk are unlikely to have a plane of cleavage.

A meta-analysis by Li et al. reported that the maintenance of the pituitary stalk may reduce the alterations in endocrine function and the occurrence of diabetes insipidus. However, it is not likely to enhance the recurrence rate of craniopharyngioma. This meta-analysis contains mostly adult series and only one paediatric study was included [43]. The paediatric study in this meta-analysis was by Jung et al. They concluded that paediatric craniopharyngiomas had high recurrence rates and low pituitary functional preservation despite anatomical stalk preservation. This might be due to pre-operative invasion of the pituitary. Therefore, maximal tumour resection might be more important than anatomical stalk preservation in paediatric craniopharyngiomas [44]. Since then, one further study was published by Jing Chen et al. In this study they report a series of 82 CPs from a pituitary stalk origin from a total of 103 paediatric CPs. They concluded for children with craniopharyngioma of pituitary stalk origin, preserving the pituitary stalk has a significant effect on the early and persistent diabetes insipidus rates. When intraoperative exploration showed excessive adhesion between the tumour and pituitary stalk, they opted to preserve the pituitary stalk, which reportedly reduced the early and persistent post-operative diabetes insipidus rates, without significantly increasing the relapse or mortality rate [42]. However, it has to be noted in that study an astonish rate of conservation of the pituitary stalk for a tumour arising from.

It has been demonstrated that surgical intervention, either transcranial or endoscopic trans-sphenoidal routes, has a higher rate of post-operative endocrinological dysfunction than minimally invasive approaches such as Ommaya reservoir placement for repeated aspiration and/or intracystic treatment [45]. Within the surgical group a recent meta-analysis by Qiao demonstrated no significant difference in endocrinology outcomes between endoscopic and transcranial approaches [46]. Irreversible central diabetes insipidus follows after 80–93% of all complete resections, and GH deficiency occurs in 75% of cases. There was a clinical concern that growth hormone replacement in patients with craniopharyngiomas may lead to increased recurrence. Several meta-analyses have demonstrated no significant increase in the rate of recurrence of craniopharyngioma in the paediatric population with growth hormone replacement at physiological levels; however, long-term follow-up is always recommended [47–49].

To try and reduce the impact on the endocrine development in children, several techniques have been developed to reduce the volume of cystic craniopharyngiomas, thereby decompressing surrounding structures such as the visual apparatus, the endocrine system and freeing up the CSF pathways. These temporary measures can delay surgery and avoid any damage to the remaining pituitary gland and stalk as well as other possible complications associated with treatment. These strategies include endoscopic fenestration into the ventricle, stereotactic or endoscopic cyst drainage, endoscopic or stereotactic placement of a catheter into the cystic component of the CP. This catheter is then connected to a subcutaneous reservoir which allows repeated aspiration of the cyst contents to reduce the size of the tumour.

Within the last 20 years, simultaneous instillation of agents to reduce the growth rate of the tumour has been used as intracystic therapies. Such agents include interferon alpha, bleomycin, and radioisotopes like phosphorous 32. Recently, the efficacy of interferon has been proposed over other agents due to its low toxicity profile. This strategy can delay the definitive surgical removal of the tumour or treatment with radiotherapy by up to 6 years thus postponing the risks of endocrinological defects as well or other possible complications [50]. This is especially important in children who have many cyclical growth spurts before the significant endocrinological event of puberty where an intact and functioning neuroendocrine axis is critical in the child's physical and neurocognitive development [51, 52].

11.4   Residual and Recurrence Management

Residual tumour is either intentional or unintentional. The neurosurgical edict of "maximal safe surgical resection" applies especially to CPs. Preservation of the hypothalamic/pituitary, visual, and vascular structures is of utmost importance. For the last 20 years, awareness of hypothalamic involvement, damage, and hypothalamic syndrome has been an increasing predominant factor in surgical decision-making. It is widely accepted that when pre-operative hypothalamic involvement is identified, hypothalamic sparing surgery should be performed. Likewise, adhesion to important neurovascular structures such as the optic nerves and chiasm or the circle of Willis where a plane of cleavage is not possible will necessitate residual CP. Biological factors that influence CP recurrence include histology (more common in aCPs), molecular profile, and macroscopic appearance. Beta-catenin, Ep-CAM, PTTG-1, cystic tumours with calcifications and whorl like structures all demonstrated a higher incidence of recurrence. These are also the features of the adamantinomatous tumours [53, 54].

Recurrence rates are usually reported as three groups for analysis: Gross total resection (GTR), subtotal resection (STR) and radiotherapy (XRT), and STR. A meta-analysis from Danuard et al. reports the rate of recurrence of adult CPs as GTR = 17%, STR + XRT = 27%, and STR = 45% [55]. This compares sharply with the meta-analysis on paediatric onset CPs by Clark et al. which found the rate of recurrence was significantly increased across all treatment groups at GTR = 35%, STR + XRT = 50%, STR = 65% [56]. This difference is probably explained by the histological mixed of the adult CPs cohort which contains both aCPs and pCPs and where pCPs have favourable features for GTR and recurrence.

Surgery for recurrence is plagued in both age groups by loss of arachnoid planes, fibrosis and gliosis, impaired wound healing which can lead to an increase in complications such as infections and CSF leaks.

The vast majority of recurrent craniopharyngiomas is at the local site; however, there are approximately 60 reports of ectopic sites of recurrence described in the literature to date. The recurrences have occurred either along the surgical tract or hypothesised to have occurred by dissemination through the CSF pathways [57].

Conventional treatment strategies such as surgery and radiotherapy are similar in both age groups. Surgical issues in children are discussed below and there is obvious restriction on cranial irradiation on the developing neural axis.

There are numerous molecular targets or antagonists for the Wnt/beta-catenin pathway none of which have been tried in craniopharyngioma [29]. In the pCPs both inhibitors of BRAF V600E (dabrafenib) and MAP kinase (trametinib) have been used with considerable success by both an adult and a child [19, 40].

Future studies on recurrence need to standardise the reporting of the variables that influence recurrence such as histology/molecular profile, location, growth pattern, and adherence to surrounding neurovascular structures.

11.5   Surgical Issues in Children

Numerous metaphors have always been used to help highlight the need for the paediatric specialty such as "children are not small adults." [58]. However, there is no other paediatric brain tumour that exemplifies the need for a paediatric multidisciplinary team approach than the craniopharyngioma. This team must have high-throughput experience and members should include a paediatric neurosurgeon, neurologist, general paediatrician, endocrinologist, ophthalmologist, oncologist, radiation oncologist, neuro-psychologist, and dietician.

Surgical issues in children with respect to craniopharyngioma can be split into two categories. The first issue is the general surgical, anaesthetic, and post-operative issues that are common to all paediatric surgical specialities. There obvious physiological difference between the paediatric and adults including total body water/blood volume/ventilation air spaces and age-related variation in physiological parameters such heart rate, rate of respiration, arterial blood pressure that have always necessitated paediatrics as a speciality.

The second issue is the neurosurgical corridor for access to the CP and the age of the child. The numerous transcranial approaches are the same in both age groups such as subfrontal (midline or fronto-lateral) or the pterional approaches. Large or giant forms of CP may identify one approach as preferable over the others by opening up a corridor. One must consider that it is usually the cyst that opens up the corridor and that cysts can be easily decompressed. One must also consider origin, growth pattern, and possible adherence to critical neurovascular structures when selecting a surgical approach. The obvious difference of smaller age-related anatomical spaces in the child and perhaps more generous arachnoid or cisternal spaces in the adult are also important factors. It is with respect to the endoscopic endonasal trans-sphenoidal route that these two age groups differ. The endoscopic endonasal trans-sphenoidal route is the most recent addition to the neurosurgeons armamentarium. Due to the small anatomical space of the nostril, nose, and age-related pneumatisation of the sphenoidal air sinus, it was previously thought that this method was not suitable in children. There have been increasingly recent publications of case series demonstrating the efficacy of the endoscopic endonasal trans-sphenoidal route in children as young as 3 years [59–61]. This corresponds to the imaging study by Jang et al. who demonstrated that pneumatisation of the sphenoid air sinus was noted as young as 2 months on axial imaging and pneumatised air sinuses were identified in 100% of 3 years olds [62].

Because of these surgical issues, the initial management on cystic CPs by intra-cystic interferon may allow disease control while waiting for further growth and development in the child before subjecting them to a surgical procedure.

11.6   Weight Control Issues in Children

Hypothalamic involvement represents the most important risk factor for a restricted long-term prognosis in patients with CP. The hypothalamic region of the diencephalon contains various nuclei that link the central nervous system to the endocrinological system which in turn controls a wide range of physiological homeostatic functions such temperature, sleep/circadian cycle, thirst/water balance, and satiety/energy stores.

Patients with CP are at a higher risk from co-morbid conditions such as type 2 diabetes mellitus, cerebrovascular and cardiovascular disease, severe infections, fractures, and respiratory disease which all influence mortality. Female sex, childhood-onset craniopharyngioma, hydrocephalus, and tumour recurrence are important risk factors. Children with CP are at a substantially higher risk of mortality than adult-onset CP. Death due to cerebrovascular diseases was increased five-fold. Hypopituitarism and diabetes insipidus were negative prognostic factors for mortality and morbidity [63, 64].

Obesity in patients with CP is due to a combination of hypothalamic dysfunction, leading to hyperphagia, decreased resting energy expenditure/basal metabolic rate, insulin resistance, and a distorted day–night rhythm, resulting in daytime somnolence and decreased activity/energy expenditure and obesity related to anterior pituitary dysfunction, for which adequate timing and dosing of growth hormone, thyroxine, glucocorticoids, and sex steroid treatment is essential for bodily homeostasis.

Obesity rates in children with craniopharyngiomas vary from 6 to 30% at diagnosis and increase to 40–60% after surgery [65]. It is therefore imperative to identify hypothalamic involvement pre-operatively both clinically and radiologically. Van Leserel et al. demonstrated that hypothalamic obesity is more prevalent in children as well as anterior pituitary dysfunction. These two factors, when combined, help explain why children with CP have a higher risk of mortality than adults [66]. Clinical pre-operative hypothalamic involvement is a poor prognostic indication of long-term outcomes [67]. This can be compounded by treatment related hypothalamic damage [65]. Currently, as hypothalamic obesity is difficult to treat, prevention remains the best strategy to date. This necessitates accurate pre-operative and intraoperative assessment.

Several pre-operative analysis of location and attachment to the hypothalamus have been described. One of the earliest grading systems to grade hypothalamic involvement was described by Puget et al. They proposed three grades, 0–2.

Grade 0 has no hypothalamic involvement, grade 1 the hypothalamus is displaced or compressed, and in grade 2 the hypothalamus is involved or unidentifiable. Using this grading scheme they recommended modifying the extent of resection by a hypothalamic sparing surgical strategy [68]. Since then, several other radiological classification schemes have been proposed. Van Gompel proposed to extend this grading system by including T2 changes in the hypothalamus and enhancement without a smooth interface as surrogate radiological markers of invasion [69]. There are two systems based on the mammillary bodies. The KRANIOPHARYNGEOM multi-centre research group who propose anatomical system based on the mammillary bodies providing a radiological landmark for the boundary between the anterior and posterior hypothalamus. Grade 1 involves anterior hypothalamic damage, whereas grade 2 involves damage to both the anterior and posterior hypothalamus [70, 71]. The other is based on mammillary body displacement as measured by the mammillary body angle [72].

A recent study by Prieto et al. attempts to predict the degree of adherence by the CP to the hypothalamus by analysing 3 components, the first component are the specific structures attached to the tumour, the second is the morphologic pattern or extent of the attachment, and the third is the adhesion strength which was reported intra-operatively. Combination of these 3 components determines 5 hierarchical levels of adherence severity with gradually increasing surgical risk of hypothalamic injury. They conclude that the position of the hypothalamus around the middle portion of the tumour, an amputated or infiltrated appearance of the pituitary stalk, and the elliptical shape of the tumour are reliable predictors of strong and extensive CP adhesions to the hypothalamus [73].

Tumours originating from the tubero-infundibular area or sub-arachnoid area will grow within the ventricle and form adhesions to the hypothalamus where no plane of dissection will be evident and can present with pre-operative hypothalamic findings [65]. ACPs have been described as more adhesive to surrounding neural structures based on the higher incidence of interdigitations that form at the brain–tumour interface. Other factors that may lead to ACPs being more strongly adherent are molecular derangements in the Wnt/β-catenin and claudin-1 pathways [12]. CPs arising from other origins may grow upwards distorting the floor of the third ventricle and there may be some layers of lepto-meninges at the brain/tumour interface.

Treatment of hypothalamic related obesity remains difficult. Prevention of hypothalamic damage remains the best strategy to date. However considering a significant number of patients present with pre-operative hypothalamic dysfunction treatment of hypothalamic obesity is required. Treatment options can include any or all the strategies employed in the treatment of conventional obesity such as life style modification, pharmacologic and surgical strategies.

However, in the hypothalamic obesity group these methods do not have the same outcomes as the successful management options in conventional obesity [74]. This is especially true of paediatric craniopharyngiomas. Studies involving life style modifications alone in craniopharyngioma-related hypothalamic obesity have consistently provided disappointing results [75]. To understand the possible reasons for this, one needs to understand how the hypothalamus regulates energy stores/metabolism/satiety and hunger and the complex interconnections and feedback systems involved with each mechanism and interplay with the circadian rhythm. Hypothalamic control of energy and energy stores in liver and adipose tissue is the result of a balance between lipolysis/lipogenesis and glycaemic control. This is mediated by the autonomic nervous system with both parasympathetic(PNS) and sympathetic(SNS) control originating from the paraventricular nucleus in the hypothalamus and projecting to the dorsal motor nucleus of the vagus (PNS) and lateral medulla and pre-locus coeruleus (SNS) [76, 77]. The peripheral signals from leptin, ghrelin, insulin, and nutrients are sensed in arcuate nucleus and have a feedback and feedforward control over two groups of neurones, known as orexigenic and anorexigenic neurones. These groups of neurones have inhibitory or excitatory effects on the paraventricular nucleus [77]. The suprachiasmatic nucleus is the main regulator of the circadian rhythm, via melatonin, and also has a balancing influence on autonomic nervous system. This coupled with reduced energy expenditure leads to hypothalamic obesity [78, 79]. This complex network provides the rationale of some of the attempts to pharmacologically treat hypothalamic obesity such as octreotide, diazoxide, metformin, glucagon like peptide 1, and beloranib [80–82]. Patients with hypothalamic obesity tend to have more risk and less benefit from surgical intervention for their obesity than patients with conventional or exogenous obesity. As the numbers for bariatric surgery for patient with CP are small, the first large meta-analysis to date was performed by Breault et al. in 2013. This is an individual level meta-analysis of 21 cases (6 Roux-en-Y gastric bypass, 8 sleeve gastrectomy, 6 adjustable banding, and 1 with biliopancreatic diversion). They demonstrated important weight loss after 1 year of follow-up. Since then, and a recent meta-analysis by Ni et al. in 2018 which include other more recent small series confirmed the benefit of bariatric surgery and that gastric bypass in the form of Roux-en-Y is the preferred treatment option [82].

11.7 Visual Outcomes

Visual loss is present in both age groups due to the close relationship of the tumour to the anterior visual pathway. Visual dysfunction is a cause of significant morbidity that has a profound impact on overall survival and quality of life. It has been demonstrated in adults with just mild visual impairment, mortality is increased twofold [83]. Visual symptoms can include blurring of vision and visual field defects. Ophthalmological findings include papilledema, optic nerve atrophy, reduction in visual acuity, and visual field defects [84]. Approximately 30% of paediatric CPs have visual complaints as the presenting symptom compared to approximately 95% of adults [55]. In the paediatric cohort, approximately 42% had optic nerve oedema, 41% with pallor compared to 6% and 14%, respectively, in adults. Up to 71.5% of children will have visual field defects compared to 60–84% of adults [55, 85–87].

Pre-operative factors that predict a good visual outcome are early surgery (within a week of presentation) and papilledema without optic nerve atrophy (OA).

Papilledema is a reversible process, whereas optic nerve atrophy is not [84]. Age at diagnosis has also been shown to influence visual outcome. Abrams et al. found the age less than 6 and visual symptoms on presentation were associated with a significantly poorer visual outcome [88], while Wan et al. found that age less than 10 at presentation was associated with visual decline [86]. Pre-operative factors that predict a poor outcome are OA, initial visual field defect, and tumour recurrence [84, 89]. Prieto et al. found that type of pre-operative and post-operative optic chiasmatic distortions on MRI can predict visual outcome. They defined 6 separate pre-operative and post-operative morphological categories. They found that a pre-operative compressed forward and stretched chiasms accounted for >80% of patients with visual loss. Post-operative finding of a thinned and displaced chiasm predicted no post-operative improvement [90].

As mentioned above, age at diagnosis is a predictor of visual outcome. This may be related to the child's ability to communicate or even appreciate the visual symptoms. Also, the younger the child the more difficult it can be for visual assessment of patient, as this requires a communicative and co-operative patient. Optical coherence tomography (OCT) is a relatively new technique whereby the thickness of the retinal nerve fibre layer (RNFL) can be measured with sub-micrometre precision. This is achieved by measuring the echo time delay of back-scattered infrared light using an interferometer and a low-coherence light source. This method provides an objective measure of optic nerve atrophy. Danesh-Meyer et al. established that patients with measurable reduction in RNFL pre-operatively from compressive chiasmatic lesions were less likely to have return of VA and VF post-operatively. In patients with significant pre-operative VA and VF deficits and normal RNFL thickness, post-operative visual function showed large improvements following decompression. Whereas patients with thin RNFL and advanced VF defect demonstrate significantly less improvement [91]. Both Mediero et al. and Bialer et al. have demonstrated the utility of OCT specifically in the use of paediatric craniopharyngiomas [92, 93].

11.8   Neurocognitive and Quality of Life Outcomes

When one considers that patients with craniopharyngioma may have morbidity associated with any or all of the vital structures such as hypothalamic, pituitary, visual and CSF pathways, it is invariable that the combination of these morbidities will have a significant impact on neurocognitive and quality of life for patients with craniopharyngioma. Morbidity can result from the tumour invading critical structures directly or from collateral damage to the same structures from intervention such as surgery or radiotherapy.

When one considers the dynamic nature of the developing child and the need for intact neuroendocrine, hypothalamic and visual systems in their development and the complex interplay and dependence of each system needed to achieve developmental milestones, both physical and cognitive, one can understand that the timing of intervention is critical to maximise the impact on the natural history of the disease while minimising the impact of said intervention.

Distortion or damage to the floor of the third ventricle can also cause neurocognitive issues. Structures in this area that influence cognition include the hypothalamus and its mammillary bodies.

The hypothalamus is a bilateral cluster of nuclei in the basal diencephalon occupying the walls and floor of the third ventricle. It acts as a complex nexus between the endocrine, autonomic nervous system, and limbic systems. The hypothalamus can regulate thermal and water homeostasis, sexual behaviour, integration of neuroendocrine and autonomic responses to stress, circadian rhythms, neurohypophyseal hormones, food/calorie intake and adipose homeostasis, cardiovascular and respiratory regulation, defensive and aggressive behaviours, wakefulness, motivated behaviours, and episodic memory encoding [94]. Damage to the hypothalamus can lead to both neurocognitive and neurobehavioural issues. Neurocognitive deficits can take on the form as reduced intelligent quotient (IQ). Even in patients with reduce IQ there can be impairment of memory, higher executive functioning, attention and processing speed [95, 96]. Neurobehavioural deficits can manifest as psychosocial issues such as depression, anxiety, mood disorders, and in children can limit independence [97, 98]. Pascual et al. performed a systemic review and meta-analysis psychiatric disorders caused by CPs and the hypothalamic alterations. They classified six main psychiatric disturbances (1) Korsakoff-like memory deficits (2) behavioural/personality changes (3) impaired emotional expression, (4) cognitive impairment, (5) mood alterations, and (6) psychotic symptoms. They found that coexistence of other hypothalamic symptoms favoured the emergence of psychotic disorders. They also found that there was a difference between children and adults. All types of alterations involving the emotional expression/control were significantly higher in children, whereas memory impairments predominated in adults [99]. Recently, it has been shown that there may be a role for oxytocin supplementation in children with hypothalamic obesity and behavioural problems [100, 101].

The mammillary bodies have an important role in memory formation. It functions as hippocampal relay projecting to the anterior thalamus via the unidirectional mamillothalamic tract. In turn, the anterior thalamic nuclei project to the cingulate. The mammillary bodies receive input from hippocampal formation via the descending component of the postcommissural fornix, this is referred to as the circuit of Papez. The mammillary bodies also receive input from the tegmental nuclei of Gudden via the mammillary peduncle [102, 103]. It is well established that damage to the mammillary bodies is present in such syndromes as Wernicke–Korsakoff and case reports establish that surgical lesions including craniopharyngiomas can cause damage to the mammillary bodies can also cause this or similar syndromes [104–106].

Regarding educational attainment, patients with childhood onset for the most part attended mainstream school both primary and secondary schools; however, they were noted to have more difficulties. Fewer graduated from secondary school/high school and fewer again attended third level education [107].

Memmesheimer et al. surveyed 59 adult patients with childhood-onset CP craniopharyngioma and found a relationship with age and social integration/independence. Using housing as a marker for social integration/independence they found the majority of young adults lived with their parents, whereas older adults tended to be independent. Although there is a natural growth in independence with age, this is less in patients with CP when compared to the general population [97]. Crom et al. noted that 19.6% of patients with childhood-onset CP required a special educational plan, 3.9% had a special education certificate of attendance, 25.4% received a high school diploma, 3.9% were college graduates, and only 1.9% achieved a postgraduate degree [107].

Several studies have shown that patients with craniopharyngioma rated their health-related quality of life as considerably lower than healthy controls. Parents' ratings were considerably lower than those of the patients. Poor functional outcome was associated with large tumours infiltrating or displacing the hypothalamus, the occurrence of hydrocephalus, and young age at diagnosis, but also with multiple operations due to tumour recurrence [95, 108–111].

11.9 Conclusion

The term craniopharyngioma comprises almost two distinct biological entities, aCP and pCP. Although they can arise from the same cell lineage they are different in almost every respect (see Table 11.1). The adamantinomatous variety is the most challenging of the two. It is only this type that is found in children compared to the mixture of the two found in adults. In adult-onset craniopharyngioma the aCP variety is more common than the pCP.

What should be clear is that the same insult, be it tumour or intervention, can have very different outcomes on the patients depending what stage of neurodevelopment they are at. This is due to the location of the tumour and the associated systems involved in the neurodevelopment process. As adult-onset CP cohort contains pCP with its favourable characteristics for resection and recurrence and this cohort by its nature will have completed neurodevelopment, outcome measures may naturally be better than childhood onset CP. It is for this reason that temporising measures of cyst drainage and intracystic therapies are being developed in childhood-onset CP to allow as much neurodevelopment to occur before a definitive surgical approach is taken.

References

1. Louis DN, Ohgaki H, Wiestler OD, Cavenee WK. In: Fred T. Bosman ESJ, Lakhani SR, Ohgaki H, editors. WHO classification of tumours of the central nervous system. 4th ed. Lyon: IARC; 2007. p. 309.
2. Sofela AA, et al. Malignant transformation in craniopharyngiomas. Neurosurgery. 2014;75:306.
3. Nielsen EH, et al. Incidence of craniopharyngioma in Denmark (n = 189) and estimated world incidence of craniopharyngioma in children and adults. J Neuro-Oncol. 2011;104:755.
4. Zacharia BE, et al. Incidence, treatment and survival of patients with craniopharyngioma in the surveillance, epidemiology and end results program. Neuro-Oncology. 2012;14(8):1070–8.
5. Dohrmann GJ, Farwell JR. Intracranial neoplasms in children: a comparison of North America, Europe, Africa, and Asia. Dis Nerv Syst. 1976;37(12):696–7.

6. Haupt R, et al. Epidemiological aspects of craniopharyngioma. J Pediatr Endocrinol Metab. 2006;19(Suppl 1):289–93.
7. Wang L, et al. Primary adult infradiaphragmatic craniopharyngiomas: clinical features, management, and outcomes in one Chinese institution. World Neurosurg. 2014;81(5-6):773–82.
8. Qi S, et al. Anatomic relations of the arachnoidea around the pituitary stalk: relevance for surgical removal of craniopharyngiomas. Acta Neurochir. 2011;153(4):785–96.
9. Davis SW, et al. Pituitary gland development and disease: from stem cell to hormone production. Curr Top Dev Biol. 2013;106:1–47.
10. Prabhu VC, Brown HG. The pathogenesis of craniopharyngiomas. Childs Nerv Syst. 2005;21(8-9):622–7.
11. Bao Y, et al. Origin of craniopharyngiomas: implications for growth pattern, clinical characteristics, and outcomes of tumor recurrence. J Neurosurg. 2016;125(1):24–32.
12. Prieto R, et al. Craniopharyngioma adherence: a reappraisal of the evidence. Neurosurg Rev. 2018. https://doi.org/10.1007/s10143-018-1010-9.
13. Ciappetta P, Pescatori L. Anatomic dissection of arachnoid membranes encircling the pituitary stalk on fresh, non-formalin-fixed specimens: anatomoradiologic correlations and clinical applications in craniopharyngioma surgery. World Neurosurg. 2017;108:479–90.
14. Pascual JM, Prieto R, Carrasco R. Infundibulo-tuberal or not strictly intraventricular craniopharyngioma: evidence for a major topographical category. Acta Neurochir. 2011;153(12):2403–25; discussion 2426.
15. Nielsen EH, et al. Acute presentation of craniopharyngioma in children and adults in a Danish national cohort. Pituitary. 2013;16(4):528–35.
16. Daubenbuchel AM, et al. Hydrocephalus and hypothalamic involvement in pediatric patients with craniopharyngioma or cysts of Rathke's pouch: impact on long-term prognosis. Eur J Endocrinol. 2015;172(5):561–9.
17. Elliott RE, Wisoff JH. Surgical management of giant pediatric craniopharyngiomas. J Neurosurg Pediatr. 2010;6(5):403–16.
18. Schlaffer SM, et al. Rathke's cleft cyst as origin of a pediatric papillary craniopharyngioma. Front Genet. 2018;9:49.
19. Borrill R, et al. Papillary craniopharyngioma in a 4-year-old girl with BRAF V600E mutation: a case report and review of the literature. Childs Nerv Syst. 2019;35:169.
20. Apps JR, Martinez-Barbera JP. Molecular pathology of adamantinomatous craniopharyngioma: review and opportunities for practice. Neurosurg Focus. 2016;41(6):E4.
21. Sekine S, et al. Expression of enamel proteins and LEF1 in adamantinomatous craniopharyngioma: evidence for its odontogenic epithelial differentiation. Histopathology. 2004;45(6):573–9.
22. Larkin SJ, Ansorge O. Pathology and pathogenesis of craniopharyngiomas. Pituitary. 2013;16(1):9–17.
23. Schweizer L, et al. BRAF V600E analysis for the differentiation of papillary craniopharyngiomas and Rathke's cleft cysts. Neuropathol Appl Neurobiol. 2015;41(6):733–42.
24. Brastianos PK, Santagata S. Endocrine tumors: BRAF V600E mutations in papillary craniopharyngioma. Eur J Endocrinol. 2016;174(4):R139–44.
25. Malgulwar PB, et al. Study of beta-catenin and BRAF alterations in adamantinomatous and papillary craniopharyngiomas: mutation analysis with immunohistochemical correlation in 54 cases. J Neuro-Oncol. 2017;133(3):487–95.
26. Holsken A, et al. Adamantinomatous and papillary craniopharyngiomas are characterized by distinct epigenomic as well as mutational and transcriptomic profiles. Acta Neuropathol Commun. 2016;4:20.
27. Hussain I, et al. Molecular oncogenesis of craniopharyngioma: current and future strategies for the development of targeted therapies. J Neurosurg. 2013;119(1):106–12.
28. Yoshimoto K, et al. High-resolution melting and immunohistochemical analysis efficiently detects mutually exclusive genetic alterations of adamantinomatous and papillary craniopharyngiomas. Neuropathology. 2018;38(1):3–10.

29. Gao C, et al. Exon 3 mutations of CTNNB1 drive tumorigenesis: a review. Oncotarget. 2018;9(4):5492–508.
30. Yang Y. Wnt signaling in development and disease. Cell Biosci. 2012;2(1):14.
31. Apps JR, et al. Tumour compartment transcriptomics demonstrates the activation of inflammatory and odontogenic programmes in human adamantinomatous craniopharyngioma and identifies the MAPK/ERK pathway as a novel therapeutic target. Acta Neuropathol. 2018;135(5):757–77.
32. Preda V, et al. The Wnt signalling cascade and the adherens junction complex in craniopharyngioma tumorigenesis. Endocr Pathol. 2015;26(1):1–8.
33. Burghaus S, et al. A tumor-specific cellular environment at the brain invasion border of adamantinomatous craniopharyngiomas. Virchows Arch. 2010;456(3):287–300.
34. Stache C, et al. Tight junction protein claudin-1 is differentially expressed in craniopharyngioma subtypes and indicates invasive tumor growth. Neuro-Oncology. 2014;16(2):256–64.
35. Massimi L, et al. Proteomics in pediatric cystic craniopharyngioma. Brain Pathol. 2017;27(3):370–6.
36. Martelli C, et al. Proteomic characterization of pediatric craniopharyngioma intracystic fluid by LC-MS top-down/bottom-up integrated approaches. Electrophoresis. 2014;35(15):2172–83.
37. Benveniste EN, Qin H. Type I interferons as anti-inflammatory mediators. Sci STKE. 2007;2007(416):pe70.
38. Falini B, Martelli MP, Tiacci E. BRAF V600E mutation in hairy cell leukemia: from bench to bedside. Blood. 2016;128(15):1918–27.
39. Brastianos PK, et al. Dramatic response of BRAF V600E mutant papillary craniopharyngioma to targeted therapy. J Natl Cancer Inst. 2016;108(2):djv310.
40. Himes BT, et al. Recurrent papillary craniopharyngioma with BRAF V600E mutation treated with dabrafenib: case report. J Neurosurg. 2018;130:1299–303.
41. Jung TY, et al. Adult craniopharyngiomas: surgical results with a special focus on endocrinological outcomes and recurrence according to pituitary stalk preservation. J Neurosurg. 2009;111(3):572–7.
42. Cheng J, Fan Y, Cen B. Effect of preserving the pituitary stalk during resection of craniopharyngioma in children on the diabetes insipidus and relapse rates and long-term outcomes. J Craniofac Surg. 2017;28(6):e591–5.
43. Li K, et al. Association of pituitary stalk management with endocrine outcomes and recurrence in microsurgery of craniopharyngiomas: a meta-analysis. Clin Neurol Neurosurg. 2015;136:20–4.
44. Jung TY, et al. Endocrinological outcomes of pediatric craniopharyngiomas with anatomical pituitary stalk preservation: preliminary study. Pediatr Neurosurg. 2010;46(3):205–12.
45. Steinbok P, Hukin J. Intracystic treatments for craniopharyngioma. Neurosurg Focus. 2010;28(4):E13.
46. Qiao N. Endocrine outcomes of endoscopic versus transcranial resection of craniopharyngiomas: a system review and meta-analysis. Clin Neurol Neurosurg. 2018;169.107–15.
47. Alotaibi NM, et al. Physiologic growth hormone-replacement therapy and craniopharyngioma recurrence in pediatric patients: a meta-analysis. World Neurosurg. 2018;109:487–496. e1.
48. Smith TR, et al. Physiological growth hormone replacement and rate of recurrence of craniopharyngioma: the Genentech National Cooperative Growth Study. J Neurosurg Pediatr. 2016;18(4):408–12.
49. Shen L, et al. Growth hormone therapy and risk of recurrence/progression in intracranial tumors: a meta-analysis. Neurol Sci. 2015;36(10):1859–67.
50. Kilday JP, et al. Intracystic interferon-alpha in pediatric craniopharyngioma patients: an international multicenter assessment on behalf of SIOPE and ISPN. Neuro-Oncology. 2017;19(10):1398–407.
51. Bock RD. Multiple prepubertal growth spurts in children of the Fels Longitudinal Study: comparison with results from the Edinburgh Growth Study. Ann Hum Biol. 2004;31(1):59–74.

52. Butler GE, McKie M, Ratcliffe SG. The cyclical nature of prepubertal growth. Ann Hum Biol. 1990;17(3):177–98.
53. Guadagno E, et al. Can recurrences be predicted in craniopharyngiomas? beta-catenin coexisting with stem cells markers and p-ATM in a clinicopathologic study of 45 cases. J Exp Clin Cancer Res. 2017;36(1):95.
54. Coury JR, et al. Histopathological and molecular predictors of growth patterns and recurrence in craniopharyngiomas: a systematic review. Neurosurg Rev. 2018. https://doi.org/10.1007/s10143-018-0978-5.
55. Dandurand C, et al. Adult craniopharyngioma: case series, systematic review, and meta-analysis. Neurosurgery. 2018;83:631.
56. Clark AJ, et al. A systematic review of the results of surgery and radiotherapy on tumor control for pediatric craniopharyngioma. Childs Nerv Syst. 2013;29(2):231–8.
57. Du C, et al. Ectopic recurrence of pediatric craniopharyngiomas after gross total resection: a report of two cases and a review of the literature. Childs Nerv Syst. 2016;32(8):1523–9.
58. Gillis J, Loughlan P. Not just small adults: the metaphors of paediatrics. Arch Dis Child. 2007;92(11):946–7.
59. Patel VS, et al. Outcomes after endoscopic endonasal resection of craniopharyngiomas in the pediatric population. World Neurosurg. 2017;108:6–14.
60. Alalade AF, et al. Suprasellar and recurrent pediatric craniopharyngiomas: expanding indications for the extended endoscopic transsphenoidal approach. J Neurosurg Pediatr. 2018;21(1):72–80.
61. Cavallo LM, et al. The endoscopic endonasal approach for the management of craniopharyngiomas: a series of 103 patients. J Neurosurg. 2014;121(1):100–13.
62. Jang YJ, Kim SC. Pneumatization of the sphenoid sinus in children evaluated by magnetic resonance imaging. Am J Rhinol. 2000;14(3):181–5.
63. Wijnen M, et al. Excess morbidity and mortality in patients with craniopharyngioma: a hospital-based retrospective cohort study. Eur J Endocrinol. 2018;178(1):95–104.
64. Olsson DS, et al. Excess mortality and morbidity in patients with craniopharyngioma, especially in patients with childhood onset: a population-based study in Sweden. J Clin Endocrinol Metab. 2015;100(2):467–74.
65. Park SW, et al. Tumor origin and growth pattern at diagnosis and surgical hypothalamic damage predict obesity in pediatric craniopharyngioma. J Neuro-Oncol. 2013;113(3):417–24.
66. van Iersel L, et al. The development of hypothalamic obesity in craniopharyngioma patients: a risk factor analysis in a well-defined cohort. Pediatr Blood Cancer. 2018;65(5):e26911.
67. Muller HL. Hypothalamic involvement in craniopharyngioma-Implications for surgical, radiooncological, and molecularly targeted treatment strategies. Pediatr Blood Cancer. 2018;65(5):e26936.
68. Puget S, et al. Pediatric craniopharyngiomas: classification and treatment according to the degree of hypothalamic involvement. J Neurosurg. 2007;106(1 Suppl):3–12.
69. Van Gompel JJ, et al. Magnetic resonance imaging–graded hypothalamic compression in surgically treated adult craniopharyngiomas determining postoperative obesity. Neurosurg Focus. 2010;28(4):E3.
70. Muller HL, et al. Post-operative hypothalamic lesions and obesity in childhood craniopharyngioma: results of the multinational prospective trial KRANIOPHARYNGEOM 2000 after 3-year follow-up. Eur J Endocrinol. 2011;165(1):17–24.
71. Muller HL, et al. Xanthogranuloma, Rathke's cyst, and childhood craniopharyngioma: results of prospective multinational studies of children and adolescents with rare sellar malformations. J Clin Endocrinol Metab. 2012;97(11):3935–43.
72. Pascual JM, et al. Displacement of mammillary bodies by craniopharyngiomas involving the third ventricle: surgical-MRI correlation and use in topographical diagnosis. J Neurosurg. 2013;119(2):381–405.
73. Prieto R, et al. Preoperative assessment of craniopharyngioma adherence: magnetic resonance imaging findings correlated with the severity of tumor attachment to the hypothalamus. World Neurosurg. 2018;110:e404–26.

74. Colquitt JL, et al. Surgery for weight loss in adults. Cochrane Database Syst Rev. 2014(8):Cd003641. https://doi.org/10.1002/14651858.CD003641.pub4.
75. Holmer H, et al. Reduced energy expenditure and impaired feeding-related signals but not high energy intake reinforces hypothalamic obesity in adults with childhood onset craniopharyngioma. J Clin Endocrinol Metab. 2010;95(12):5395–402.
76. Geerling JC, et al. Paraventricular hypothalamic nucleus: axonal projections to the brainstem. J Comp Neurol. 2010;518(9):1460–99.
77. Haliloglu B, Bereket A. Hypothalamic obesity in children: pathophysiology to clinical management. J Pediatr Endocrinol Metab. 2015;28(5-6):503–13.
78. Nagai K, et al. SCN output drives the autonomic nervous system: with special reference to the autonomic function related to the regulation of glucose metabolism. Prog Brain Res. 1996;111:253–72.
79. Harz KJ, et al. Obesity in patients with craniopharyngioma: assessment of food intake and movement counts indicating physical activity. J Clin Endocrinol Metab. 2003;88(11):5227–31.
80. Castro-Dufourny I, Carrasco R, Pascual JM. Hypothalamic obesity after craniopharyngioma surgery: treatment with a long acting glucagon like peptide 1 derivated. Endocrinol Diabetes Nutr (English ed). 2017;64(3):182–4.
81. Hamilton JK, et al. Hypothalamic obesity following craniopharyngioma surgery: results of a pilot trial of combined diazoxide and metformin therapy. Int J Pediatr Endocrinol. 2011;2011:1–7.
82. Ni W, Shi X. Interventions for the treatment of craniopharyngioma-related hypothalamic obesity: a systematic review. World Neurosurg. 2018;118:e59.
83. McCarty CA, Nanjan MB, Taylor HR. Vision impairment predicts 5 year mortality. Br J Ophthalmol. 2001;85(3):322–6.
84. Jacobsen MF, et al. Predictors of visual outcome in patients operated for craniopharyngioma - a Danish national study. Acta Ophthalmol. 2018;96(1):39–45.
85. Drimtzias E, et al. The ophthalmic natural history of paediatric craniopharyngioma: a long-term review. J Neuro-Oncol. 2014;120(3):651–6.
86. Wan MJ, et al. Long-term visual outcomes of craniopharyngioma in children. J Neuro-Oncol. 2018;137(3):645–51.
87. Astradsson A, et al. Visual outcome, endocrine function and tumor control after fractionated stereotactic radiation therapy of craniopharyngiomas in adults: findings in a prospective cohort. Acta Oncol. 2017;56(3):415–21.
88. Abrams LS, Repka MX. Visual outcome of craniopharyngioma in children. J Pediatr Ophthalmol Strabismus. 1997;34(4):223–8.
89. Lee MJ, Hwang J-M. Initial visual field as a predictor of recurrence and postoperative visual outcome in children with craniopharyngioma. J Pediatr Ophthalmol Strabismus. 2012;49:38.
90. Prieto R, Pascual JM, Barrios L. Optic chiasm distortions caused by craniopharyngiomas: clinical and magnetic resonance imaging correlation and influence on visual outcome. World Neurosurg. 2015;83(4):500–29.
91. Danesh-Meyer HV, et al. In vivo retinal nerve fiber layer thickness measured by optical coherence tomography predicts visual recovery after surgery for parachiasmal tumors. Invest Ophthalmol Vis Sci. 2008;49(5):1879–85.
92. Bialer OY, et al. Retinal NFL thinning on OCT correlates with visual field loss in pediatric craniopharyngioma. Can J Ophthalmol. 2013;48(6):494–9.
93. Mediero S, et al. Visual outcomes, visual fields, and optical coherence tomography in paediatric craniopharyngioma. Neuroophthalmology. 2015;39(3):132–9.
94. Barbosa DAN, et al. The hypothalamus at the crossroads of psychopathology and neurosurgery. Neurosurg Focus. 2017;43(3):E15.
95. Ozyurt J, Muller HL, Thiel CM. A systematic review of cognitive performance in patients with childhood craniopharyngioma. J Neuro-Oncol. 2015;125(1):9–21.
96. Fjalldal S, et al. Hypothalamic involvement predicts cognitive performance and psychosocial health in long-term survivors of childhood craniopharyngioma. J Clin Endocrinol Metab. 2013;98(8):3253–62.

97. Memmesheimer RM, et al. Psychological well-being and independent living of young adults with childhood-onset craniopharyngioma. Dev Med Child Neurol. 2017;59(8):829–36.

98. Ondruch A, et al. Cognitive and social functioning in children and adolescents after the removal of craniopharyngioma. Childs Nerv Syst. 2010;27(3):391–7.

99. Pascual JM, et al. Craniopharyngiomas primarily involving the hypothalamus: a model of neurosurgical lesions to elucidate the neurobiological basis of psychiatric disorders. World Neurosurg. 2018;120:e1245.

100. Hoffmann A, et al. First experiences with neuropsychological effects of oxytocin administration in childhood-onset craniopharyngioma. Endocrine. 2017;56(1):175–85.

101. Daubenbuchel AM, et al. Oxytocin in survivors of childhood-onset craniopharyngioma. Endocrine. 2016;54(2):524–31.

102. Dillingham CM, et al. How do mammillary body inputs contribute to anterior thalamic function? Neurosci Biobehav Rev. 2015;54:108–19.

103. Vann SD, Nelson AJ. The mammillary bodies and memory: more than a hippocampal relay. Prog Brain Res. 2015;219:163–85.

104. Tanaka Y, et al. Amnesia following damage to the mammillary bodies. Neurology. 1997;48(1):160–5.

105. Savastano LE, et al. Korsakoff syndrome from retrochiasmatic suprasellar lesions: rapid reversal after relief of cerebral compression in 4 cases. J Neurosurg. 2018;128(6):1731–6.

106. Kahn EA, Crosby EC. Korsakoff's syndrome associated with surgical lesions involving the mammillary bodies. Neurology. 1972;22(2):117–25.

107. Crom DB, et al. Health status in long-term survivors of pediatric craniopharyngiomas. J Neurosci Nurs. 2010;42(6):323–8.

108. Poretti A, et al. Outcome of craniopharyngioma in children: long-term complications and quality of life. Dev Med Child Neurol. 2004;46(4):220–9.

109. Pedreira CC, et al. Health related quality of life and psychological outcome in patients treated for craniopharyngioma in childhood. J Pediatr Endocrinol Metab. 2006;19(1):15.

110. Laffond C, et al. Quality-of-life, mood and executive functioning after childhood craniopharyngioma treated with surgery and proton beam therapy. Brain Inj. 2012;26(3):270–81.

111. Heinks K, et al. Quality of life and growth after childhood craniopharyngioma: results of the multinational trial KRANIOPHARYNGEOM 2007. Endocrine. 2018;59(2):364–72.

Elham Rostami, Olivera Casar-Borota,
and Olafur Gudjonsson

12.1   Introduction

Harvey Cushing described craniopharyngiomas (CP) as "the most baffling problem which confronts the neurosurgeon" [1]. The current standard treatment for these histologically benign, but clinically aggressive tumours is surgery followed by adjuvant radiation therapy. However, there is a high recurrence rate [2], with additional morbidity. The histological distinction between the adamantinomatous (ACP) and papillary (PCP) subtype of craniopharyngioma has been known for decades. However, recent developments in molecular and genetic analysis have identified specific mutations in each, β-catenin in ACP and BRAF mutation in PCP [3, 4] and also a distinct methylation pattern [5]. This has also shed more light on the heterogeneity and pathology of this tumour and opened a new field of treatment opportunities [6]. Furthermore, findings indicating connection between stem cells and ACP have postulated the paracrine model in which pituitary stem cells drive neoplastic proliferation of nearby epithelial cells through growth factor signalling [7, 8]. The increased

E. Rostami (✉)
Department of Neuroscience, Uppsala University, Uppsala, Sweden

Department of Neurosurgery, Uppsala University Hospital, Uppsala, Sweden

Department of Neuroscience, Karolinska Institutet, Stockholm, Sweden
e-mail: Elham.rostami@neuro.uu.se

O. Casar-Borota
Department of Clinical Pathology, Uppsala University Hospital, Uppsala, Sweden

Department of Immunology, Genetics and Pathology, Uppsala University, Uppsala, Sweden
e-mail: olivera.casar-borota@igp.uu.se

O. Gudjonsson
Department of Neuroscience, Uppsala University, Uppsala, Sweden

Department of Neurosurgery, Uppsala University Hospital, Uppsala, Sweden
e-mail: olafur.gudjonsson@Akademiska.se

© Springer Nature Switzerland AG 2020   209
E. Jouanneau, G. Raverot (eds.), *Adult Craniopharyngiomas*,
https://doi.org/10.1007/978-3-030-41176-3_12

interest in molecular and genetic alterations in CPs has identified several biomarkers that have paved the way for new possibility to predict the biological behaviour of this tumour as well as early diagnosis of recurrence and new treatment options.

12.2   Adamantinomatous Craniopharyngioma

12.2.1 Histopathology

ACP is a cystic tumour composed of cords and lobules of squamous, frequently whorled epithelium bordered by palisading columnar basal cells. The epithelium has a looser structure in the areas designated as stellate reticulum. Islands of the so-called wet keratin representing anucleate degenerative remnants of tumour epithelial cells are easily recognized in the majority of cases. The tumour epithelium protrudes into surrounding brain tissue that usually demonstrates gliosis, Rosenthal fibres and lymphocytic inflammatory reaction. Less frequently, granulomatous reaction and cholesterol clefts may be seen. Occasionally, groups of adenohypophyseal cells can be identified in the inflammatory infiltrates.

12.2.2 CTNNB1

Two-thirds of human ACP shows a mutation in the regulatory gene encoding β-catenin CTNNB1 [3, 4, 9]. β-catenin is a cytoplasmic protein that regulates gene transcription in Wingless–Int (Wnt) signalling and plays an important role in stem cell renewal and organ regeneration [10]. Levels of cytoplasmic β-catenin are kept low by a protein inhibitory complex comprising of adenomatous polyposis coli/glycogen synthase kinase-3β (GSK-3β)/axin that induces proteasomal degradation. The mutant form of β-catenin that is expressed following mutation in CTNNB1 results in enhanced degradation resistance and accumulation of β-catenin [11].

Abnormal expression of β-catenin induces neoplastic transformation of normal cells. Immunohistochemical analysis with anti-β-catenin antibody reveals membrane expression of the protein in the epithelial cells with nucleocytoplasmic accumulation in the cell clusters forming whorled structures. The nucleocytoplasmic accumulation of β-catenin is a hallmark of ACP [12]. It has been shown that stronger β-catenin immunostaining is positively associated with tumour progression and recurrence [13].

When Wnt signalling is activated, the GSK-3β is phosphorylated leading to dissociation of the inhibitory complex. This inhibits the degradation of β-catenin and levels of β-catenin increase in the cytoplasm. This, in turn, induces transcription factor, T-cell factor/lymphoid enhancer-binding factor, and mutations along this pathway are associated with several diseases and cancer types [11]. This wide range involvement of Wnt/β-catenin signalling pathway provides alternative points for therapeutic interventions and has made this pathway a prime target for pharmacological research and development [14].

Histological, immunohistochemical and molecular features of ACP are illustrated in Fig. 12.1.

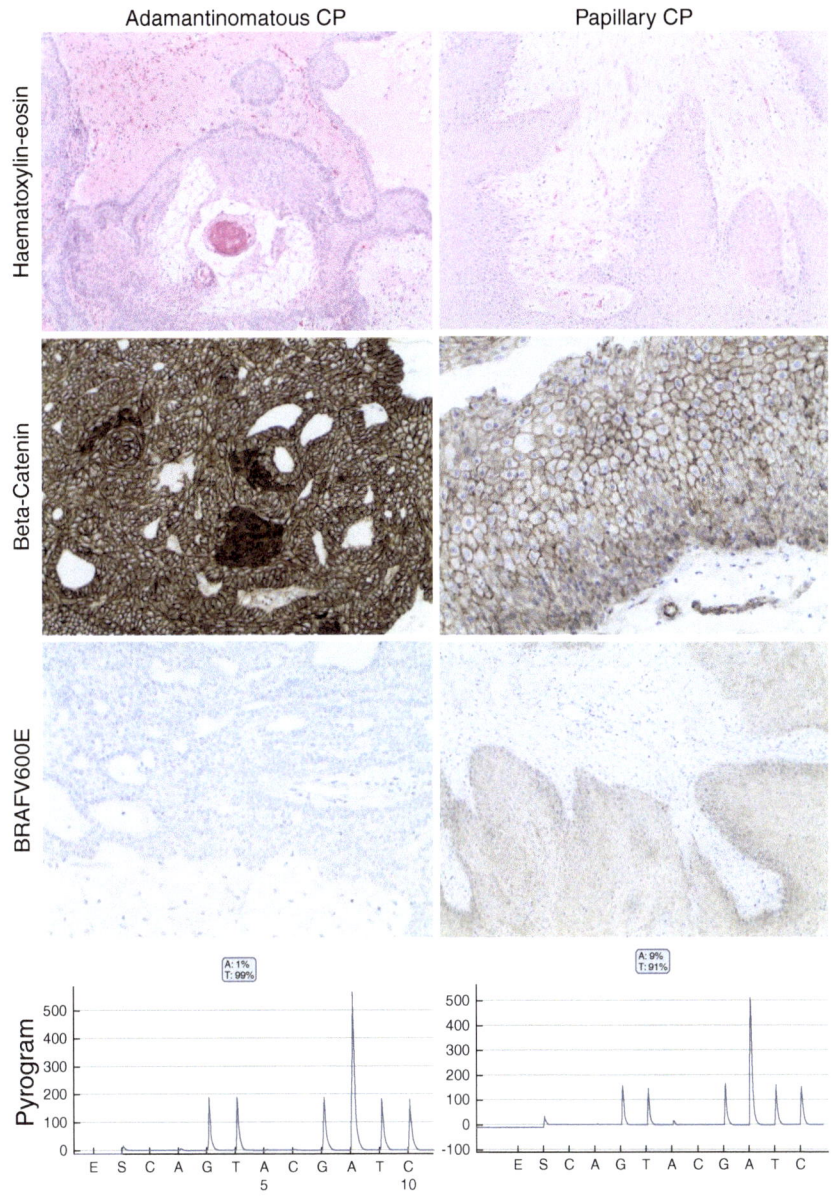

Fig. 12.1 Histopathological and molecular genetic features of adamantinomatous and papillary craniopharyngioma. Haematoxylin-eosin staining demonstrates epithelial cords with "stellate reticulum" and "wet keratin" in ACP and papillary epithelial protrusions in PCP (×100). Beta-catenin shows nucleocytoplasmic accumulation in whorled tumour cell clusters in ACP and membranous expression in epithelial tumour cells of PCP (×200). Immunohistochemistry for BRAFV600E shows no immunolabeling in ACP and usually weak intracytoplasmic immunolabeling in epithelial tumour cells in PCP (×100). Pyrogram generated from the BRAF wild-type ACP specimen and from the PCP specimen demonstrating c.1799 T > A mutation resulting in the V600E mutant BRAF protein

12.2.3 Growth Factors

Disruption of several growth factor pathways has been demonstrated in ACP. Overexpression of epidermal growth factor receptor (EGFR) has been shown both on mRNA and protein level. EGFR plays a role in Wnt signalling activation through direct interaction with β-catenin. Fascin, a β-catenin target gene, is involved in cellular motility upon activation and is also increased in ACP. Activated EGFR has shown to significantly promote tumour cell migration in vitro and nuclear coexpression of activated EGFR, β-catenin, and fascin has been detected in infiltrating cell aggregates [15]. Both EGFR activation and fascin expression was significantly decreased by gefitinib, an EGFR inhibitor. This indicates that EGFR signalling may play a role in cell migration and brain parenchyma infiltration often seen in ACP [15].

Vascular endothelial growth factor (VEGF) is important in angiogenesis and tumour growth and Wnt/β-catenin signalling regulates its transcription. In APC with constitutively active β-catenin and Wnt signalling there is an overexpression of VEGF. VEGF overexpression has also been associated with recurrence of ACP [16]. Thus, there is a potential for VEGF-inhibitors such as bevacizumab that is in use as first-line therapy in a variety of cancers to be tested in ACP.

Additional growth factors that have shown increased expression in ACP are fibroblast growth factor (FGF), growth hormone receptor (GHR) and insulin-like growth factor 1 receptor (IGF-1R).

12.3 Papillary Craniopharyngioma

12.3.1 Histopathology

PCP is characterized by a papillary growth pattern with mature nonkeratinizing squamous epithelium lining fibrovascular cores. This histological subtype typically lacks "wet keratin" and whorled epithelial cell clusters. β-catenin is expressed in the cell membrane without nucleocytoplasmic aggregates characteristic for ACP.

12.3.2 BRAFV600E

The BRAF gene is coding for a cytosolic serine/threonine kinase that is part of the mitogen-activated protein kinase (MAPK) pathway. It is activated by a somatic point mutation in human cancer and upregulates MAPK pathway [17]. This promotes transcription of prosurvival and growth genes. This hyperactivity disrupts hormone-producing cells development and encourages the proliferation of pituitary stem cells. BRAFV600E mutation is present in more than 95% of PCP cases [3, 18] and no other recurrent mutations or genomic aberrations have been reported so far.

Immunohistochemical analysis with antibody towards mutated BRAFV600E shows cytoplasmic immunolabeling of the epithelial tumour cells in PCPs. As immunolabeling with antibody toward BrafV600E mutated BRAF can be observed even without the presence of the mutation [19, 20], molecular genetic analysis is highly recommended to confirm the mutation and should be obligatory when pharmacological therapy targeted the mutant BRAF is considered. Craniopharyngioma cases with uncertain histological pattern can be subcategorised into specific variants following targeted sequencing for BRAFV600E and immunohistochemical analysis for β-catenin [21]. Rarely, BRAFV600E mutation can coexist with CTNNB1 mutations in adamantinomatous craniopharyngioma [22], which motivates at least immunohistochemical analysis of BRAFV600E even in ACPs. Pathologists should be aware of strong BRAFV600E immunolabeling not related to the BRAF mutation in a subset of adenohypophyseal cells in the surgical specimens containing the islands of anterior pituitary tissue [20].

Histological, immunohistochemical and molecular features of PCP are illustrated in Fig. 12.1.

12.4   Transitional and Mixed CP

Although craniopharyngiomas are divided into adamantinomatous and papillary type based on their histological features, cases with combined and transitional type have been reported [21, 23–26]. Reports on the coexistence of CTNNB1 and BRAF mutations in CPs further support the true existence of mixed CPs [22, 27].

The proposed hypotheses are that either the tumour may have developed from two different sources at the same time, or a cystic area of ACP may have undergone squamous metaplasia with the development of PCP. The first hypothesis and the embryological origin are supported by the histological and genetic overlapping [22] and also described in a foetal autopsy case of embryonal craniopharyngioma [28]. There is also a suggestion that the combined features in ACP are the result of squamous metaplasia mediated by inflammation [25]; however, the evidence for this is currently very weak. The resemblance of Rathke's cleft cyst (RCC) and PCP has been suggested to support the hypothesis that PCP is a histopathological continuum with RCC [23]. The mixed cases tend to have a higher recurrence rate [21, 24].

Although there are evidence of mixed CP in the literature, the origin and clinical course of these rare CPs remains unclear.

12.5   Postnatal Pituitary Progenitor/Stem Cells

Recently, there has been a high interest in the connection between stem cells and CP. Embryonic stem cells express specific genes and molecular markers, and several of these have been detected in the marginal zone of human pituitary [29]. Furthermore, several molecular markers shared by pluripotent embryonic stem cells and adult pituitary stem cells, such as SOX2, SOX9, CD44, DLL4, OCT4 have been found in β-catenin accumulating cells in human ACPs [30, 31]. Immunohistochemical and molecular genetic profile of stem cell markers with a predominance of SOX9 and CD44 in ACP in comparison to pituitary adenomas suggest that ACP may originate from a more undifferentiated cell cluster. Wingless (Wnt)/β-catenin is a critical regulator of stem cells and mutant β-catenin expression in undifferentiated Rathke's pouch progenitors has shown to lead to tumours resembling human ACPs; however, this does not seem to happen in already differentiated cells [7]. Moreover, SOX9 overexpression seems to be correlated with recurrent growth of ACP [32]. Studies in PCP have also shown that SOX2 plays an important role in the pathogenesis of PCP [33]. Hyperactivation of the MAPK pathway resulted in expression of the gain-of-function alleles BRAFV600E and KrasG12D in the developing mouse pituitary, consequently leading to severe hyperplasia and abnormal morphogenesis of the gland by the end of gestation [33]. These markers could help to understand and predict the biological behaviour of CPs and hopefully be targets for chemotherapy.

12.6   CP Recurrence and Molecular Markers

The recurrence of CP is a challenging task for most neurosurgeons due to adherence and difficulty of resection is associated with significant morbidity. There is a high interest to predict the recurrence of these tumours and several biomarkers have been identified as presented in Table 12.1. Variation in miRNAs expression have been observed in cell proliferation and apoptosis, but also involved in neoplastic transformation. It is believed that for ACP, a number of miRNAs also participate in its recurrence via regulating several target genes [34, 35].

Rapid recurrence has been observed in CPs with high expression of Ki-67 and p53 reflecting high proliferative and apoptotic activity in tumour cells [36, 37] but there are also reports that failed to detect this correlation [38]. Markers contributing to higher local invasion of tumour and increased recurrence rate have been

Table 12.1 Biomarkers associated with recurrence of craniopharyngiomas

Biomarker	Expression profile
miRNA	Increased in ACP
Ki-67	Increased in CP
p53	Increased in CP
CD166	Increased in CP
β-catenin	Increased in CP
Retinoic acid receptor	Increased in CP
MMP-9	Increased in ACP
Cathepsins	Increased in ACP
VEGF	Increased in ACP
Collagen IV	Increased in ACP
CXCL12/CXCR4	Increased in ACP
SHH-pathway	Increased in ACP
SOX9	Increased in ACP
BRAF/CTNNB1	BRAF mutation lower recurrence rate

identified in ACP such as collagen IV, MMP-9 [39], SHH [40] and Cathepsins, while RAR and β-catenin was detected in both ACP and PCP [41–43].

Moreover, increased expression of chemokines has been associated with a high recurrence rate. Chemokines CXCR4 and CXCL12 are believed to increase the risk of recurrence through the increased potential for local invasion and angiogenesis [44, 45]. VGEFVGEF is an additional marker that may affect angiogenesis and recurrence rate, but the results are not yet conclusive [46, 47].

There are also reports on higher recurrence rate in mixed cases of CP [21, 24].

One of the drawbacks of these results and the limitation in the application of them is the fact that most of them do not report on tumour remnants, which is currently the most important factor contributing to recurrent tumour growth.

12.7 Inflammation and Immune Response

The brain parenchyma surrounding CP is often infiltrated by inflammatory cells and rich in cytokines produced by tumour cells [48]. Chemokines are a family of small pro-inflammatory chemoattractant cytokines that bind to specific G- protein-coupled transmembrane receptors and play an important role in tumour growth, angiogenesis and metastasis.

They may also play a key role in tissue reaction and adherence of tumour to the surrounding tissue. Craniopharyngiomas usually consist of a cystic and solid component. The cyst is filled with secreted fluid, cholesterol crystals, and epithelial cells and is associated with a major risk of recurrence. Furthermore, it has pro-inflammatory properties as the cyst rupture may lead to chemical meningitis detected also in the CSF [49]. Analysis of the cystic fluid has shown a ten-fold increase in IL-1, TNF-a and a >5000 fold increase in IL-6 [50] and intracystic injection of INF-a has the highest benefit to risk ratio compared to bleomycin or radioisotopes [51]. Microarray analysis of the cyst fluid revealed significantly increased expression of both pro-inflammatory mediators IL-6, CXCL8 (IL-8), and CXCL1 (GRO) as well as immunosuppressive IL-10 [48]. Analysis of the solid tumour component of ACP has also shown increased expression of cyto- and chemokines such as CXCL12 and its receptor CXCR4, pro-inflammatory mediators IL-6, CXCL8 (IL-8) and CXCL1 (GRO) as well as immunosuppressive IL-10 and IDO-1.

Majority of the studies have been performed on ACP with little information on the inflammatory processes in PCP. However, preoperative inflammatory markers from peripheral blood samples have been measured in both and it was shown that WBC and lymphocyte are increased in both ACP and PCP compared to other sellar region tumours [52]. The PCP group had higher neutrophil count and neutrophil-lymphocyte ratio than the ACP and healthy control groups. What has been recently seen in both types of CPs is the expression of programmed cell death protein 1/ programmed death-ligand 1 (PD-1/PD-L1) immune checkpoint pathway [53]. In this study, both ACP and PCP contained significant numbers of PD-L1 expressing immune cells. Available PD-1/PD-L1 inhibitors such as Nivolumab and

Atezolizumab, may be a new avenue for the systemic treatment of recurrent craniopharyngioma.

Current studies indicate the importance of the immune response in CP. This together with the successful utilization of directed therapies against inflammatory mediators in other tumour types and other diseases such as monoclonal antibodies directed against human IL-6R (tocilizumab) and IL-6 (siltuximab) opens a new field of treatment possibilities for craniopharyngiomas.

12.8   Pharmaceutical Agents and Molecular Targets

The deepened insight into the pathology of CPs has identified pathways of importance and possible molecular targets for treatment (Table 12.2). Several of these targets have previously been identified in other cancer and disease types and could thereby readily be applied to CPs. The importance of Wnt/β-catenin signalling pathway has generated more than 40 different substances where several of them are in clinical trials for other types of cancer treatment [14]. Currently, the CTNNB1 mutation in ACP is not readily targetable but further understanding of its role in tumorigenesis could make therapeutic implications possible [55].

Disturbed growth factor signalling has shown to be a hallmark of ACPs and several inhibitors are available and have successfully been used in cancer treatment such as treatment of lung- and breast cancer with Bevacizumab [56]. However, it failed to show any benefit in overall survival of patients with newly diagnosed glioblastoma [57]. Thus, its effect in ACPs remains to be elucidated.

The V600E point mutation in BRAF found in PCPs leads to a direct therapeutic potential with Dabrafenib since this was already used in melanoma [58]. This has been successfully tested as dual therapy with MEK-inhibitors (Trametinib) due to the development of acquired resistance and fewer side effects [59]. First encouraging case report was published by Brastianos et al. [60] where they used this treatment in a 39-year-old male with PCP and BRAFV600E mutation. The tumour had decreased by 85% after 35 days of treatment. Interestingly, the authors could detect

Table 12.2 Pharmaceutical agents and molecular targets

Molecular target	Drug
Wnt/β-catenin signalling	>40 substances
PD-1 inhibitors	Nivolumab
PD-L1 inhibitors	Atezolizumab
SHH-inhibitors	Vismodegib
EGFR-inhibitors	Gefitinib
VEGF-inhibitors	Bevacizumab
BRAF-inhibitor	Dabrafenib
MEK-inhibitor	Trametinib
IL-6	Siltuximab
IL-6R	Tocilizumab

The table presents one drug in each category but there are currently several drugs for each molecular target

Month 0-diagnosis   Month 5-Preoperative   Month 5-Postoperative   Month 7-tumor recur   Month 12- 15w treatment

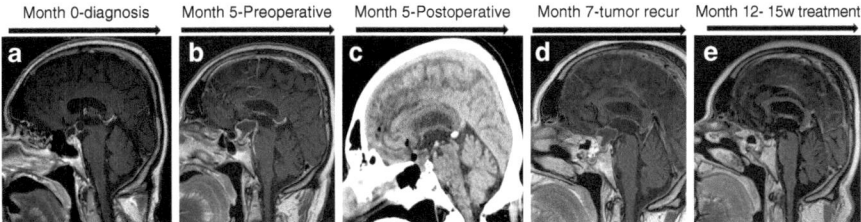

Fig. 12.2 A 65-year-old male diagnosed with CP (**a**) that progressed (**b**) and the patients underwent surgery (**c**), the histopathology showed a PCP with BRAFV600E mutation. The tumour recurred at 2 months postoperatively (**d**). At this time treatment with Dabrafenib (Tafinlar) 150 mg twice daily was initiated. After 3 weeks, Trametinib (Mekinist) 2 mg once daily was added, and the treatment lasted for a total of 7 weeks. MRI during the last week of treatment (15 weeks) showed a 91% reduction of the tumour (**e**) [54]. Reprinted with permission from Rostami et al. Acta Neurochir (Wien) 2017;159:2217–21 [54]

BRAFV600E in peripheral blood, but since the patient had been operated several times it was unclear if the surgery related tissue trauma caused DNA release into the peripheral blood.

We have so far treated one recurrent PCP with this dual therapy with significantly reduced tumour volume, but the treatment had to be halted after 15 weeks due to pyrexia [54] (Fig. 12.2). There are currently three additional case reports on achieving good response when using BRAF-targeted therapy for patients with PCP [61–63]. Although these reports are promising, many issues remain to be elucidated such as agents used, timing and duration of use, the response durability and potential use as neoadjuvant therapy to improve resection outcome. Hopefully, these questions can be addressed in ongoing clinical Phase II Alliance A071601 trial (NCT03224767).

Interestingly, in a recent study using explant cultures of both human and mouse ACP, MAPK/ERK pathway inhibitor trametinib, reduced proliferation and increased apoptosis [64]. Further studies are though needed to evaluate the clinic though needed to evaluate the clinical role of MEK-inhibitors in ACP.

Currently, the CTNNB1 mutation in ACP is not readily targetable and there are no ongoing clinical trials evaluating existing or new pharmaceutical agents.

12.8.1 Future Perspective

During recent years, the advancement of molecular biology and genetics have enabled a deeper insight into the underlying pathology of craniopharyngiomas and the more detailed characterization of ACP, PCP and mixed craniopharyngiomas. Several pathways, genes and proteins have been identified to play an important role in the pathogenesis and tumour behaviour of CPs and are being investigated as targets of treatment. Several markers have also been proposed for diagnosis of the recurrence of CP. Although the new biomarkers open a new avenue of studies on early diagnosis and prediction of recurrence none of them can currently be reliably used. One of the pitfalls is the inconsistency in reporting on important surgical variables when genetic and molecular profiling is correlated to outcome and recurrence. Future studies should take this into consideration, in particular the variables such as tumour remnants, which is currently the most important risk factor for recurrence. Emerging treatments may be applied to reduce the tumour size and facilitate total surgical removal of the tumours potentially improving the outcome.

Currently, the most successful adjuvant treatment is offered by dual therapy with BRAF and MEK inhibitors in PCPs expressing BRAFV600E mutation. However, these are case studies and ongoing and coming larger clinical trials will provide more information on this treatment option and its long-term efficacy. New findings on the role of inflammatory mediators and immune checkpoint pathways in ACPs may initiate new treatment options with already available pharmaceutical agents.

It might be possible that in the future, analysis of tumour markers in serum and/or cerebrospinal fluid in combination with MR imaging would provide sufficient information on diagnosis and available targeted therapy could be applied precluding any surgical intervention.

Acknowledgments The authors thank Magnus Sundström, PhD, for his kind help with DNA analyses and for generating the pyrograms illustrating BRAF mutational status in the presented cases.

References

1. Cushing H. Intracranial tumors. Notes upon series of two thousand verified cases with surgical mortality percentages pertaining thereto. Springfield, IL: Thomas; 1932.
2. Bulow B, Attewell R, Hagmar L, Malmstrom P, Nordstrom CH, Erfurth EM. Postoperative prognosis in craniopharyngioma with respect to cardiovascular mortality, survival, and tumor recurrence. J Clin Endocrinol Metab. 1998;83:3897–904.
3. Brastianos PK, Taylor-Weiner A, Manley PE, et al. Exome sequencing identifies BRAF mutations in papillary craniopharyngiomas. Nat Genet. 2014;46:161–5.
4. Goschzik T, Gessi M, Dreschmann V, et al. Genomic alterations of adamantinomatous and papillary craniopharyngioma. J Neuropathol Exp Neurol. 2017;76:126–34.
5. Holsken A, Sill M, Merkle J, et al. Adamantinomatous and papillary craniopharyngiomas are characterized by distinct epigenomic as well as mutational and transcriptomic profiles. Acta Neuropathol Commun. 2016;4:20.
6. Martinez-Gutierrez JC, D'Andrea MR, Cahill DP, Santagata S, Barker FG 2nd, Brastianos PK. Diagnosis and management of craniopharyngiomas in the era of genomics and targeted therapy. Neurosurg Focus. 2016;41:E2.
7. Gaston-Massuet C, Andoniadou CL, Signore M, et al. Increased wingless (Wnt) signaling in pituitary progenitor/stem cells gives rise to pituitary tumors in mice and humans. Proc Natl Acad Sci U S A. 2011;108:11482–7.
8. Martinez-Barbera JP. 60 Years of neuroendocrinology: biology of human craniopharyngioma: lessons from mouse models. J Endocrinol. 2015;226:T161–72.
9. Sekine S, Shibata T, Kokubu A, et al. Craniopharyngiomas of adamantinomatous type harbor beta-catenin gene mutations. Am J Pathol. 2002;161:1997–2001.
10. Logan CY, Nusse R. The Wnt signaling pathway in development and disease. Annu Rev Cell Dev Biol. 2004;20:781–810.
11. Polakis P. The many ways of Wnt in cancer. Curr Opin Genet Dev. 2007;17:45–51.

12. Hofmann BM, Kreutzer J, Saeger W, et al. Nuclear beta-catenin accumulation as reliable marker for the differentiation between cystic craniopharyngiomas and Rathke cleft cysts: a clinico-pathologic approach. Am J Surg Pathol. 2006;30:1595–603.
13. Juca CEB, Colli LM, Martins CS, et al. Impact of the canonical Wnt pathway activation on the pathogenesis and prognosis of adamantinomatous craniopharyngiomas. Horm Metab Res. 2018;50:575–81.
14. Voronkov A, Krauss S. Wnt/beta-catenin signaling and small molecule inhibitors. Curr Pharm Des. 2013;19:634–64.
15. Holsken A, Gebhardt M, Buchfelder M, Fahlbusch R, Blumcke I, Buslei R. EGFR signaling regulates tumor cell migration in craniopharyngiomas. Clin Cancer Res. 2011;17:4367–77.
16. Olsen JJ, Pohl SO, Deshmukh A, et al. The role of Wnt signalling in angiogenesis. Clin Biochem Rev. 2017;38:131–42.
17. Davies H, Bignell GR, Cox C, et al. Mutations of the BRAF gene in human cancer. Nature. 2002;417:949–54.
18. La Corte E, Younus I, Pivari F, et al. BRAF V600E mutant papillary craniopharyngiomas: a single-institutional case series. Pituitary. 2018;21:571–83.
19. Sperveslage J, Gierke M, Capper D, et al. VE1 immunohistochemistry in pituitary adenomas is not associated with BRAF V600E mutation. Acta Neuropathol. 2013;125:911–2.
20. Mordes DA, Lynch K, Campbell S, et al. VE1 antibody immunoreactivity in normal anterior pituitary and adrenal cortex without detectable BRAF V600E mutations. Am J Clin Pathol. 2014;141:811–5.
21. Weiner HL, Wisoff JH, Rosenberg ME, et al. Craniopharyngiomas: a clinicopathological analysis of factors predictive of recurrence and functional outcome. Neurosurgery. 1994;35:1001–10; discussion 10–11.
22. Larkin SJ, Preda V, Karavitaki N, Grossman A, Ansorge O. BRAF V600E mutations are characteristic for papillary craniopharyngioma and may coexist with CTNNB1-mutated adamantinomatous craniopharyngioma. Acta Neuropathol. 2014;127:927–9.
23. Crotty TB, Scheithauer BW, Young WF Jr, et al. Papillary craniopharyngioma: a clinicopathological study of 48 cases. J Neurosurg. 1995;83:206–14.
24. Szeifert GT, Sipos L, Horvath M, et al. Pathological characteristics of surgically removed craniopharyngiomas: analysis of 131 cases. Acta Neurochir. 1993;124:139–43.
25. Okada T, Fujitsu K, Ichikawa T, et al. Coexistence of adamantinomatous and squamous-papillary type craniopharyngioma: case report and discussion of etiology and pathology. Neuropathology. 2012;32:171–3.
26. Miller DC. Pathology of craniopharyngiomas: clinical import of pathological findings. Pediatr Neurosurg. 1994;21(Suppl 1):11–7.
27. Bi WL, Greenwald NF, Ramkissoon SH, et al. Clinical identification of oncogenic drivers and copy-number alterations in pituitary tumors. Endocrinology. 2017;158:2284–91.
28. Yamada H, Haratake J, Narasaki T, Oda T. Embryonal craniopharyngioma. Case report of the morphogenesis of a craniopharyngioma. Cancer. 1995;75:2971–7.
29. Garcia-Lavandeira M, Quereda V, Flores I, et al. A GRFa2/Prop1/stem (GPS) cell niche in the pituitary. PLoS One. 2009;4:e4815.
30. Garcia-Lavandeira M, Saez C, Diaz-Rodriguez E, et al. Craniopharyngiomas express embryonic stem cell markers (SOX2, OCT4, KLF4, and SOX9) as pituitary stem cells but do not coexpress RET/GFRA3 receptors. J Clin Endocrinol Metab. 2012;97:E80–7.
31. Holsken A, Stache C, Schlaffer SM, et al. Adamantinomatous craniopharyngiomas express tumor stem cell markers in cells with activated Wnt signaling: further evidence for the existence of a tumor stem cell niche? Pituitary. 2014;17:546–56.
32. Chang CV, Araujo RV, Cirqueira CS, et al. Differential expression of stem cell markers in human adamantinomatous craniopharyngioma and pituitary adenoma. Neuroendocrinology. 2017;104:183–93.
33. Haston S, Pozzi S, Carreno G, et al. MAPK pathway control of stem cell proliferation and differentiation in the embryonic pituitary provides insights into the pathogenesis of papillary craniopharyngioma. Development. 2017;144:2141–52.

34. Samis J, Vanin EF, Sredni ST, et al. Extensive miRNA expression analysis in craniopharyngiomas. Childs Nerv Syst. 2016;32:1617–24.
35. Campanini ML, Colli LM, Paixao BM, et al. CTNNB1 gene mutations, pituitary transcription factors, and MicroRNA expression involvement in the pathogenesis of adamantinomatous craniopharyngiomas. Horm Cancer. 2010;1:187–96.
36. Tena-Suck ML, Salinas-Lara C, Arce-Arellano RI, et al. Clinico-pathological and immuno-histochemical characteristics associated to recurrence/regrowth of craniopharyngiomas. Clin Neurol Neurosurg. 2006;108:661–9.
37. Nishi T, Kuratsu J, Takeshima H, Saito Y, Kochi M, Ushio Y. Prognostic significance of the MIB-1 labeling index for patient with craniopharyngioma. Int J Mol Med. 1999;3:157–61.
38. Prieto R, Pascual JM, Subhi-Issa I, Jorquera M, Yus M, Martinez R. Predictive factors for craniopharyngioma recurrence: a systematic review and illustrative case report of a rapid recurrence. World Neurosurg. 2013;79:733–49.
39. Xia Z, Liu W, Li S, et al. Expression of matrix metalloproteinase-9, type IV collagen and vascular endothelial growth factor in adamantinous craniopharyngioma. Neurochem Res. 2011;36:2346–51.
40. Gomes DC, Jamra SA, Leal LF, et al. Sonic hedgehog pathway is upregulated in adamantinomatous craniopharyngiomas. Eur J Endocrinol. 2015;172:603–8.
41. Lefranc F, Mijatovic T, Decaestecker C, et al. Monitoring the expression profiles of integrins and adhesion/growth-regulatory galectins in adamantinomatous craniopharyngiomas: their ability to regulate tumor adhesiveness to surrounding tissue and their contribution to prognosis. Neurosurgery. 2005;56:763–76.
42. Lubansu A, Ruchoux MM, Brotchi J, Salmon I, Kiss R, Lefranc F. Cathepsin B, D and K expression in adamantinomatous craniopharyngiomas relates to their levels of differentiation as determined by the patterns of retinoic acid receptor expression. Histopathology. 2003;43:563–72.
43. Guadagno E, de Divitiis O, Solari D, et al. Can recurrences be predicted in craniopharyngiomas? Beta-catenin coexisting with stem cells markers and p-ATM in a clinicopathologic study of 45cases. J Exp Clin Cancer Res. 2017;36:95.
44. Gong J, Zhang H, Xing S, et al. High expression levels of CXCL12 and CXCR4 predict recurrence of adamanti-nomatous craniopharyngiomas in children. Cancer Biomark. 2014;14:241–51.
45. Yin X, Liu Z, Zhu P, et al. CXCL12/CXCR4 promotes proliferation, migration, and invasion of adamantinomatous craniopharyngiomas via PI3K/AKT signal pathway. J Cell Biochem. 2019;120(6):9724–36. https://doi.org/10.1002/jcb.28253. Epub 2018 Dec 23.
46. Vidal S, Kovacs K, Lloyd RV, Meyer FB, Scheithauer BW. Angiogenesis in patients with craniopharyngiomas: correlation with treatment and outcome. Cancer. 2002;94:738–45.
47. Xu J, You C, Zhang S, et al. Angiogenesis and cell proliferation in human craniopharyngioma xenografts in nude mice. J Neurosurg. 2006;105:306–10.
48. Donson AM, Apps J, Griesinger AM, et al. Molecular analyses reveal inflammatory mediators in the solid component and cyst fluid of human adamantinomatous craniopharyngioma. J Neuropathol Exp Neurol. 2017;76:779–88.
49. Satoh H, Uozumi T, Arita K, et al. Spontaneous rupture of craniopharyngioma cysts. A report of five cases and review of the literature. Surg Neurol. 1993;40:414–9.
50. Mori M, Takeshima H, Kuratsu J. Expression of interleukin-6 in human craniopharyngiomas: a possible inducer of tumor-associated inflammation. Int J Mol Med. 2004;14:505–9.
51. Bartels U, Laperriere N, Bouffet E, Drake J. Intracystic therapies for cystic craniopharyngioma in childhood. Front Endocrinol (Lausanne). 2012;3:39.
52. Chen M, Zheng SH, Yang M, Chen ZH, Li ST. The diagnostic value of preoperative inflammatory markers in craniopharyngioma: a multicenter cohort study. J Neuro-Oncol. 2018;138:113–22.
53. Coy S, Rashid R, Lin JR, et al. Multiplexed immunofluorescence reveals potential PD-1/PD-L1 pathway vulnerabilities in craniopharyngioma. Neuro-Oncology. 2018;20:1101–12.

54. Rostami E, Witt Nystrom P, Libard S, Wikstrom J, Casar-Borota O, Gudjonsson O. Recurrent papillary craniopharyngioma with BRAFV600E mutation treated with neoadjuvant-targeted therapy. Acta Neurochir. 2017;159:2217–21.
55. Gao C, Wang Y, Broaddus R, Sun L, Xue F, Zhang W. Exon 3 mutations of CTNNB1 drive tumorigenesis: a review. Oncotarget. 2018;9:5492–508.
56. Pavlidis ET, Pavlidis TE. Role of bevacizumab in colorectal cancer growth and its adverse effects: a review. World J Gastroenterol. 2013;19:5051–60.
57. Gilbert MR, Dignam JJ, Armstrong TS, et al. A randomized trial of bevacizumab for newly diagnosed glioblastoma. N Engl J Med. 2014;370:699–708.
58. Long GV, Stroyakovskiy D, Gogas H, et al. Dabrafenib and trametinib versus dabrafenib and placebo for Val600 BRAF-mutant melanoma: a multicentre, double-blind, phase 3 randomised controlled trial. Lancet. 2015;386:444–51.
59. Eroglu Z, Ribas A. Combination therapy with BRAF and MEK inhibitors for melanoma: latest evidence and place in therapy. Ther Adv Med Oncol. 2016;8:48–56.
60. Brastianos PK, Shankar GM, Gill CM, et al. Dramatic response of BRAF V600E mutant papillary craniopharyngioma to targeted therapy. J Natl Cancer Inst. 2016;108
61. Aylwin SJ, Bodi I, Beaney R. Pronounced response of papillary craniopharyngioma to treatment with vemurafenib, a BRAF inhibitor. Pituitary. 2016;19:544–6.
62. Roque A, Odia Y. BRAF-V600E mutant papillary craniopharyngioma dramatically responds to combination BRAF and MEK inhibitors. CNS Oncol. 2017;6:95–9.
63. Himes BT, Ruff MW, Van Gompel JJ, et al. Recurrent papillary craniopharyngioma with BRAF V600E mutation treated with dabrafenib: case report. J Neurosurg. 2018:1–5.
64. Apps JR, Carreno G, Gonzalez-Meljem JM, et al. Tumour compartment transcriptomics demonstrates the activation of inflammatory and odontogenic programmes in human adamantinomatous craniopharyngioma and identifies the MAPK/ERK pathway as a novel therapeutic target. Acta Neuropathol. 2018;135:757–77.

Conclusions

13

Emmanuel Jouanneau and Gérald Raverot

It has been a long journey from the first description of a craniopharyngioma, by Friedrich Von Zenker in 1857, and the identification of the adiposo-genital syndrome by Frölich and Babinski in 1900.

More than a century later, this tumor continues to challenge physicians and the quote from H Cushing, "Craniopharyngiomas are the most baffling problem which confronts the Neurosurgeon," recalled by Professor Ed Laws in his preface, remains perfectly true today.

Some advances are however encouraging for the future.

It is well established that there are two peaks of incidence of craniopharyngiomas; under 15 years of age and in patients in their sixties.

The two types of craniopharyngiomas are now well characterized: An adamantinomatous form (ACP), existing both in children and in adults, and the papillary form (PCP) found only in adults. The old concept of CP arising from embryonic ectodermal remnants of the primitive mouth or *stomodeum* is now questionable if not obsolete. This concept fails to explain the two potent forms of CP and why CP may develop after decades.

Recent molecular and experimental data showed that ACP is driven by the CTNNB1 mutation/β catenin in adult SOX2 pituitary stem cell forming clusters. Those clusters promote tumor development thereafter in a paracrine manner. The location where mutations take place (infundibulum, pars tuberalis, pituitary)

E. Jouanneau
Pituitary and Skull Base Neurosurgical Department,
Neurological Hospital, Hospices Civils de Lyon, Lyon, France

Claude Bernard University Lyon 1, Lyon, France
e-mail: emmanuel.jouanneau@chu-lyon.fr

G. Raverot (✉)
Endocrinology Department, "Groupement Hospitalier Est" Hospices Civils de Lyon,
Lyon University, Lyon, France
e-mail: gerald.raverot@chu-lyon.fr

© Springer Nature Switzerland AG 2020
E. Jouanneau, G. Raverot (eds.), *Adult Craniopharyngiomas*,
https://doi.org/10.1007/978-3-030-41176-3_13

explains the different forms of CP: sellar, suprasellar, infundibular, and intraventricular.

PCPs clearly represent a different tumor, only encountered in the adult even if ACPs are the most frequent form in adults. These are driven by BRAF-V600E mutations expressed by cells throughout the tumor, a mutation that promotes the proliferation of a subpopulation of SOX2 cells.

SOX2 stem cells are therefore key cells in the development of CPs with distinct mutations.

Adult-onset CPs (AO-CP) are rare tumors which explain the very few pure adult series. Consequently, therapeutic strategies have been extrapolated from mixed or pediatric series.

However, pediatric CP and AO-CP are quite different in terms of their clinical presentation, the location of the tumor (mainly sellar-suprasellar in adults), and the therapeutic strategies employed, these being perhaps more conservative in children as the consequences of lesions in the immature hypothalamus may be more dramatic.

For AO-CP, important concepts are:

– Firstly, the data from the literature joined to our own experience showed that hypothalamic syndrome is frequent at diagnosis with the classical overweight issues. Further studies are warranted to obtain more precise data on cognitive function.
– Secondly, regarding surgery, the surgical innovation is clearly the development of the endoscopic endonasal extended approach over the last two decades. Surgically, approaching from below clearly allows a better exposure of the hypothalamus. Even though we have no randomized studies, pituitary surgeons agree that such an approach results in either an improvement in surgical outcomes or a diminution in morbidity.

After the publication of the results of pediatric neurosurgery, the rule was to avoid GTR in MRI grade II CP. In adults, this does not appear to be as true, but we still do not understand why some patients get better while some do not, while the post-operative MRI results seem to show very similar appearance of a hole in the third ventricle. As has been nicely described by R Prieto, a thorough study of the MR criteria helps surgeons to plan the surgical route and predict likely difficulties of surgery. In the end, it is the surgeon in theater who will decide how far he/she can go without endangering the patient. The key point for us is the degree of adhesion to the hypothalamus or optic chiasma as well as the location of invasion. As soon as a sharp dissection is obligatory, we must take the decision to end surgery especially when it is extended posteriorly. Indeed, damage to mammillary bodies has been implicated in behavioral, memory, and obesity issues. Cystic walls also have to be frequently kept in place. Interestingly, for cystic AO-CP, recent data supports conservative treatment with large opening of the cyst alone (*i.e.,* without upfront radiotherapy) in the ventricle that may control the tumor for years with minimal morbidity.

All decisions need experience, training and perhaps even more so in the case of pituitary adenomas, particularly considering the rarity of such tumors, meaning dedicated surgeons and referral centers are of paramount importance.

The place of radiotherapy remains open to debate. When a gross total removal is performed, a wait-and-see attitude could be the recommended approach. In the case of subtotal removal the key point is whether to treat upfront or not. In the absence of randomized studies, this point remains open to debate. In the case of a significant tumor residue, the progression free survival PFS has improved in pediatric series after STR and radiotherapy. Therefore, it would be recommended in the young or middle-aged population, whereas a wait-and-see approach would be used in the oldest patients. Regarding the technique to be employed, the standard technique is IRMT. Evidence is missing for an additional benefit for proton-therapy and radiosurgery. Once again, clinical trials are ongoing but will probably take time.

Overweight issues remain the major side effect for patients, altering their quality of life. The underlying mechanisms for this are numerous and not perfectly understood. Medical therapies have been disappointing although GLP-1 and oxytocin trials are ongoing. Bariatric surgery can be proposed in the adult with fewer ethical issues than for children. Non-reversible methods (sleeve or other techniques) may be more efficient. The key point is to deal with this metabolic risk at the very beginning with dietary measures, exercise programs, and strict follow-up. Both patients and physicians need to be alert to this issue as, in many situations, ignorance or negligence can lead to dramatic and irreversible outcomes. In addition to metabolic consequences, hypopituitarism is a common finding in adult patients with CP, occurring both pre- and post-operatively. In the case of hypopituitarism, it is important not to underdiagnose and undertreat, but at the same time not to overtreat. Key advice is presented, in this book, to help clinicians to optimize pre-and post-operative endocrinological management.

Despite surgery and radiotherapy, in almost 30% of cases, recurrence can be observed. The most interesting recent advance in therapy is the use of targeted therapies that are based on molecular data. Promising results have been reported with a combination of BRAF and MEK-inhibitors, but data on the long-term control are lacking. A phase II study (NCT03224767) is ongoing. CTNNB1 inhibitors are currently unavailable but immunotherapy drugs, such as PD-L1 inhibitors, present another innovative option.

Finally, CPs have a very bad reputation for being benign but recurrent tumors. We have all experienced dramatic cases; however, this is not the usual profile. Indeed, we were pleasantly surprised when we considered the outcomes of our adult patients (more than 50 treated in the modern era). Certainly, we have cases of recurrence, overweight issues (mostly starting before treatment), but very few difficult situations and most of them resume normal life after diagnosis and treatment. This point remains to be confirmed in large multicenter studies.

As we conclude this book, focused on adult CP, many questions remain unresolved. In view of the rarity of such tumors, international multicenter trials will be required. To this end a European Task Force is now emerging to address this challenging topic.

Index

© Springer Nature Switzerland AG 2020
E. Jouanneau, G. Raverot (eds.), *Adult Craniopharyngiomas*,
https://doi.org/10.1007/978-3-030-41176-3